Comprehensive Atlas of Dermatoscopy Cases

Horacio Cabo • Aimilios Lallas
Editors

Comprehensive Atlas of Dermatoscopy Cases

Springer

Editors
Horacio Cabo
Instituto de Investigaciones Medicas
"A. Lanari". Dermatology Section
University of Buenos Aires
Buenos Aires
Argentina

Aimilios Lallas
First Department of Dermatology
Aristotle University of Thessaloniki
Thessaloniki
Greece

ISBN 978-3-030-08328-1 ISBN 978-3-319-76932-5 (eBook)
https://doi.org/10.1007/978-3-319-76932-5

Softcover re-print of the Hardcover 1st edition 2018

Printed on acid-free paper

This Springer imprint is published by the registered company Springer International Publishing AG part of Springer Nature.
The registered company address is: Gewerbestrasse 11, 6330 Cham, Switzerland

Foreword

It's my great pleasure and honor to write a few words to comment on this last endeavor in the field of dermoscopy. Horacio and Aimilios are not only among the world leaders of this technique but also represent the past, present, and future of our beloved field of interest.

I met Horacio for the first time in Rome in 2001, at the first World Congress of Dermoscopy, and since then there was no project or major event in the field of dermoscopy in which he was not present and deeply involved. Aimilios represents the new blood, the one who took dermoscopy to the next step and who will contribute to the further development of the technique in the near future. In sum, dermoscopy is in their genes and, therefore, this atlas is a "must-read" book.

The concept behind this book is to provide the reader with exceptional examples of the vast majority of skin conditions, of which dermoscopy may facilitate the diagnosis or management. I am sure this book will definitely contribute to the body of knowledge in dermoscopy and further expand the didactic material, which will help our young clinicians to improve their ability to recognize pigmented and non-pigmented skin tumors, as well as many other dermatologic conditions.

Giuseppe Argenziano
Dermatology Unit
University of Campania
Naples, Italy

Preface

Dear friends and colleagues,

The book you hold in your hands (or see on your screen) is not one more textbook on dermoscopy. It is rather a collection…

A collection of exemplar cases with high didactic value, highlighting how dermoscopy improves our everyday work as clinicians.

A collection of experience from several years we spent on practicing and teaching dermoscopy.

A collection of good friends and excellent colleagues—most of them already famous experts in the field, who contributed with their cases.

The book includes cases of numerous entities (mostly, but not exclusively, skin tumors) of different levels of diagnostic difficulty.

Presented in an easy-to-read way, each case consists of a short description of the clinical history, followed by macroscopic and dermatoscopic images, in a way that the readers can exercise their diagnostic capacity. Immediately afterwards, the dermatoscopic image is analyzed and the most important clues leading to the correct diagnosis are highlighted, aiming to help the reader to improve his/her diagnostic skills. Finally, a few key points on the topic are discussed.

The cases have been ordered not by diagnosis but according to the clinical presentation and the anatomic site, aiming to approach as much as possible the real clinical scenario.

Cases are presented within the chapters. Each case is specific to one or several of the chapter authors, whose initials are presented in parentheses next to the case number.

Our aim was to provide an easy-to-follow tool to practice and improve the diagnostic skills of the readers, highlight useful clues, and underline management rules that are particularly useful for the ordinary clinical practice.

We deeply thank all our friends and colleagues that contributed with their great cases, allowing us to create this beautiful collection.

We hope that you will find the book useful and that you will enjoy reading it.

Buenos Aires, Argentina — Horacio Cabo
Thessaloniki, Greece — Aimilios Lallas

Contents

Contributors

Zoe Apalla First Department of Dermatology, Aristotle University of Thessaloniki, Thessaloniki, Greece

Giuseppe Argenziano Dermatology Unit, University of Campania, Naples, Italy

Renato Marchiori Bakos Universidade Federal do Rio Grande do Sul, Porto Alegre, Brazil

Gabriella Brancaccio Dermatology Unit, University of Campania, Naples, Italy

Ralph P. Braun Department of Dermatology, University of Zürich, Zürich, Switzerland

Horacio Cabo Instituto de Investigaciones Médicas "A. Lanari". Dermatology Section, University of Buenos Aires, Buenos Aires, Argentina

Cristina Carrera Dermatology Department, University of Barcelona, Hospital Clínic de Barcelona, Barcelona, Spain

Teresa Deinlein Department of Dermatology, Medical University of Graz, Graz, Austria

Pedro Diego Zaballos Dermatology Department, Hospital Santa Tecla de Tarragona, University of Rovira i Virgili, Tarragona, Spain

Natalia Espinosa Dermatology Department, University of Barcelona, Hospital Clínic de Barcelona, Barcelona, Spain

Francesca Farnetani Department of Dermatology, University of Modena and Reggio Emilia, Modena, Italy

Fabrizio Favero Department of Dermatology and Venereology, Medical University of Graz, Graz, Austria

Roberta Giuffrida Department of Clinical and Experimental Medicine, Section of Dermatology, University of Messina, Messina, Italy

Virginia Mariana Gonzalez Hospital Alemán, Buenos Aires, Argentina

Rainer Hofmann-Wellemhof Department of Dermatology, Medical University of Graz, Graz, Austria

Manu Jain Memorial Sloan Kettering Cancer Center, New York, NY, USA

Raimonds Karls Department of Infectology and Dermatology, Riga Stradins University, Derma Clinic Riga, Ltd., Riga, Latvia

Alexander Katoulis 2nd Department of Dermatology-Venereology, National and Kapodistrian University of Athens, "ATTIKON" University Hospital, Athens, Greece

Harald Kittler Department of Dermatology, Medical University of Vienna, Vienna, Austria

Michael Kunz Department of Dermatology, University of Zürich, Zürich, Switzerland

Romana Kupsa Department of Dermatology, Medical University of Graz, Graz, Austria

Antonia Laino University of Queensland (UQ), St Lucia, QLD, Australia

Aimilios Lallas First Department of Dermatology, Aristotle University of Thessaloniki, Thessaloniki, Greece

Caterina Longo Dermatology Unit, University of Modena and Reggio Emilia, Modena, Italy

Josep Malvehy Dermatology Department, Barcelona, Spain

Ashfaq A. Marghoob Memorial Sloan Kettering Cancer Center, New York, NY, USA

Cesare Massone Department of Dermatology, Medical University of Graz, Graz, Austria

Department of Dermatology, Galliera Hospital, Genoa, Italy

Daniel Morgado Carrasco Dermatology Department, University of Barcelona, Hospital Clínic de Barcelona, Barcelona, Spain

Elvira Moscarella Dermatology and Skin Cancer Unit, Arcispedale S Maria Nuova, IRCCS, Reggio Emilia, Modena, Italy

John Paoli University of Gothenburg, Gothenburg, Sweden

Chryssoula Papageorgiou First Department of Dermatology, Aristotle University of Thessaloniki, Thessaloniki, Greece

Giovanni Pellacani Department of Dermatology, University of Modena and Reggio Emilia, Modena, Italy

Rosario Peralta Instituto de Investigaciones Medicas "A. Lanari". Dermatology Section, University of Buenos Aires, Buenos Aires, Argentina

H. Peter Soyer Department of Dermatology, The University of Queensland (UQ), St Lucia, QLD, Australia

Susana Puig Dermatology Department, Barcelona, Spain

Erika Richtig Department of Dermatology, Medical University of Graz, Graz, Austria

Georg Richtig Department of Dermatology, Medical University of Graz, Graz, Austria

Institute of Experimental and Clinical Pharmacology, Medical University of Graz, Graz, Austria

Sonia Rodriguez Saa University of Mendoza, Mendoza, Argentina

Emilia Noemi Cohen Sabban Instituto de Investigaciones Médicas "A. Lanari". Chief of Dermatology Section, University of Buenos Aires, Buenos Aires, Argentina

Gabriel Salerni Dermatologist Doctor in Medicine Universidad Nacional de Rosario and Hospital Provincial del Centenario de Rosario Santa Fe, Santa Fe, Argentina

Alon Scope Melanoma and Pigmented Lesion Clinic, Chaim Sheba Medical Center, Ramat-Gan, Israel

Faculty of Medicine, Tel Aviv University, Tel Aviv, Israel

Dimitrios Sgouros 2nd Department of Dermatology-Venereology, National and Kapodistrian University of Athens, "ATTIKON" University Hospital, Athens, Greece

Wilhem Stolz Dermatology Department, Klinikum Schwabing, Munich, Germany

Luc Thomas Department of Dermatology, Lyons Cancer Research Center (Pr Puisieux) INSERM U1052, CNRS UMR5286 Lyon 1 University Centre Hospitalier Lyon Sud, Lyon, France

Danica Tiodorovic Medical Faculty of Nis, Serbia, Clinic of Dermatology, Clinical Center Nis, Nis, Serbia

Antonella Tosti Department of Dermatology, Miller School of Medicine, University of Miami, Miami, FL, USA

Philipp Tschandl Department of Dermatology, Medical University of Vienna, Vienna, Austria

Oriol Yélamos Memorial Sloan Kettering Cancer Center, New York, NY, USA

Iris Zalaudek Department of Dermatology, Medical University of Graz, Graz, Austria

Structures, Patterns, Criteria and Colours

1

Horacio Cabo and Aimilios Lallas

Although this book is oriented to the resolution of clinical dermoscopy cases, it is our intention to provide a very brief review of the most important aspects of dermoscopy.

The dermatoscope reveals several morphologic structures that cannot be seen with the naked eye.

The multiple repetitions of a *structure* form a *pattern*. When the structures are associated with a specific diagnosis, they are called *criteria.*

For example, a roundish brown area or brown globule represents a *structure*. A lesion dermoscopically characterized by the presence of multiple brown globules is considered to display a *globular pattern*. Finally, the presence of brown globules is associated with the diagnosis of a melanocytic lesion; thus, aggregated brown globules are considered a *criterion* of melanocytic lesions (Table 1.1, Figs. 1.1, 1.2, 1.3, 1.4 and 1.5).

Table 1.1 Dermoscopic criteria for melanocytic lesions

Pigment network
Aggregated globules
Streaks or projections
Homogeneous blue pigmentation
Pattern of parallel pigmented lines

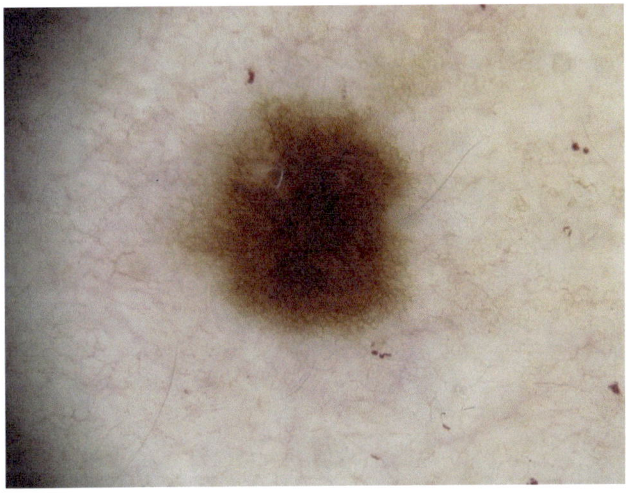

Fig. 1.1 Pigment network—reticular pattern—nevus

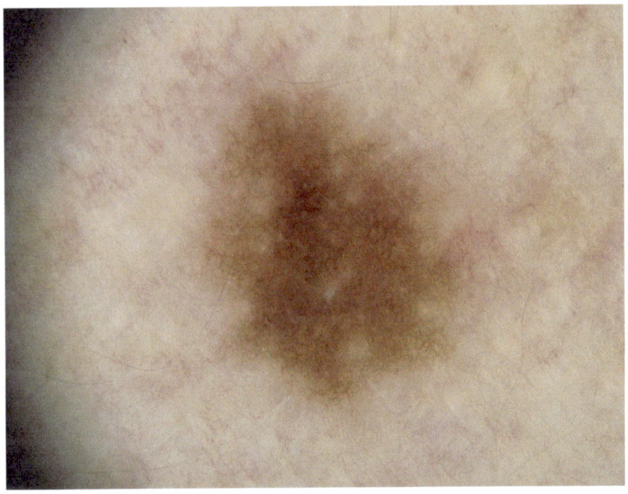

Fig. 1.2 Pigment network—reticular pattern—nevus

H. Cabo (✉)
Instituto de Investigaciones Médicas "A. Lanari". Dermatology Section, University of Buenos Aires, Buenos Aires, Argentina

A. Lallas
First Department of Dermatology, Aristotle University of Thessaloniki, Thessaloniki, Greece

H. Cabo, A. Lallas (eds.), *Comprehensive Atlas of Dermatoscopy Cases*, https://doi.org/10.1007/978-3-319-76932-5_1

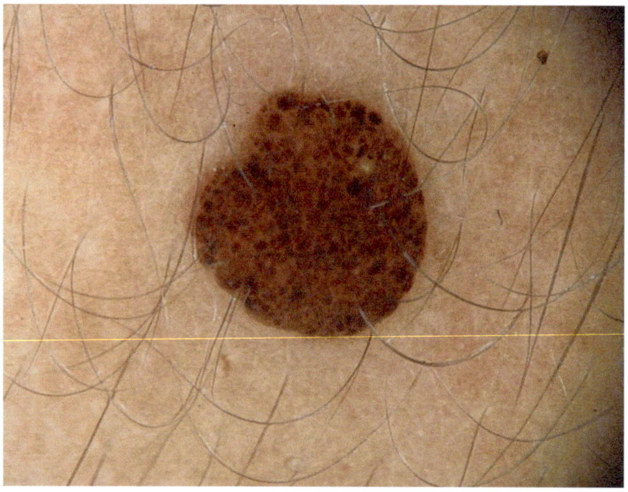

Fig. 1.3 Globules—globular pattern—nevus

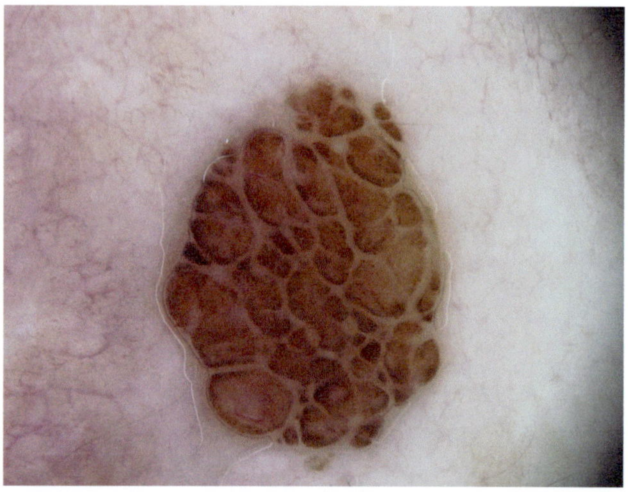

Fig. 1.4 Globules—globular pattern—nevus

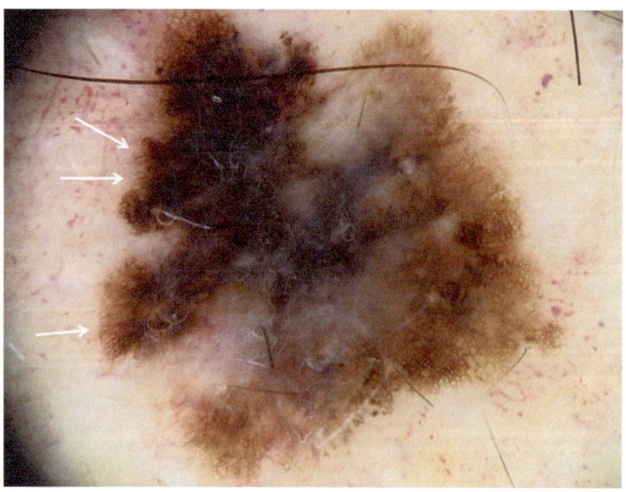

Fig. 1.5 Streaks (white arrows)—melanoma

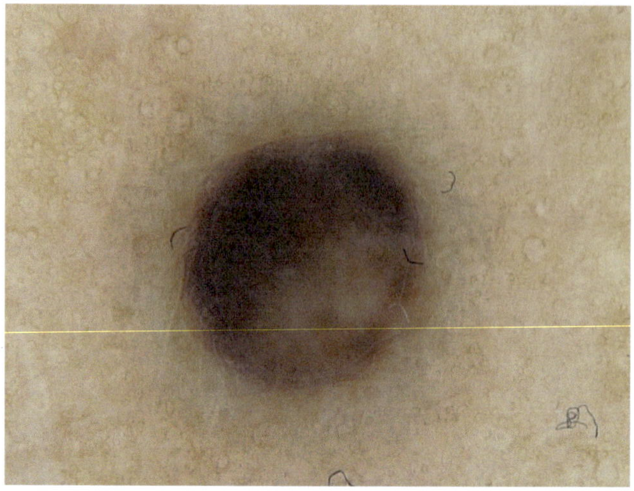

Fig. 1.6 Homogeneous blue pigmentation—blue nevus

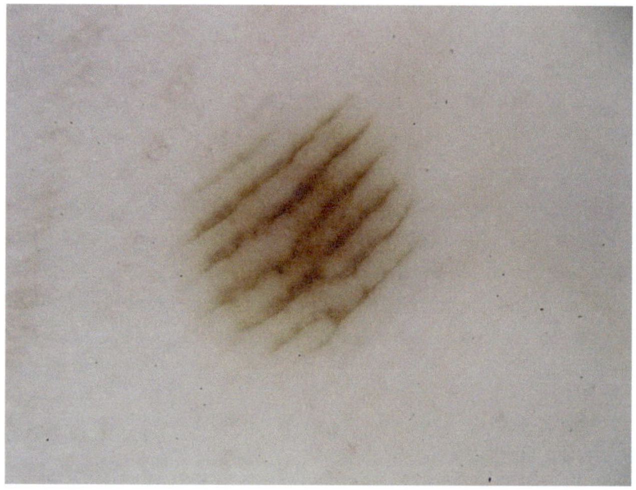

Fig. 1.7 Parallel furrow pattern—acral nevus

In addition to the morphologic structures, also colours are of paramount importance in dermoscopy (Figs. 1.6, 1.7, 1.8, 1.9 and 1.10).

Dermoscopic colours are a result of the presence of one or more of the three main chromophores of the skin: melanin, haemoglobin and keratin.

It is necessary to consider type, number and colour distribution.

The different colours that can be observed are white, red, black, blue, grey, yellow, light brown and dark brown and their combinations or variants.

Red, pink or blue-red colours are due to the vessels, haemoglobin and its degree of oxidation.

White colour results from the presence of keratin, fibrosis or atrophy.

Yellow colour corresponds to keratin or serum.

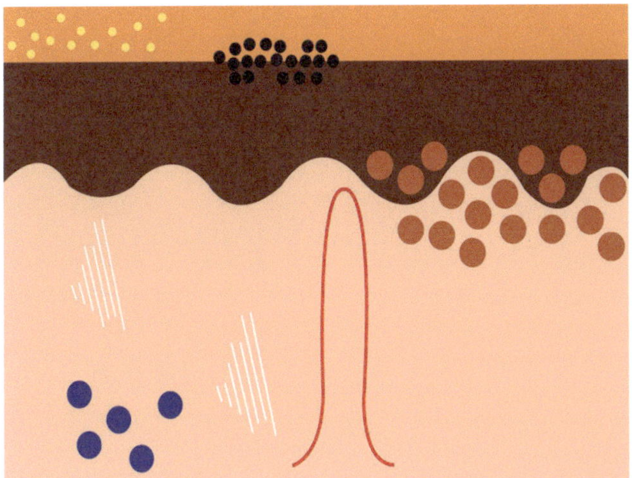

Fig. 1.8 With the dermatoscope, you can see different colours depending on the location in the skin. White colour represents lack of pigment, atrophy or fibrosis. Yellow colour corresponds to keratin. Brown colour is related to melanin; in the stratum corneum or epidermis, it looks black; in the dermoepidermal junction and in the papillary dermis, dark brown or light brown; and in the dermis, blue. Red, pink or blue-red colour is due to the vessels, haemoglobin and the degree of oxidation of this

Brown, black and blue colours are related to melanin.

- The presence of melanin in the stratum corneum or superficial epidermis projects *black.*
- Melanin at the level of the dermoepidermal junction and in the papillary dermis results in *dark brown or light brown.*
- Melanin in the dermis dermoscopically gives rise to *blue* colour.

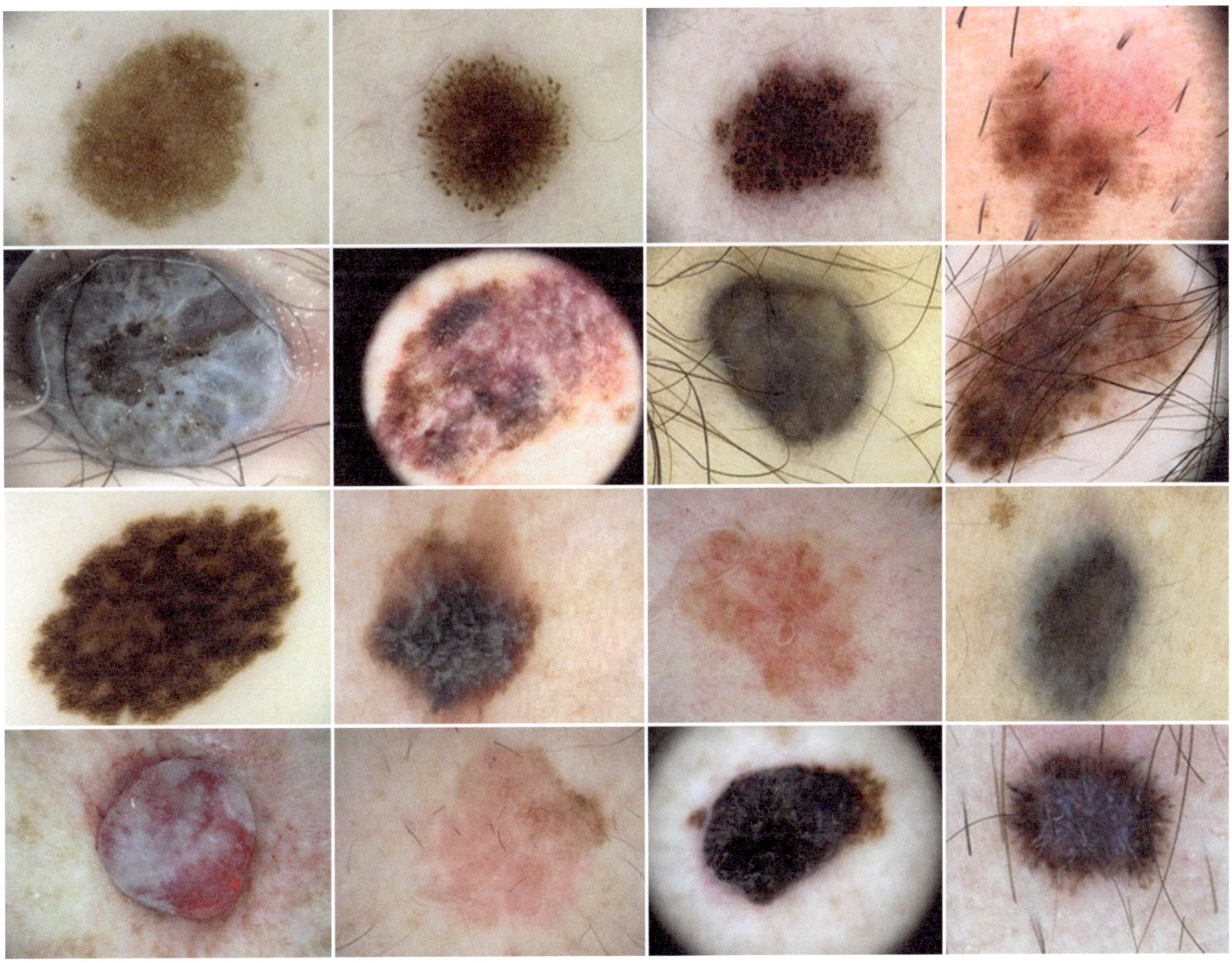

Fig. 1.9 Examples of cutaneous lesions with different colours

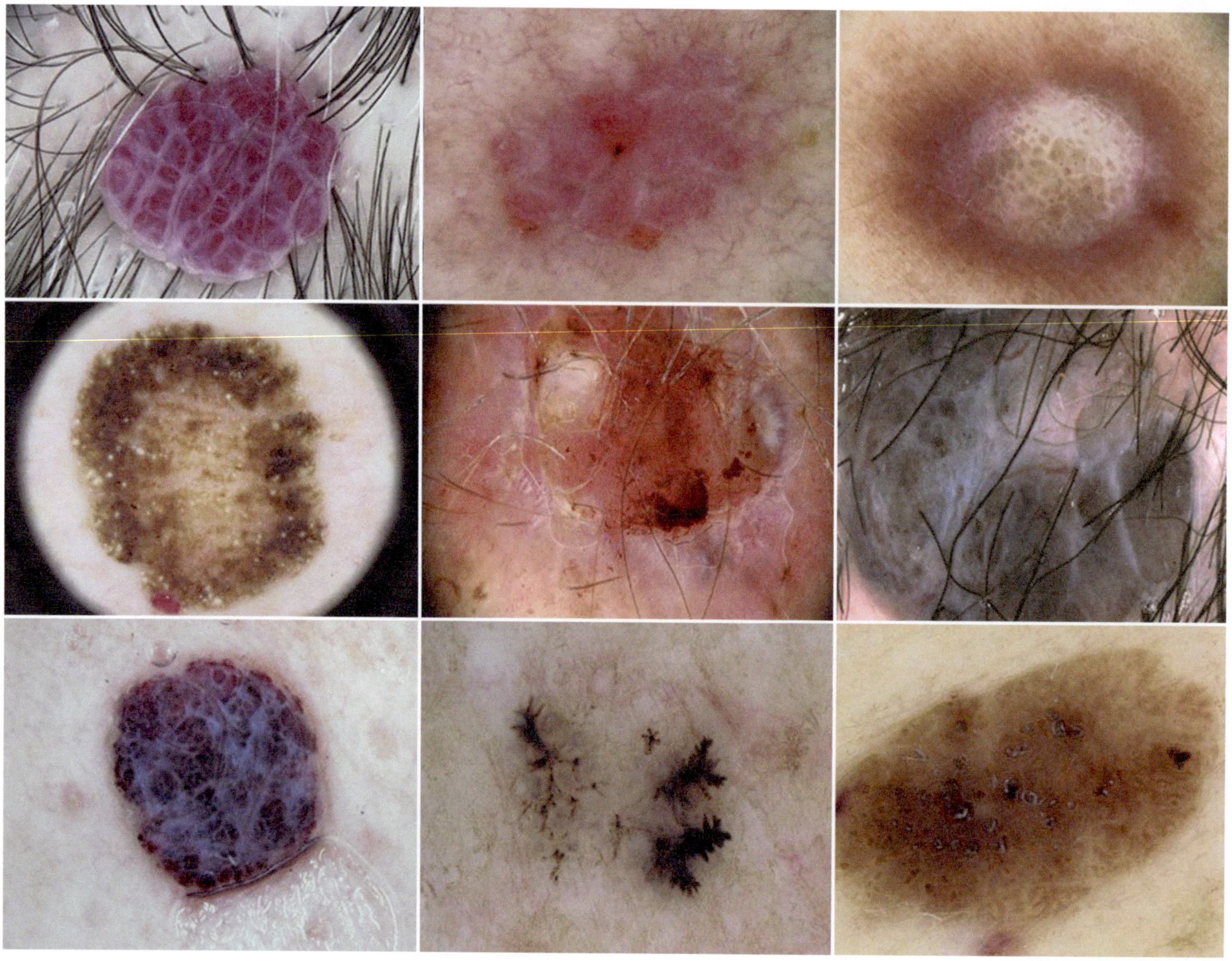

Fig. 1.10 Examples of cutaneous lesions with different colours

Nevi

2

Horacio Cabo and Aimilios Lallas

Congenital and Acquired Nevi

The term "melanocytic nevi" comprises a heterogeneous group of benign melanocytic proliferations with different epidemiologic, clinical, dermoscopic, and histopathologic characteristics. Within this spectrum, it is possible to distinguish two main categories: *congenital melanocytic nevi (CMN) and acquired melanocytic nevi (AMN).*

In general, CMN are present at birth, although they may become evident months or even years later. According to their size, they are classified into small (less than 1.5 cm), medium (1.5–20 cm), and large or giant (more than 20 cm) (Figs. 2.1, 2.2, 2.3, and 2.4).

With the exception of Spitz nevus and blue nevus that display specific dermoscopic pattern, all other nevi (congenital and acquired) may be dermoscopically classified into three main groups: nevi with a *reticular pattern,* nevi with a *globular pattern, and* nevi with a *mixed pattern (central or peripheral)* (Figs. 2.5, 2.6, 2.7, 2.8, 2.9, 2.10, 2.11, and 2.12).

Reticular pattern: the pigment network extends all over the lesion and is characterized by a relatively uniform color and line thickness. A peculiar variant is the *patched reticular pattern* where the pigment network areas alternate with areas without pigment network, usually skin-colored.

Globular pattern: globules are distributed over the lesion and are relatively uniform in terms of diameter and color. The *cobblestone pattern* represents a frequent variation, characterized by large and angulated globules.

Mixed Pattern: presence of both reticular and globular patterns in the same lesion. Globules location defines whether it is central or peripheral.

- *Central mixed pattern:* globules in the central area and pigment network in the periphery with two variants, the *hyperpigmented*, in which the central globules are highly pigmented and a brown zone can be seen in the central area, and the *hypo-pigmented*, where the central globules show little pigment and there is a central whitish or skin-colored area.
- *Peripheral mixed pattern:* globules are in the peripheral area. This variant is common in young people and related to the nevi growth. In general, there are one to three lines of globules. These should not appear in adults, since at maturity nevi must remain stable.

Other less frequent variants are *homogeneous pattern* (homogeneous brown lesions due to an even pigmentation over the entire lesion, which prevents structure distinction), *half-and-half pattern* (half globules and half pigment network), and *multicomponent pattern*, with the presence of three or more dermoscopy structures. It is associated with atypical nevi or melanoma.

H. Cabo (✉)
Instituto de Investigaciones Médicas "A. Lanari". Dermatology Section, University of Buenos Aires, Buenos Aires, Argentina

A. Lallas
First Department of Dermatology, Aristotle University of Thessaloniki, Thessaloniki, Greece

H. Cabo, A. Lallas (eds.), *Comprehensive Atlas of Dermatoscopy Cases*, https://doi.org/10.1007/978-3-319-76932-5_2

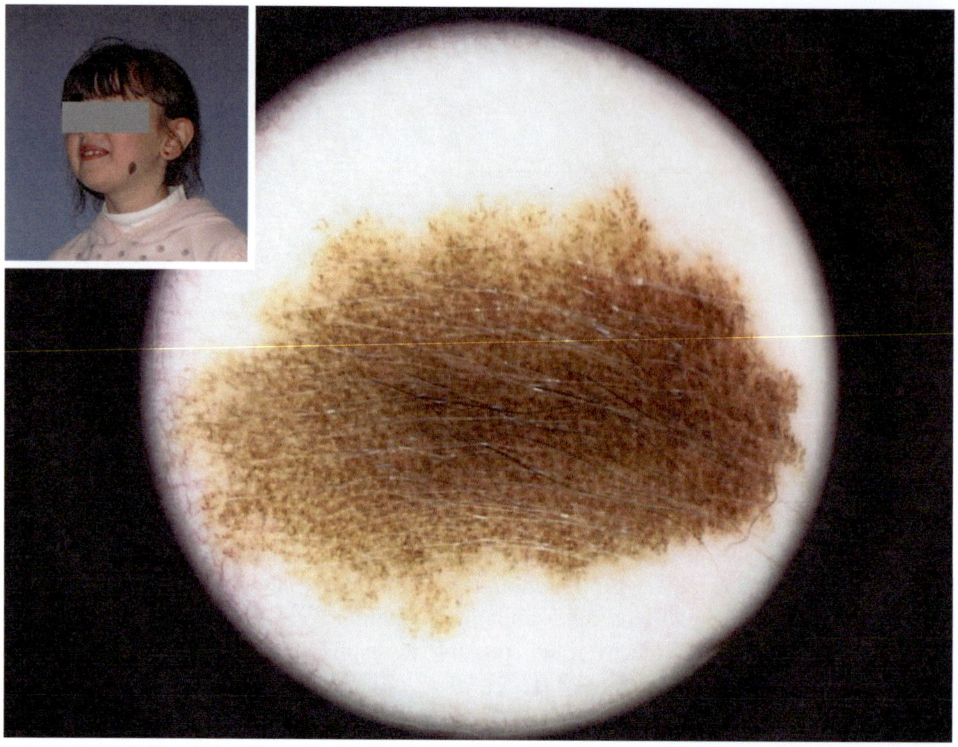

Fig. 2.1 Clinical and dermoscopy view of small melanocytic nevus on the face with reticular pattern

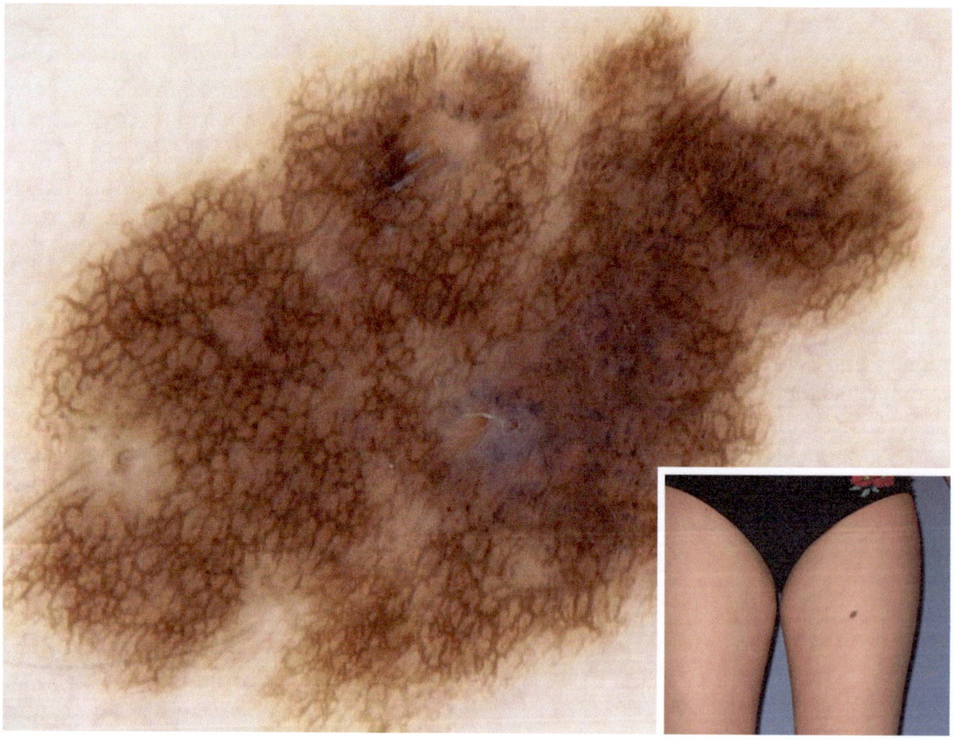

Fig. 2.2 Clinical and dermoscopy view of small melanocytic nevus on the leg with reticular pattern

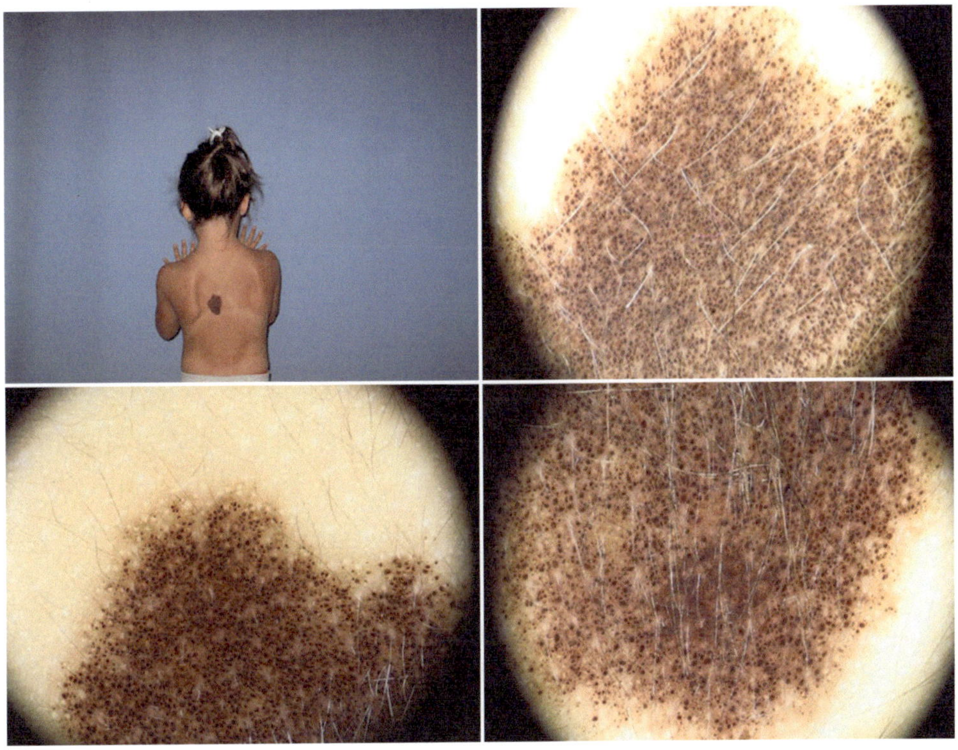

Fig. 2.3 Clinical and dermoscopy view of medium congenital melanocytic nevus on the back with reticular pattern

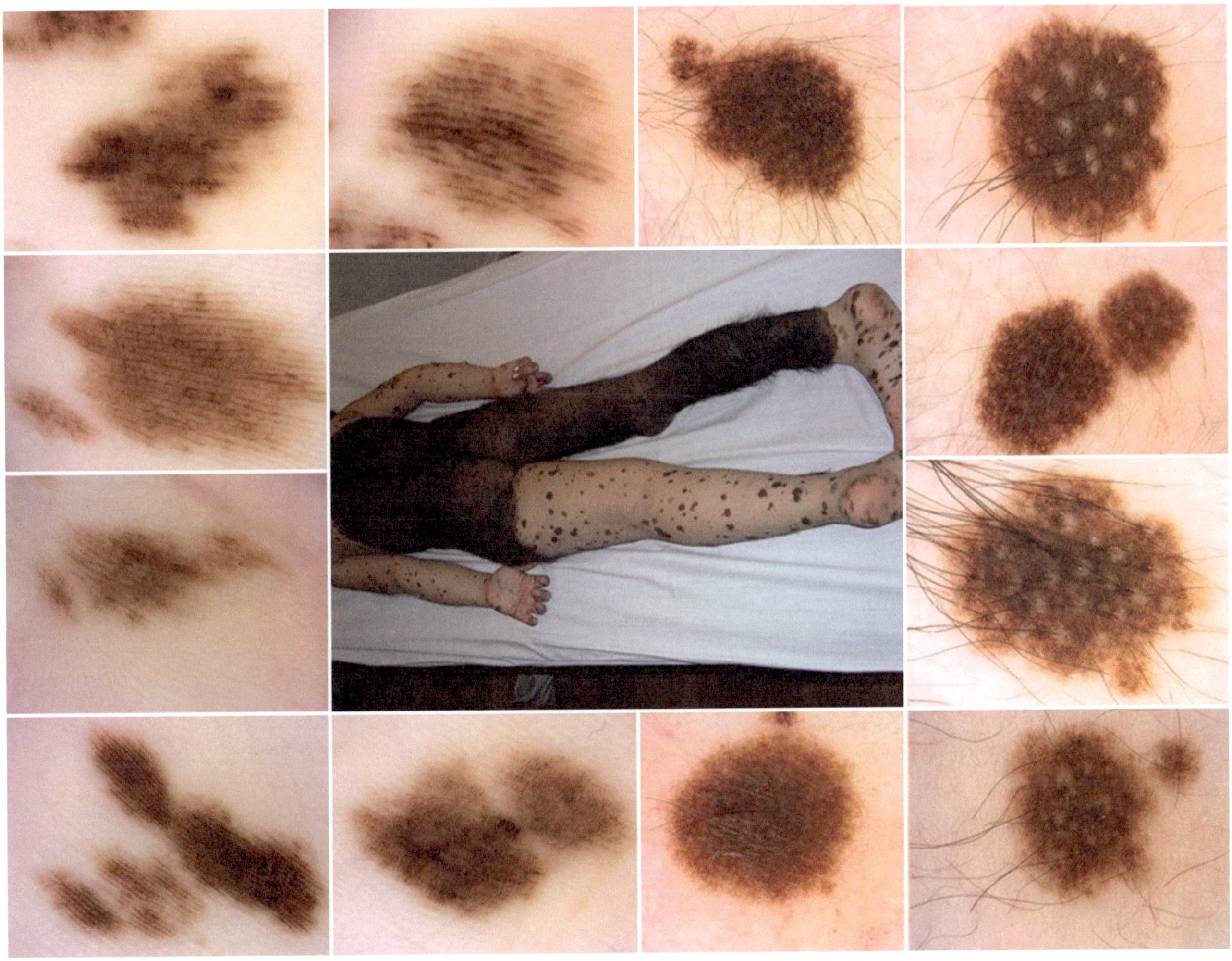

Fig. 2.4 Clinical and dermoscopy view of a giant congenital melanocytic nevus involving almost all the body sites with different dermoscopy patterns

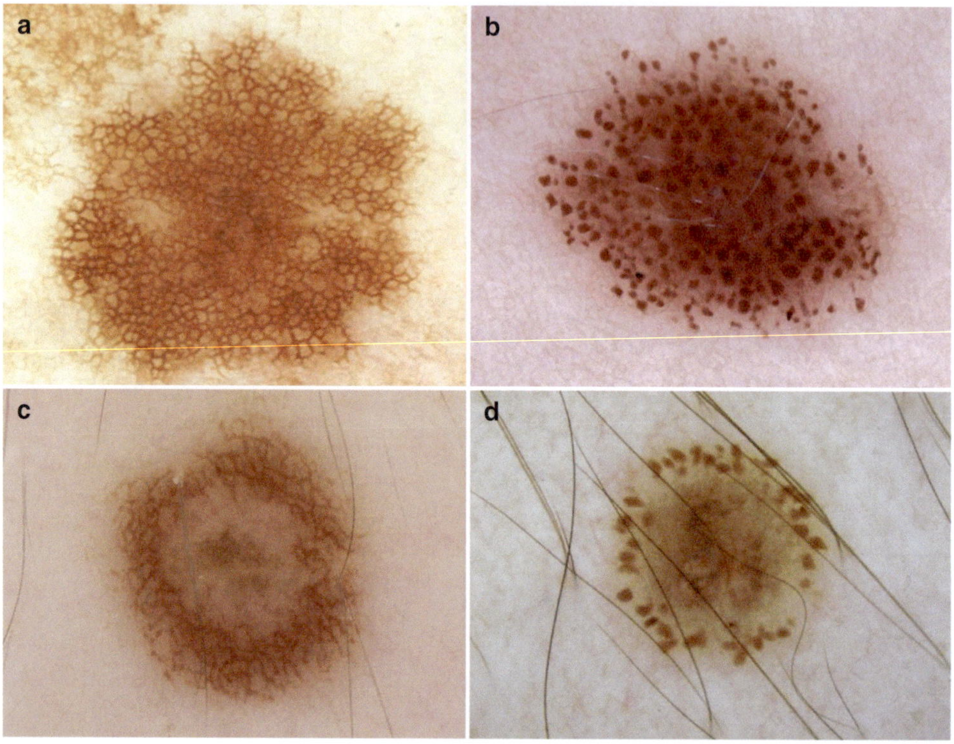

Fig. 2.5 Melanocytic nevi with (**a**) reticular pattern, (**b**) globular pattern, (**c**) mixed central pattern, (**d**) mixed peripheral pattern

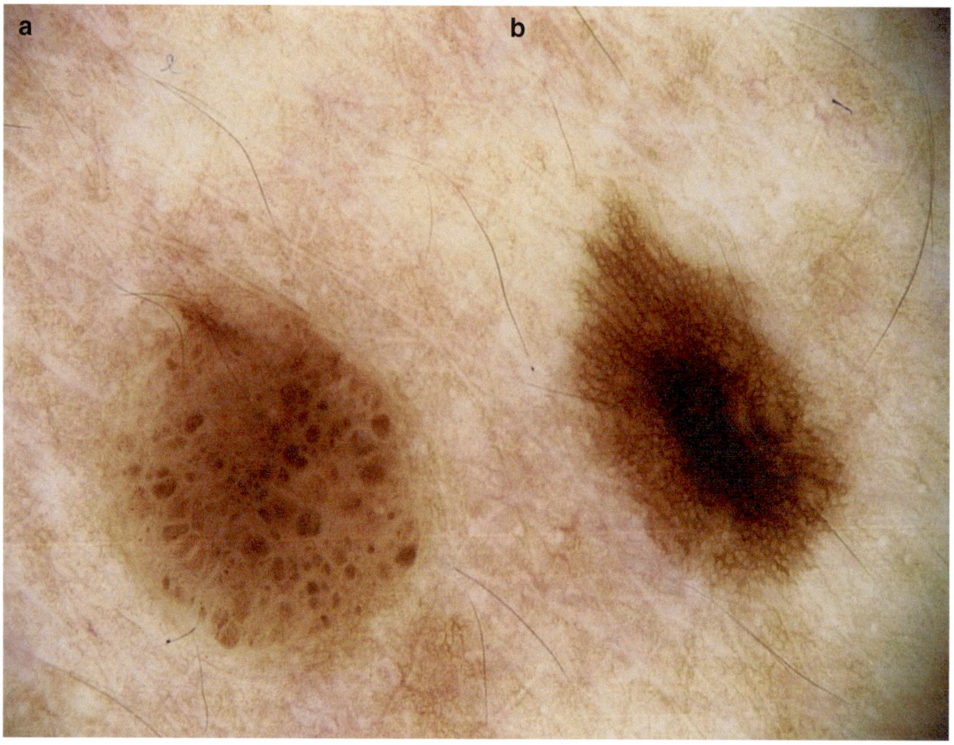

Fig. 2.6 Melanocytic nevi with (**a**) globular pattern, (**b**) reticular pattern

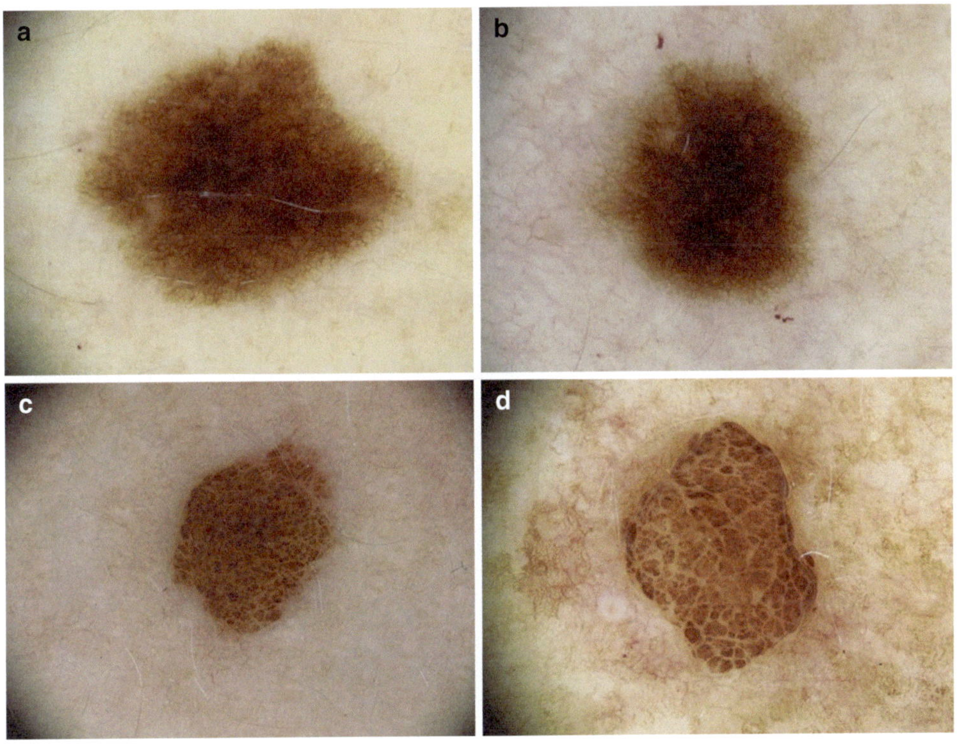

Fig. 2.7 Melanocytic nevi with (**a**, **b**) reticular pattern. (**c**, **d**) Globular pattern

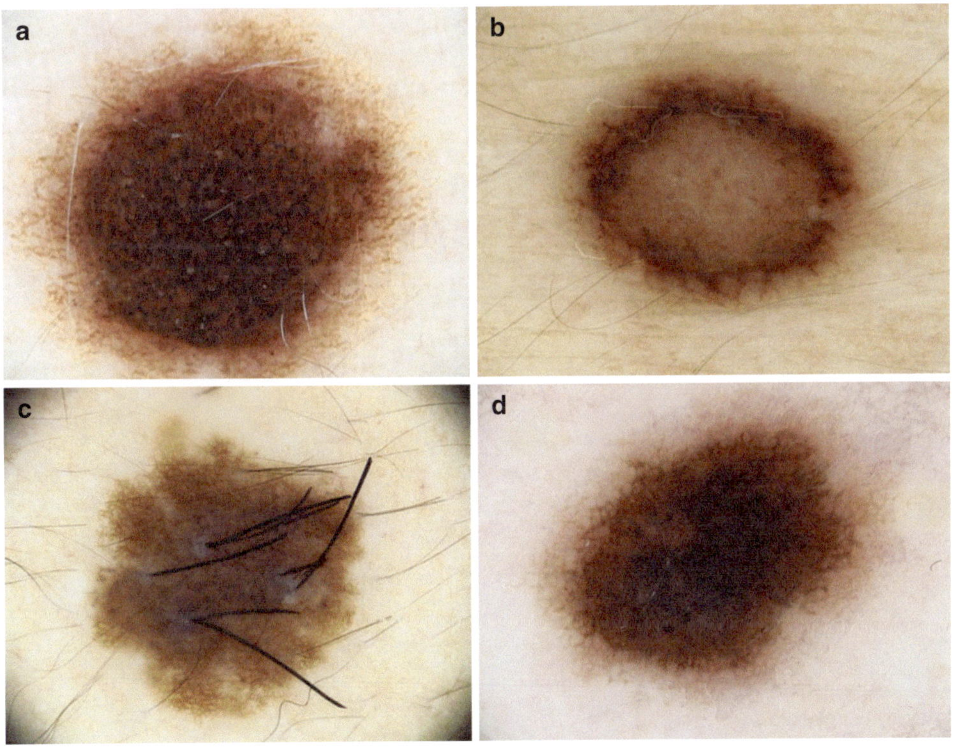

Fig. 2.8 Melanocytic nevi (**a**–**d**) with mixed central pattern

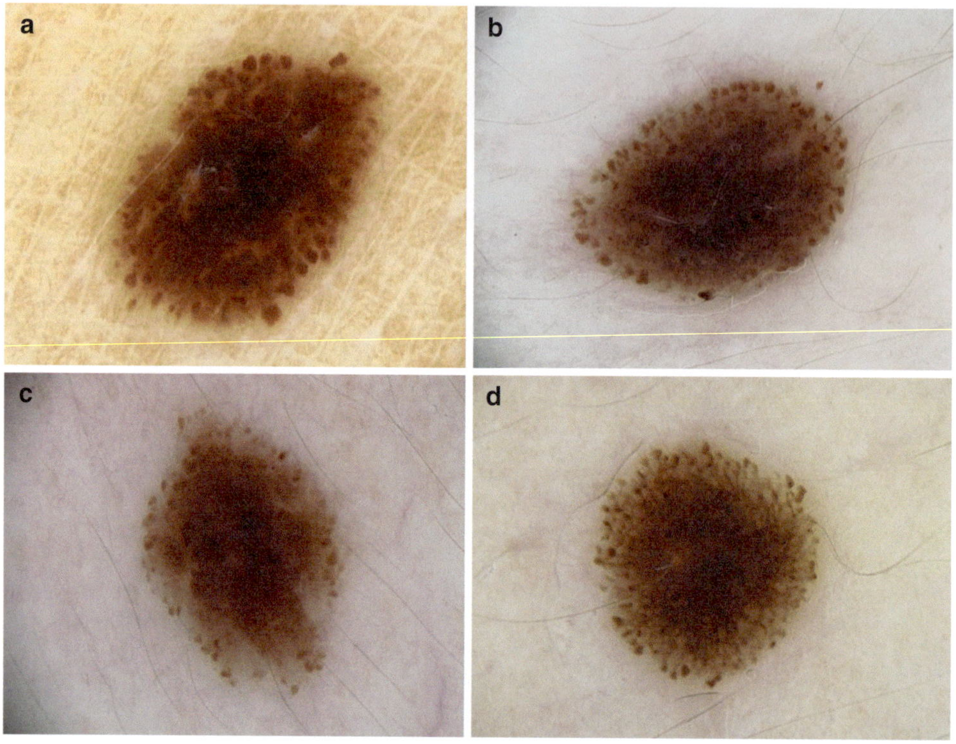

Fig. 2.9 Melanocytic nevi (**a**–**d**) with mixed peripheral pattern

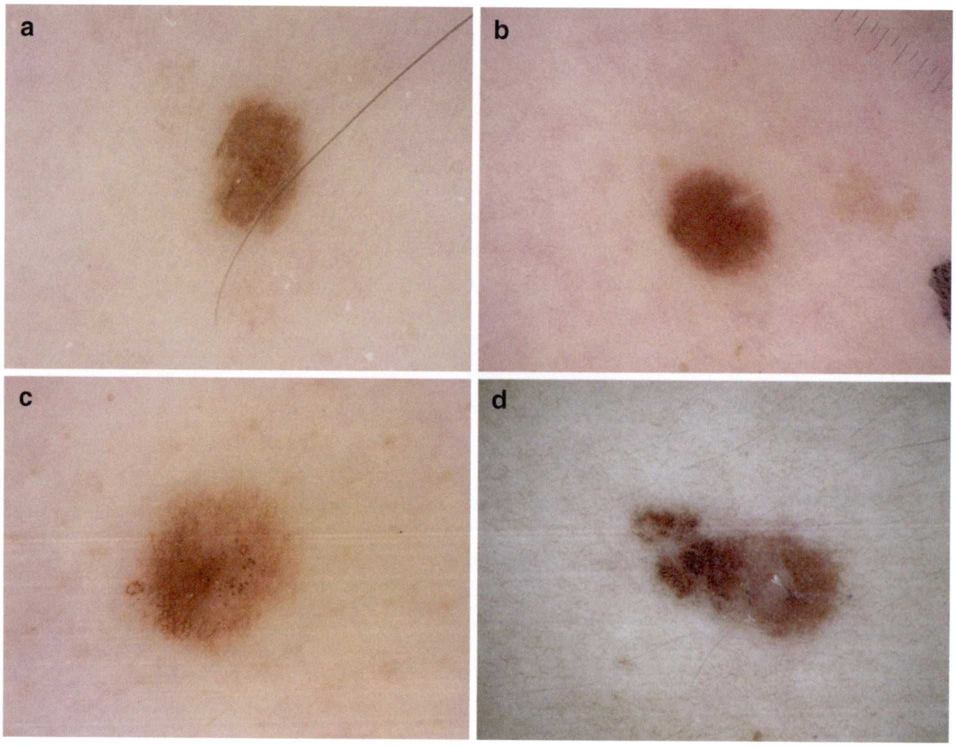

Fig. 2.10 Melanocytic nevus with homogeneous pattern (**a**–**b**) and half-and-half pattern, half globules, and half pigment network (**c**–**d**)

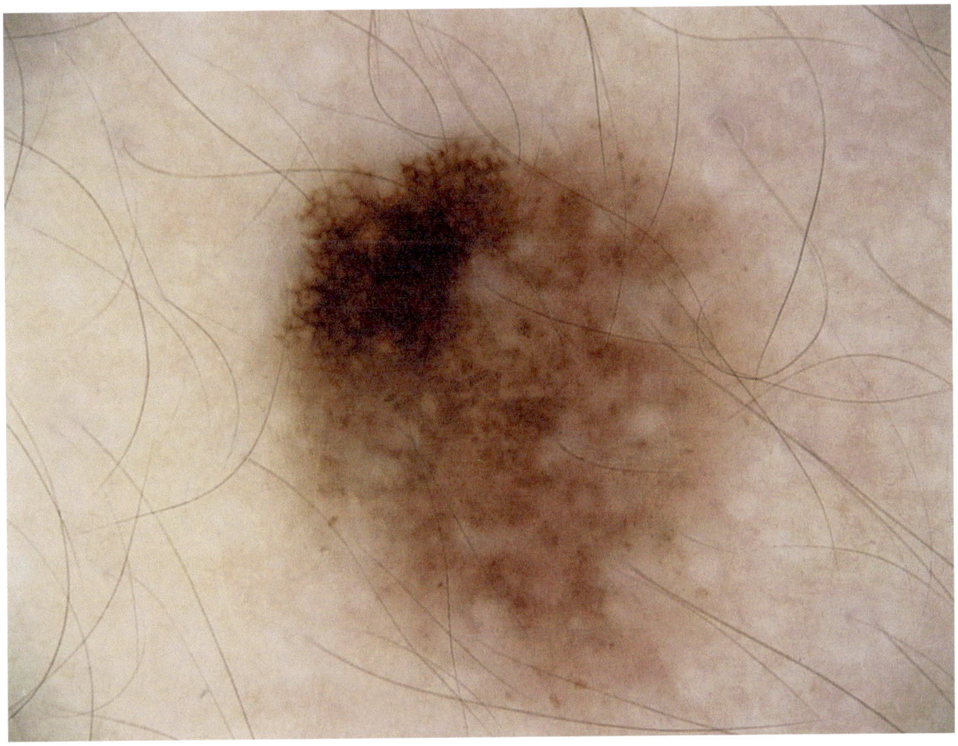

Fig. 2.11 Melanocytic nevus with multicomponent pattern

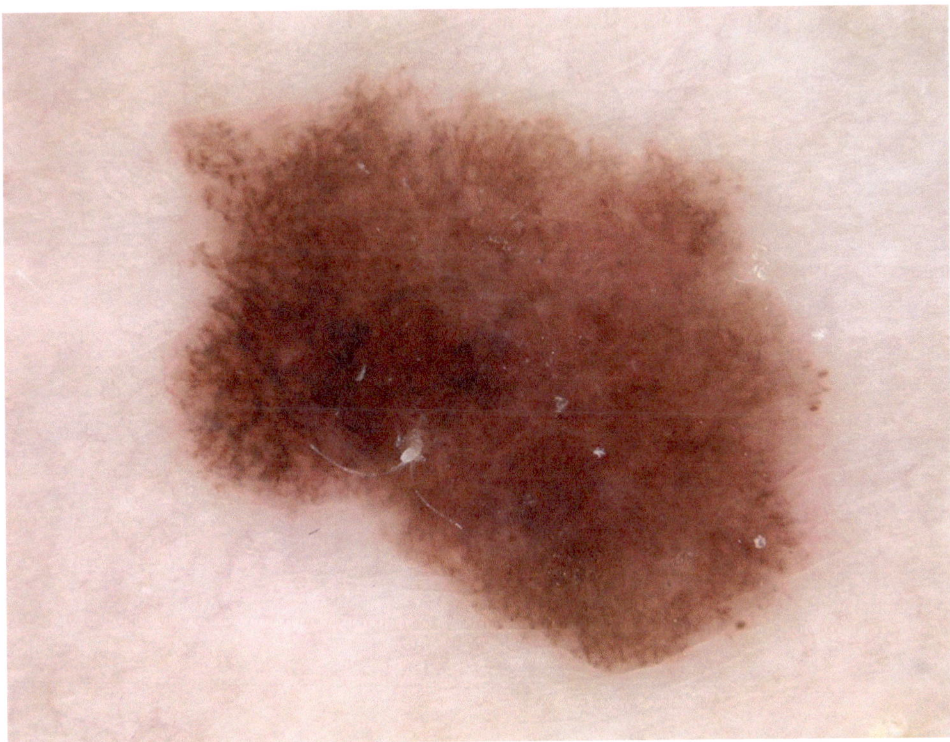

Fig. 2.12 Melanocytic nevus with multicomponent pattern

Spitz Nevus

Spitz nevi can present as macules, papules, nodules, or plaques and their size is usually smaller than 6 mm, rarely exceeding 10 mm.

The hypo-pigmented variant, the "classic" type, typically develops as a pink-reddish papule or nodule, which often is fast-growing and more frequently located in the head/neck area. However, the majority of Spitz nevi are pigmented lesions and they show a brown-to-black appearance (also called Reed nevi).

The main dermoscopy patterns of Spitz nevi are the *reticular, globular, starburst, homogenous, and atypical patterns*, for pigmented lesions, and the *vascular pattern* (homogenous pink pattern, dotted vessels, and inverse network) in hypo-pigmented or amelanotic lesions (Figs. 2.13, 2.14, 2.15, 2.16, and 2.17).

Reticular pattern has a homogeneous and regular pigment network covering most part of the lesion.

Globular pattern is with gray-brown large globules, distributed throughout the lesion or at the periphery.

Starburst pattern is the most frequent pattern and corresponds to the radial growth phase of this lesion. Peripheral black to gray globules are fused with the central body of the lesion (forming the so-called streaks, pseudopods, or radial streaming) and are responsible for the starburst appearance, similar to an exploding star.

Homogenous pattern has a diffuse, uniform, structureless, pink, dark brown, or black-bluish color, which fills most of the lesion and lacks evidence of clear-cut streaks at the periphery.

Atypical pattern has features suggestive of melanoma such as irregularity in the distribution of colors and structures and the presence of blue-white veil, black blotches, irregular streaks, and irregular globules.

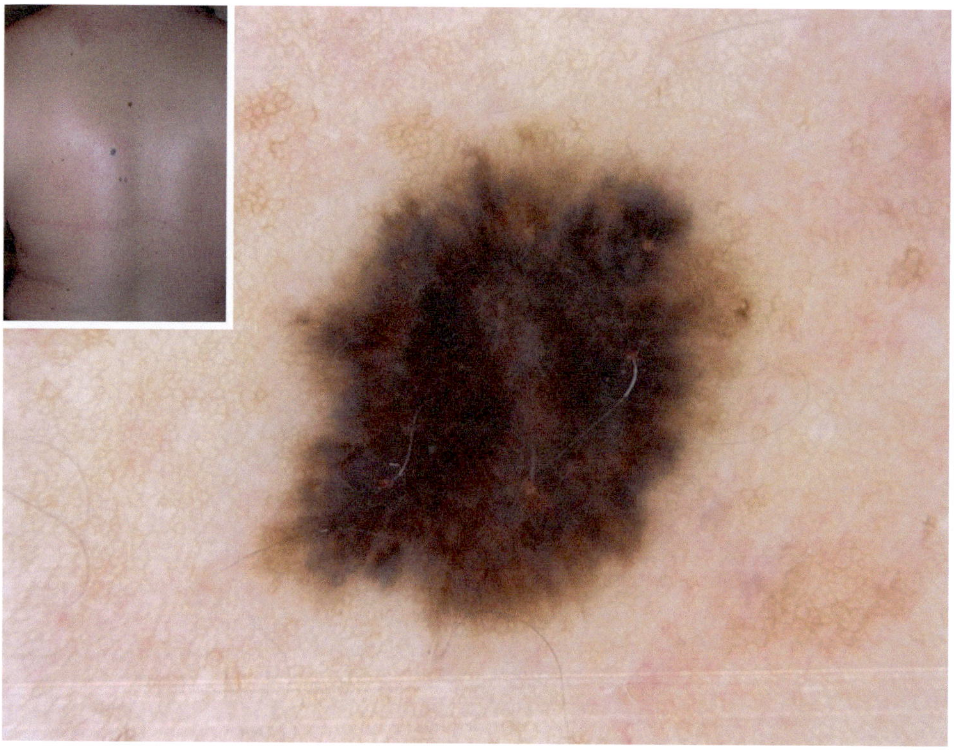

Fig. 2.13 Spitz nevus with reticular pattern

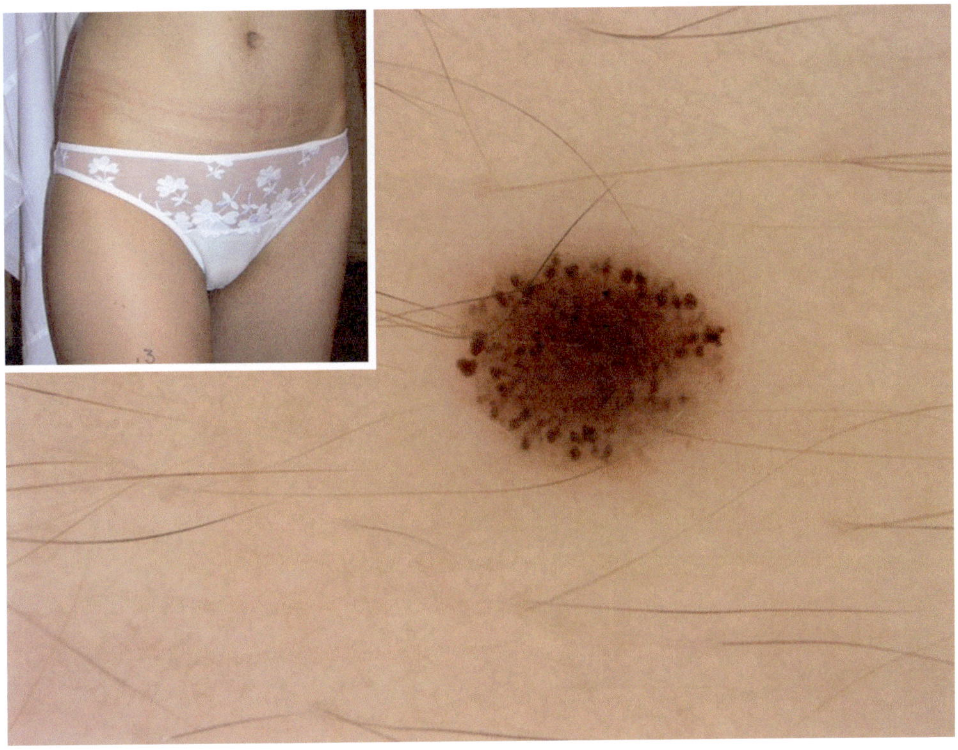

Fig. 2.14 Spitz and peripheral globules nevus with reticular pattern

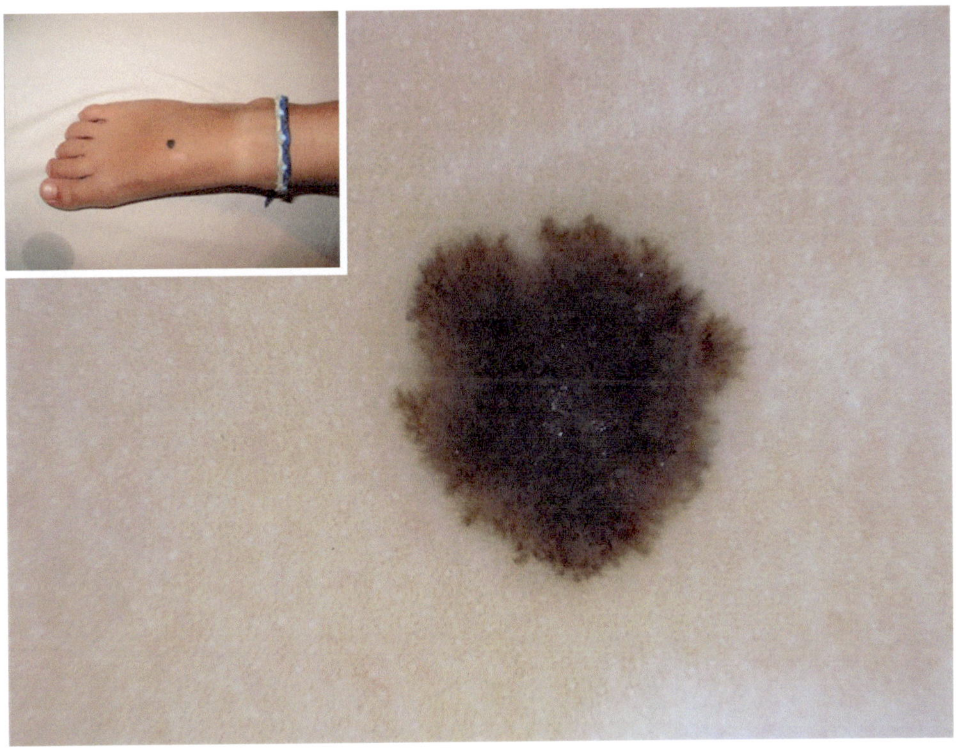

Fig. 2.15 Spitz nevus with starburst pattern

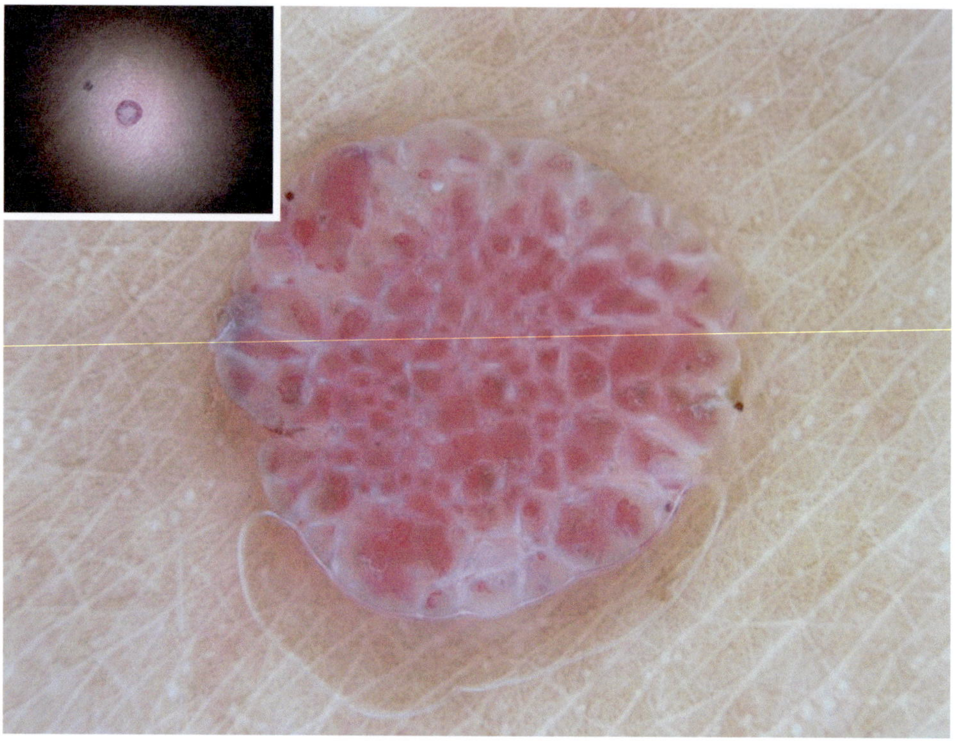

Fig. 2.16 Spitz nevus with a vascular pattern

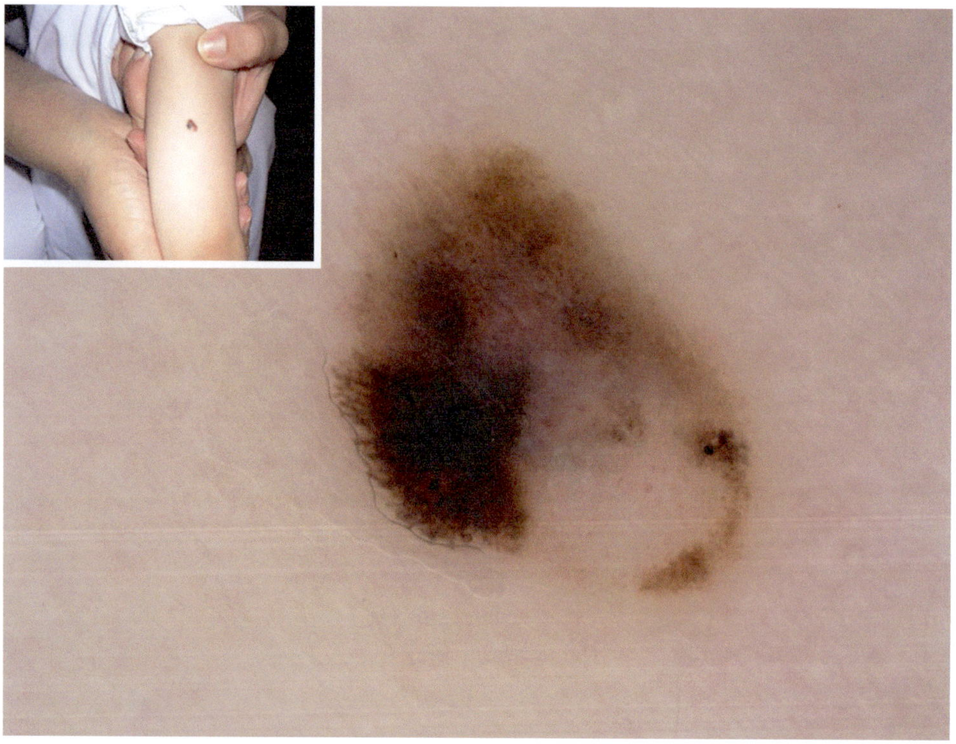

Fig. 2.17 Spitz nevus with atypical pattern

Blue Nevus and Combined Nevus (Figs. 2.18 and 2.19)

Blue nevus is a melanocytic nevus. There are two main types, common and cellular. Common blue nevus is usually a nodular lesion of bluish-gray or bluish-black color. Cellular blue nevus is typically a larger nodule, blue or black in color, which preferably develops on the sacrocoxal area or in the buttocks. It appears in infancy and manifests less frequently than the common blue nevus. Melanoma metastasis, tattoos, and radiotherapy marks are included in the differential diagnosis of common blue nevi, among others.

Dermoscopy criteria: Blue nevus is typified by a homogeneous blue coloration with generally uniform pigmentation but looks different under polarized and non-polarized light dermoscopes.

Combined nevus is a melanocytic nevus characterized by the association of a blue nevus with a dermal, compound, or junction nevus in the same lesion.

Clinically the features of the blue nevus prevail in the lesion. They may be similar to a blue nevus or present a targetoid form (combined targetoid nevus), with a blue central area and a light or dark brown coloration in the peripheral part of the lesion.

Dermoscopy criteria: They may present a homogeneous blue coloration, which makes them indistinguishable from blue nevi. There may also be combined nevi with two colors, a homogeneous blue, dark blue, or black central zone and a peripheral zone in different shades of brown with structureless areas, globules, or pigment network.

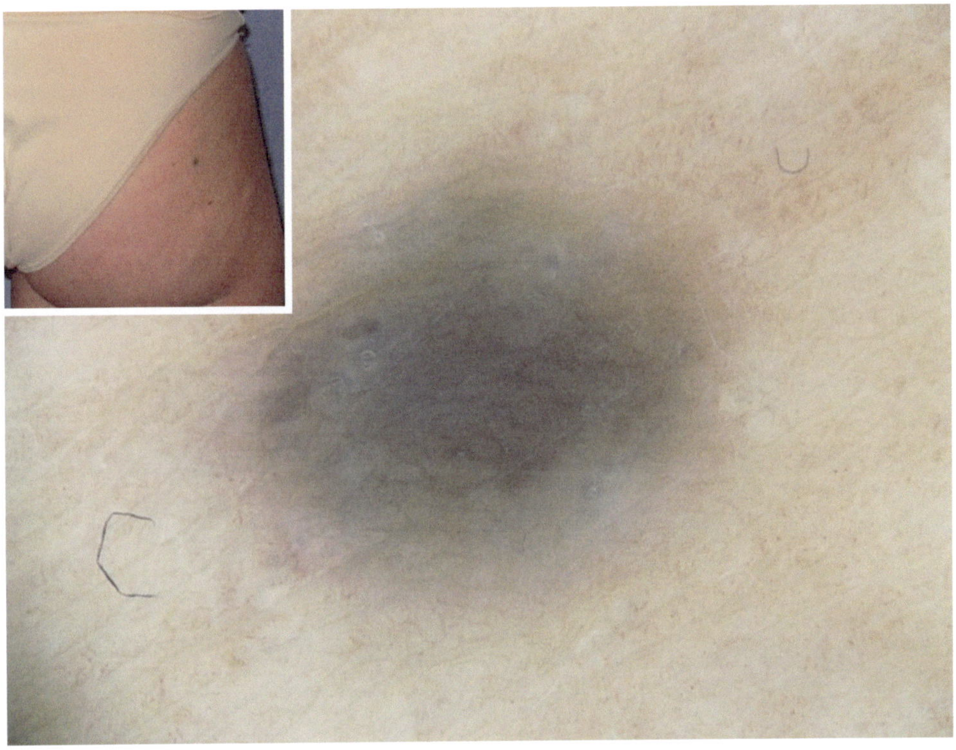

Fig. 2.18 Blue nevus

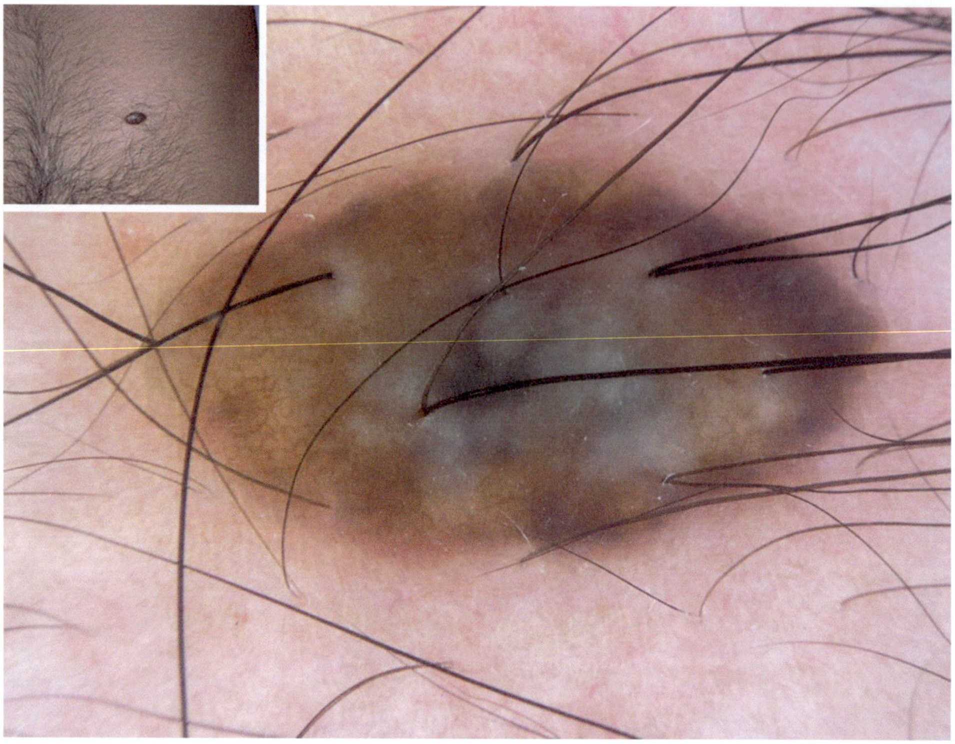

Fig. 2.19 Combined nevus (intradermal nevus + blue nevus)

Recurrent Nevus (Fig. 2.20)

Recurrent or persistent nevus (RN) results from the recurrence of pigmentation after an incomplete excision of a nevus, usually compound or intradermal. RN might appear after an incomplete surgical excision (e.g. shave excision) but also after laser surgery, radiotherapy, or nevus traumatism. The most frequent site of appearance is the trunk.

Dermoscopy of RN typically shows globules of variable size and color and that are irregularly distributed or peripheral streaks. However, the pigmentation is typically restricted within the scar of the previous excision.

Clinical Clues

- History of previous excision
- Histopathologic study, if possible
- Time span between appearance and recurrence
  - RN: 4–10 months after excision
  - Melanoma: more than a year
- Pigment location
  - NR: pigmentation within the scar
  - Melanoma: pigmented lesions spread beyond the scar

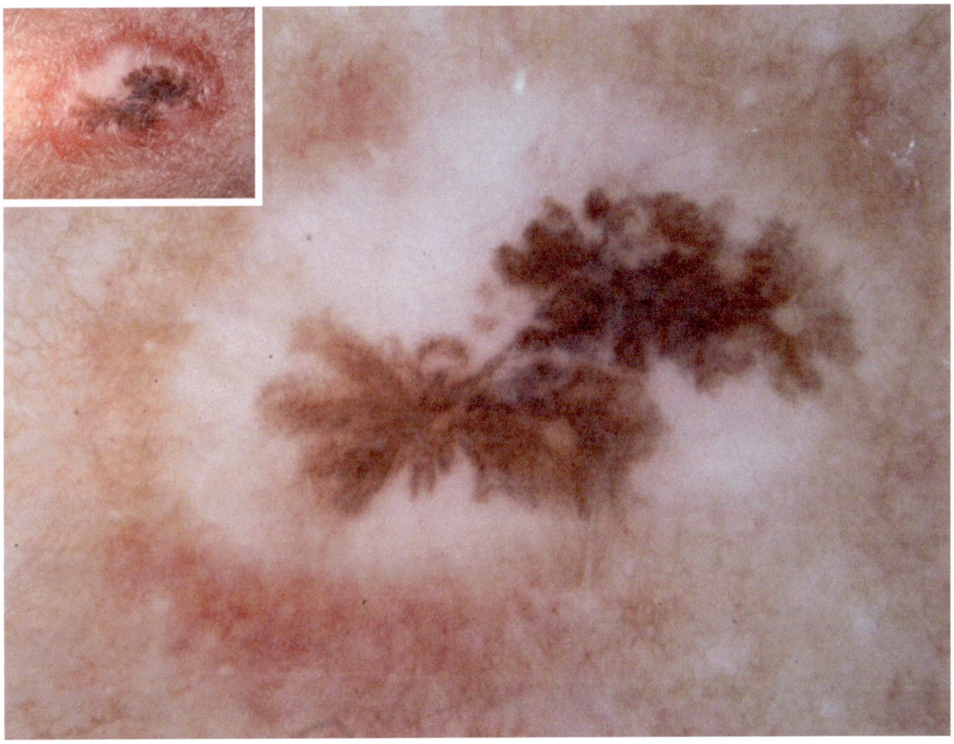

Fig. 2.20 Recurrent nevus

Melanoma

3

Horacio Cabo and Aimilios Lallas

Superficial Spreading Melanoma (SSM)

According to pattern analysis, any pigmented lesion is dermoscopically characterized by a global pattern and local features. The local features associated with melanoma are known as "melanoma-specific criteria."

Global patterns of SSM (Figs. 3.1, 3.2, 3.3, 3.4, and 3.5):

Atypical reticular pattern
Atypical globular pattern
Peripheral streak pattern
Multicomponent pattern
Unspecific pattern

Local features of SSM (Figs. 3.6, 3.7, 3.8, 3.9, 3.10, 3.11, 3.12, 3.13, and 3.14):

Atypical pigment network
Negative pigment network
Irregular streaks
Irregular dots and globules
Blue-white veil
Regression structures with white or blue areas
Irregular pigmentation
Irregular vascular pattern
Shiny white lines

H. Cabo (✉)
Instituto de Investigaciones Médicas "A. Lanari". Dermatology Section, University of Buenos Aires, Buenos Aires, Argentina

A. Lallas
First Department of Dermatology, Aristotle University of Thessaloniki, Thessaloniki, Greece

H. Cabo, A. Lallas (eds.), *Comprehensive Atlas of Dermatoscopy Cases*, https://doi.org/10.1007/978-3-319-76932-5_3

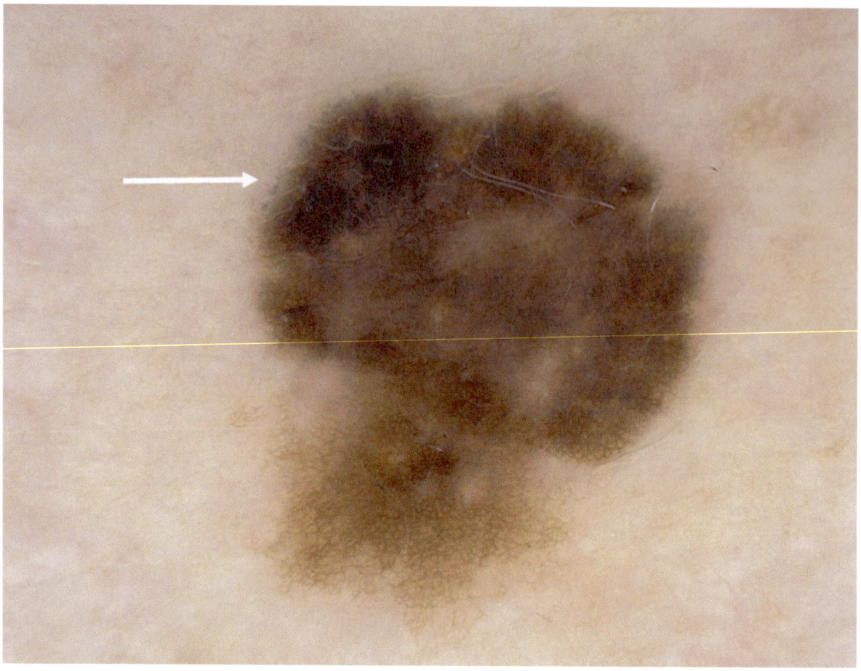

Fig. 3.1 Melanoma in situ with atypical reticular pattern (black, gray, or brown network with irregular mesh and wide lines) (white arrow)

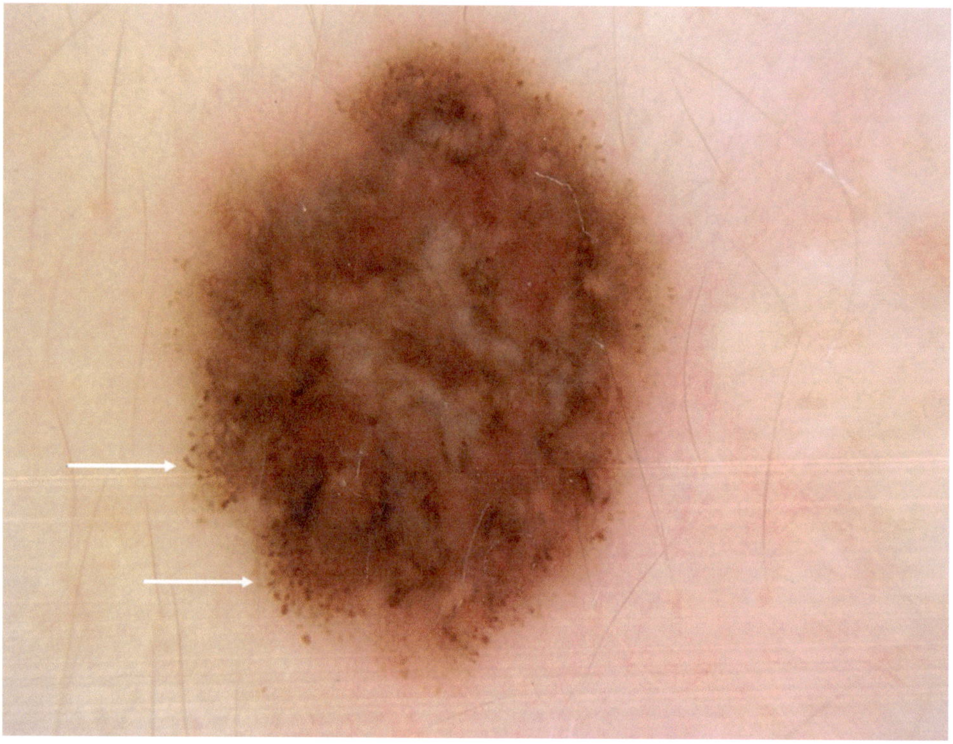

Fig. 3.2 Atypical nevus with atypical globular pattern (dots and globules of different size and color distributed irregularly over the lesion) (white arrows)

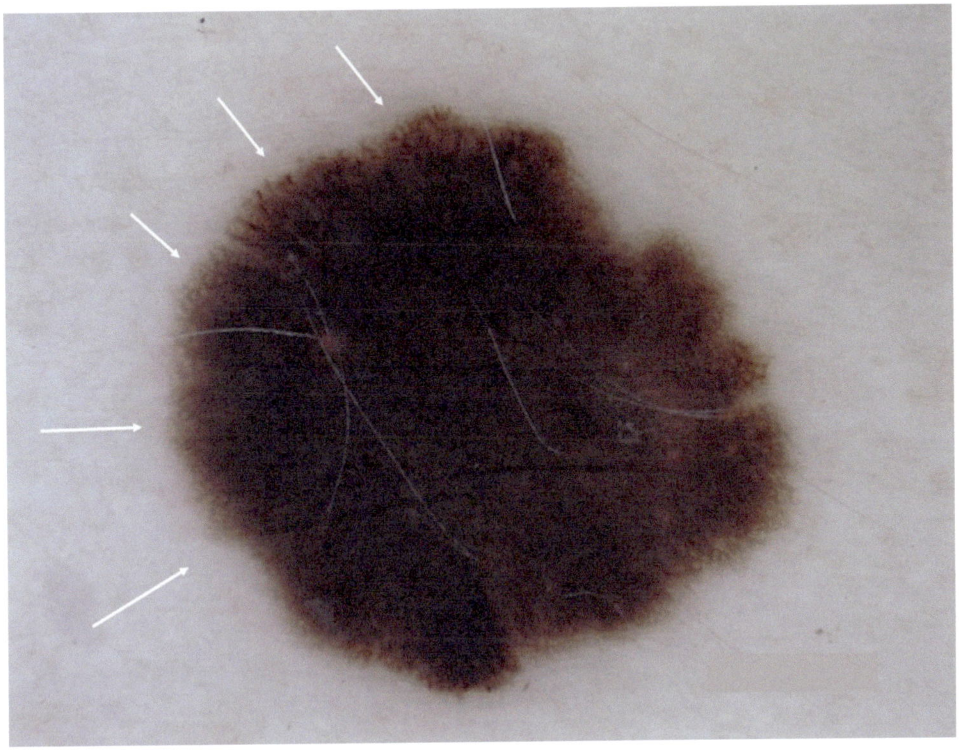

Fig. 3.3 Peripheral streak pattern. Superficial spreading melanoma with irregular streaks (irregular projections)—white arrows

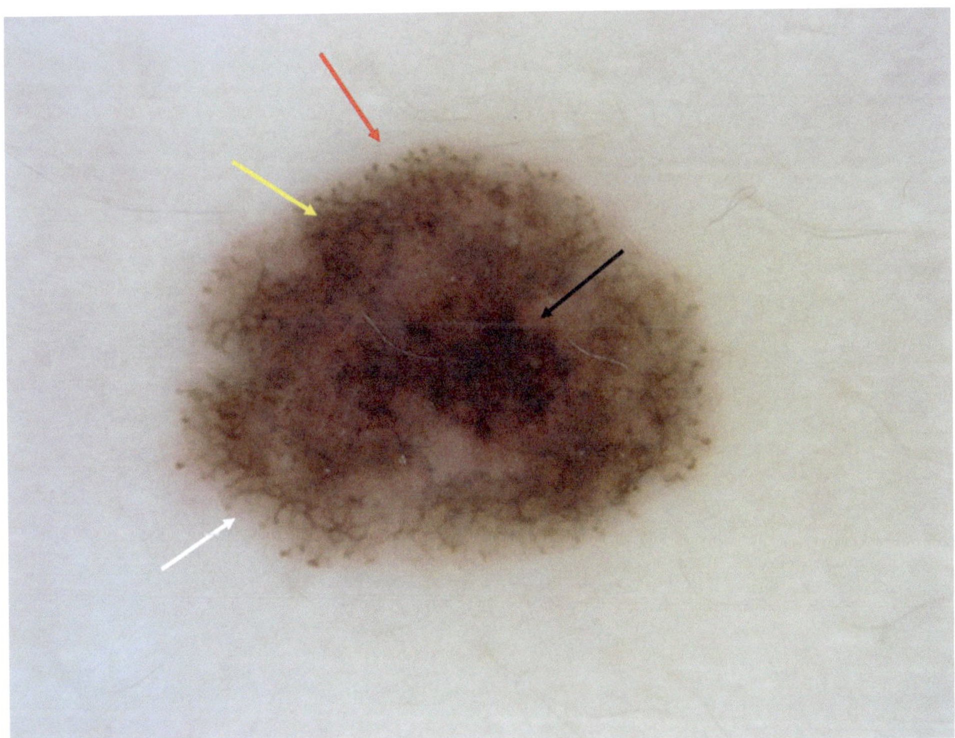

Fig. 3.4 Melanoma in situ. Multicomponent pattern: the combination of three or more dermoscopy patterns in the same lesion. This pattern is most frequently associated with the existence of melanoma (red arrow: irregular globules; white arrow: streaks; yellow arrow: atypical network; black arrow: asymmetric pigmentation)

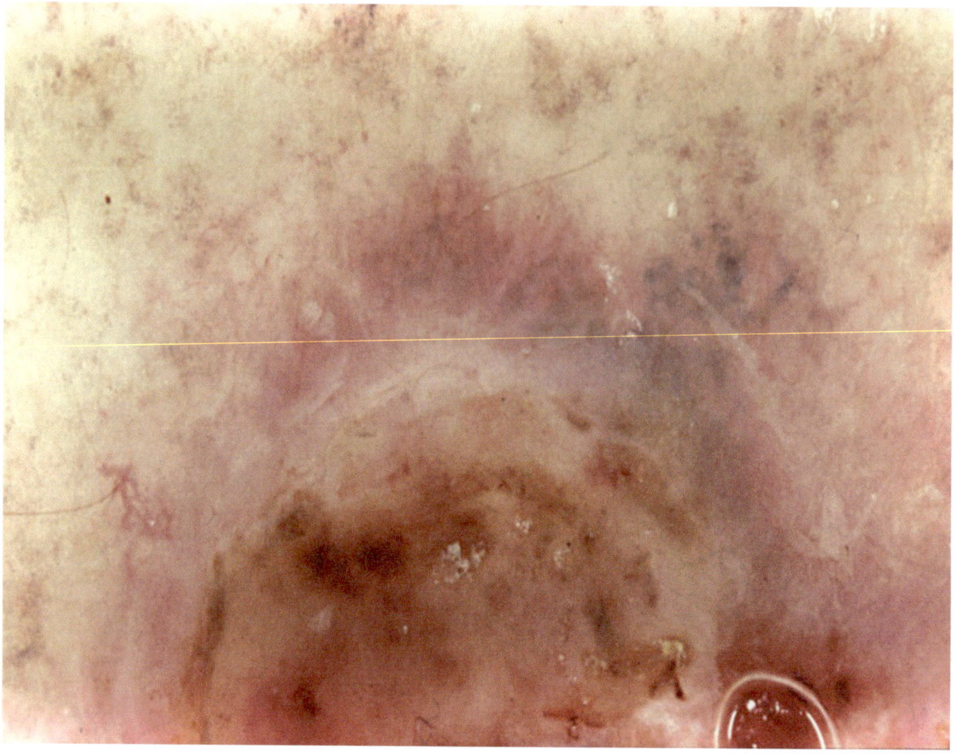

Fig. 3.5 SSM with unspecific pattern

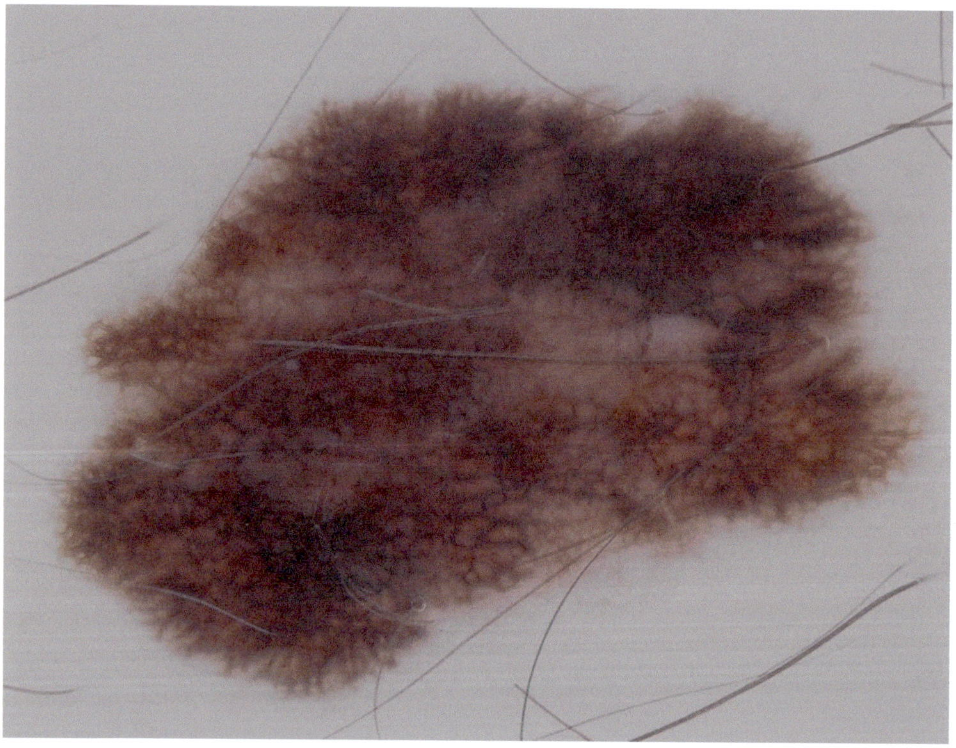

Fig. 3.6 Melanoma in situ with atypical network over the entire lesion

Fig. 3.7 Melanoma in situ with negative pigment network (white arrow)

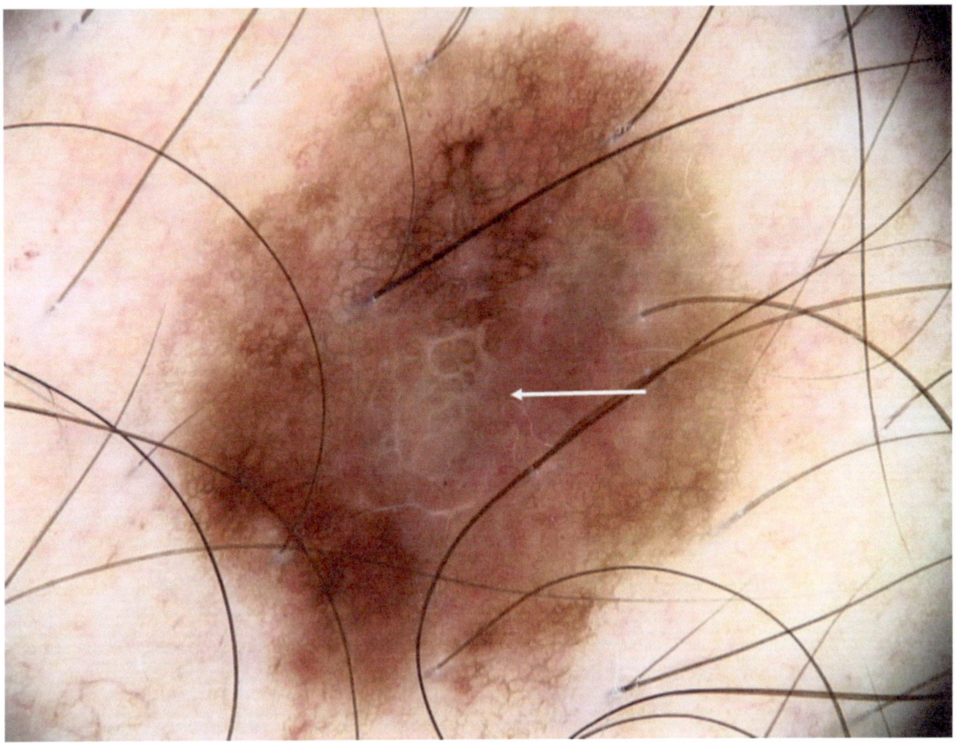

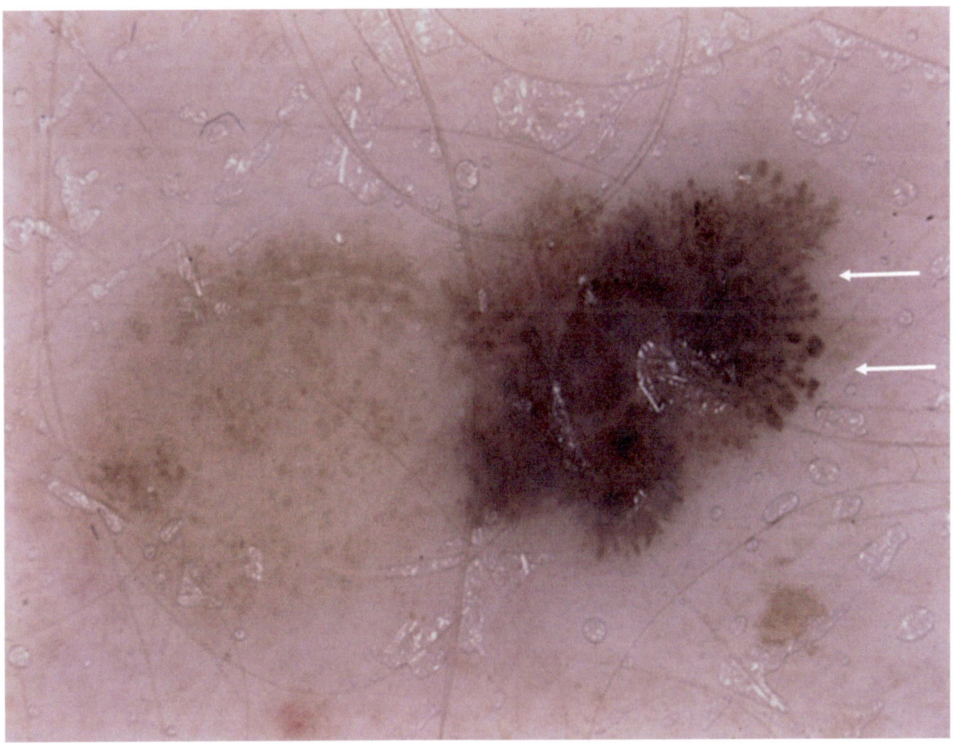

Fig. 3.8 Spreading superficial melanoma with irregular streaks (white arrows)

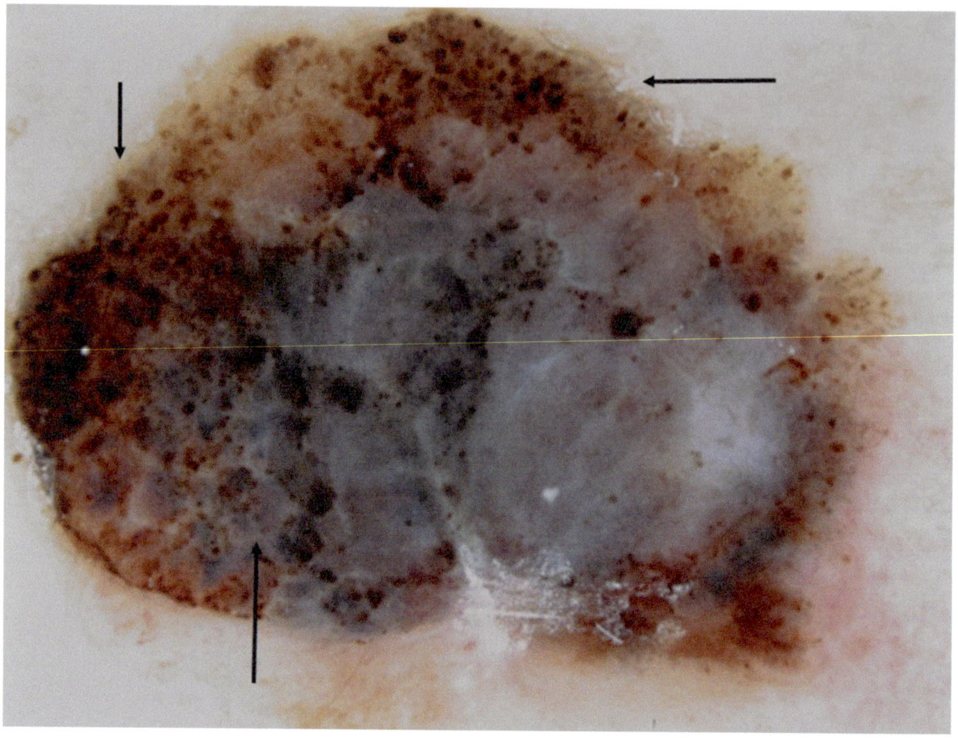

Fig. 3.9 Superficial spreading melanoma with irregular dots and globules (black arrows)

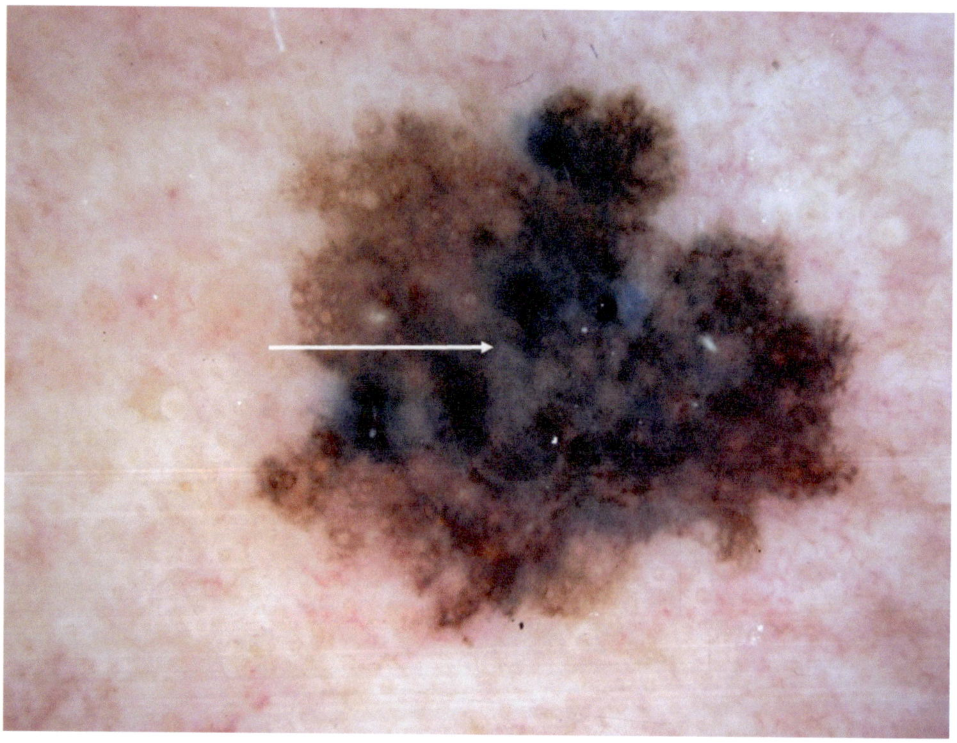

Fig. 3.10 Superficial spreading melanoma with blue-white veil (white arrow)

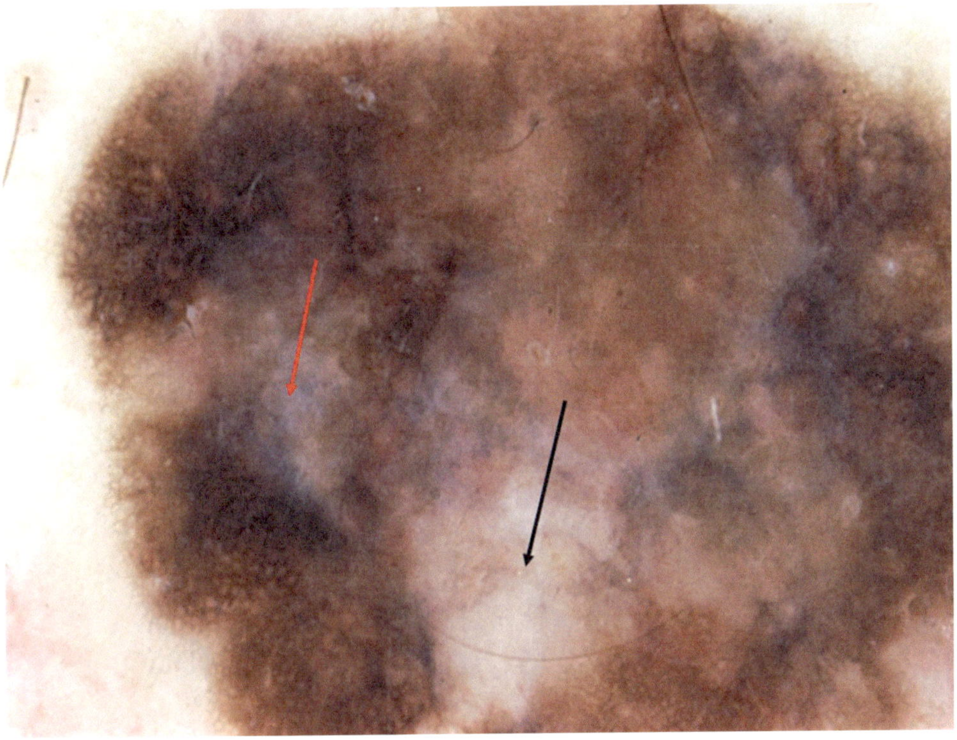

Fig. 3.11 Superficial spreading melanoma with regression, blue areas (red arrow), and white areas (black arrow)

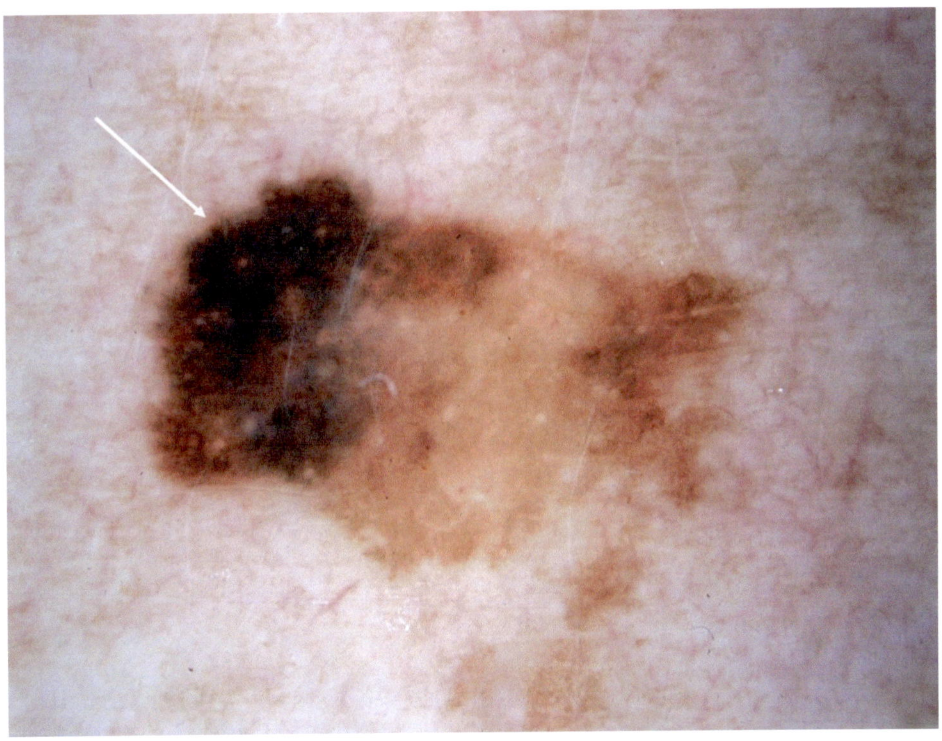

Fig. 3.12 Superficial spreading melanoma with irregular pigmentation (white arrow)

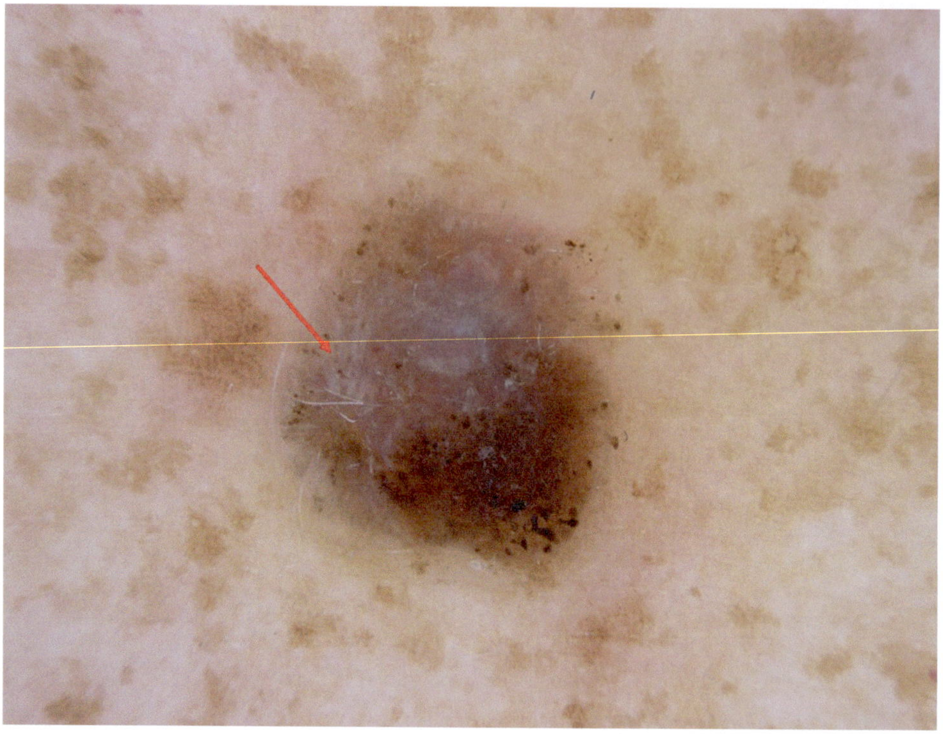

Fig. 3.14 Superficial spreading melanoma with shiny white lines (red arrow)

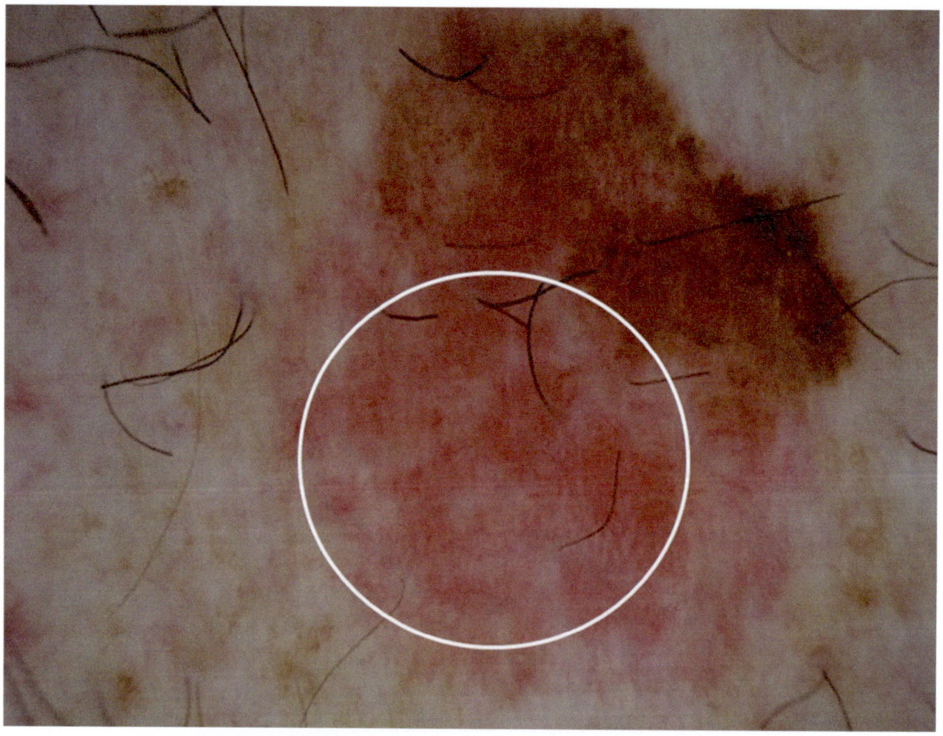

Fig. 3.13 Hypomelanotic superficial spreading melanoma with irregular random vascular pattern and polymorphous pattern (white circle)

Lentigo Maligna Melanoma (LM)

The dermoscopic features of LM are the following (Figs. 3.15 and 3.16):

Blue-gray color: Sometimes this is the only clue to suspect a LM.

Blue, gray, or black pigmented and asymmetrically pigmented follicular openings: The presence of dark brown or black follicular pigmentation indicates the irregular proliferation of atypical melanocytes within the follicles.

Two concentric circles (circle within a circle):

Slate gray dots around the follicular openings: It is an early sign of LM and it is the beginning of granular–annular pattern.

Rhomboidal structures: At a later stage, it is possible to detect dark brown or black lines or short streaks, highly specific around the follicles.

Homogeneous blue-gray areas with the hair follicles spared or obliterated.

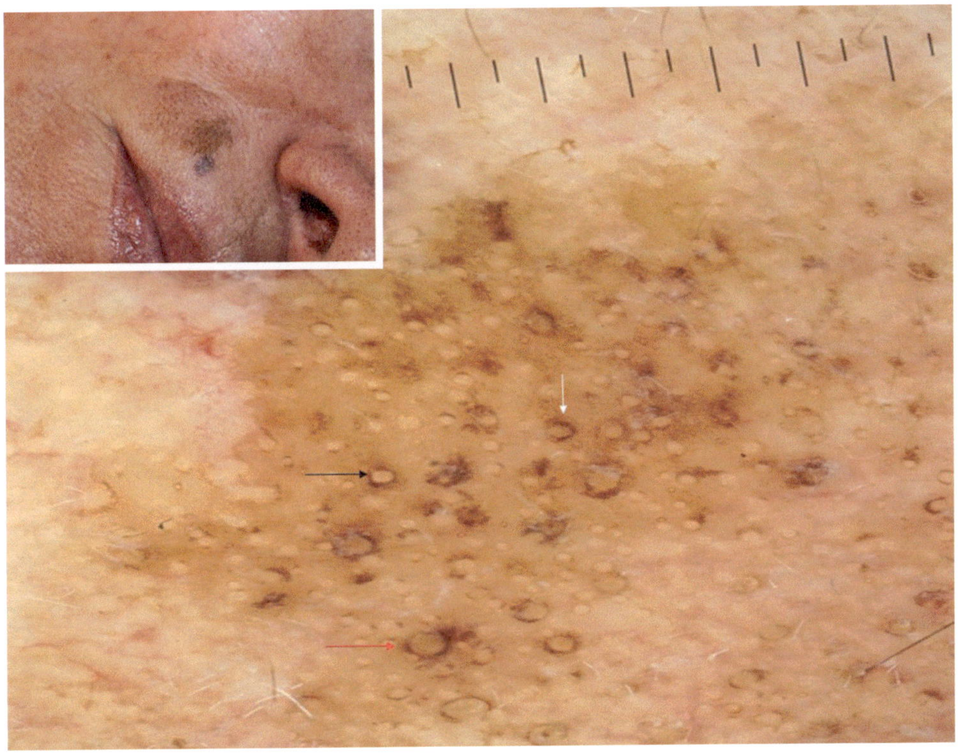

Fig. 3.15 Lentigo maligna: Blue-gray pigmented follicular openings (black arrow); asymmetric pigmentation of the follicular openings (red arrow); circle within a circle (white arrow)

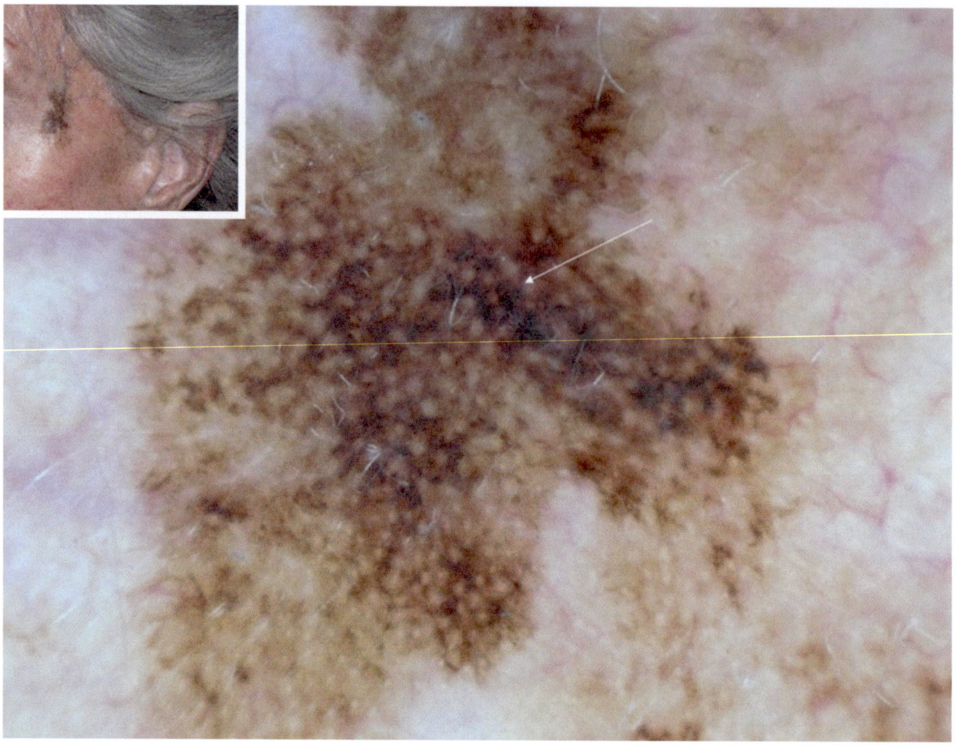

Fig. 3.16 Lentigo maligna with rhomboidal structures (white arrow)

Acral Melanoma (AM) (Fig. 3.17)

Dermoscopy features of AM are as follows:

Parallel ridge pattern (due to the special anatomical characteristics of the acral zones)

Diffuse pigmentation with varying coloration

Irregular and peripheral globules/dots

Abrupt end of pigmentation at the periphery of the lesion.

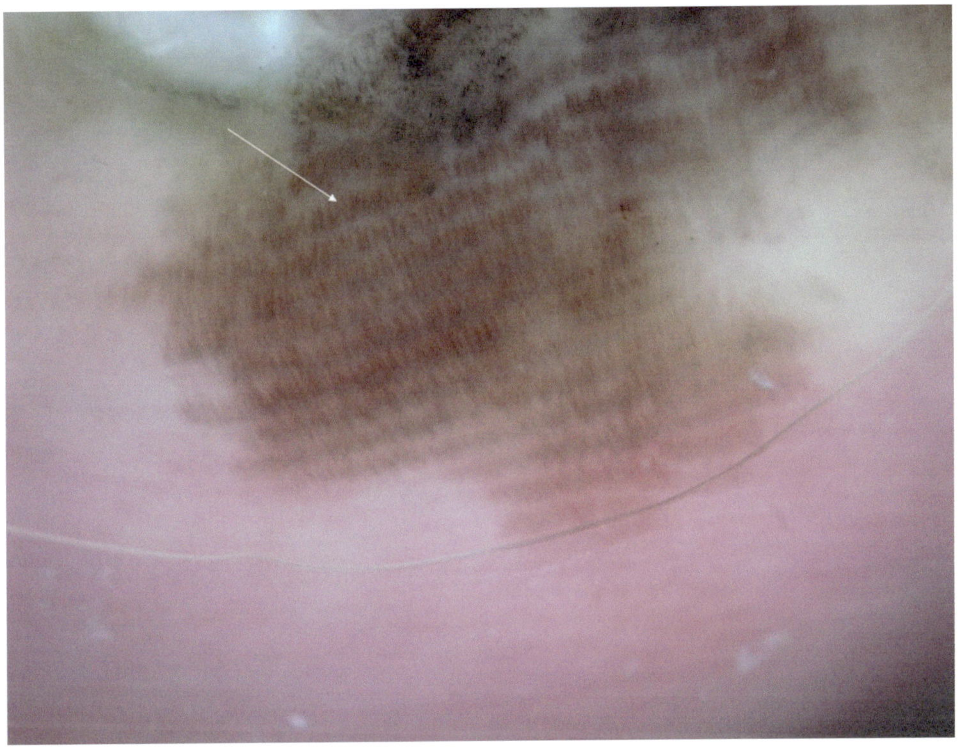

Fig. 3.17 Acral melanoma with parallel ridge pattern (white arrow)

Nodular Melanoma (NM)

Dermoscopically, NM lacks the criteria resulting from melanin deposition at the level of the dermo-epidermal junction (pigment network, brown dots/globules), the criteria related to radial growth and pagetoid spreading *(lines or streaks, black dots/globules, and multiple gray dots)*, as well as of the criteria observed in early stages of regression, such as *white areas (fibrosis)* and *multiple blue-gray dots.*

Similarly, when NM develops on specific sites (such as face, palms, and soles), it usually does not display the dermoscopic criteria seen in SSM on the same sites, since also these criteria correspond to melanin deposition at the level of the dermo-epidermal junction.

Dermoscopic examination of NM usually reveals ***multiple colors*** (black, light brown, dark brown, blue, gray, red, and white), ***blue-white veil*** (blue-white or white-grayish diffuse confluent pigmentation), and an ***atypical vascular pattern,*** which is defined by the presence of linear-irregular vessels or by the simultaneous presence of vessels of various morphologies (polymorphous vessels) (Fig. 3.18)

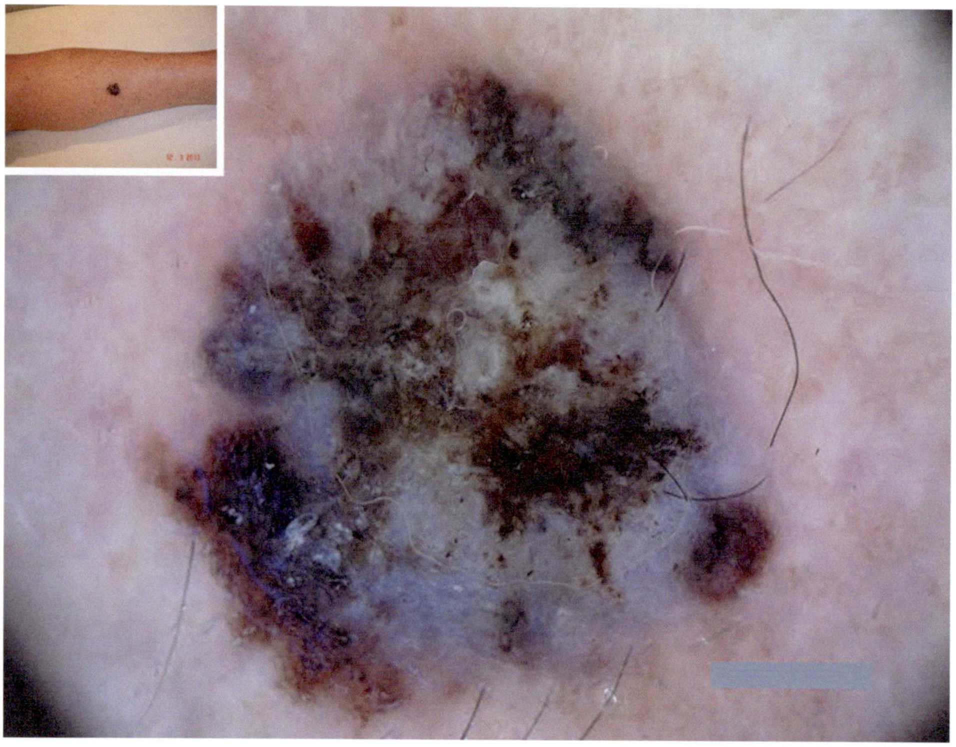

Fig. 3.18 Nodular melanoma; elevated lesion with multiple colors

Melanoma Simulators

Lesions that may simulate a melanoma, both clinically and dermoscopically, are called melanoma simulators. They can be divided into two groups, nonmelanocytic and melanocytic melanomas simulators (Figs. 3.19 and 3.20).

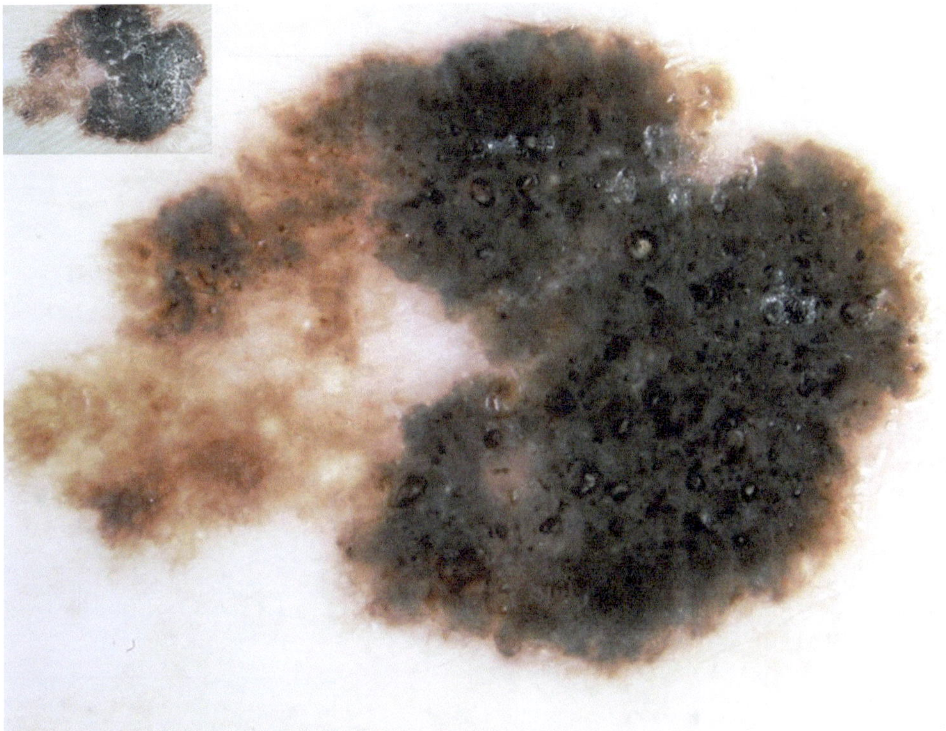

Fig. 3.19 Seborrheic keratosis simulating melanoma under clinical and dermoscopy view

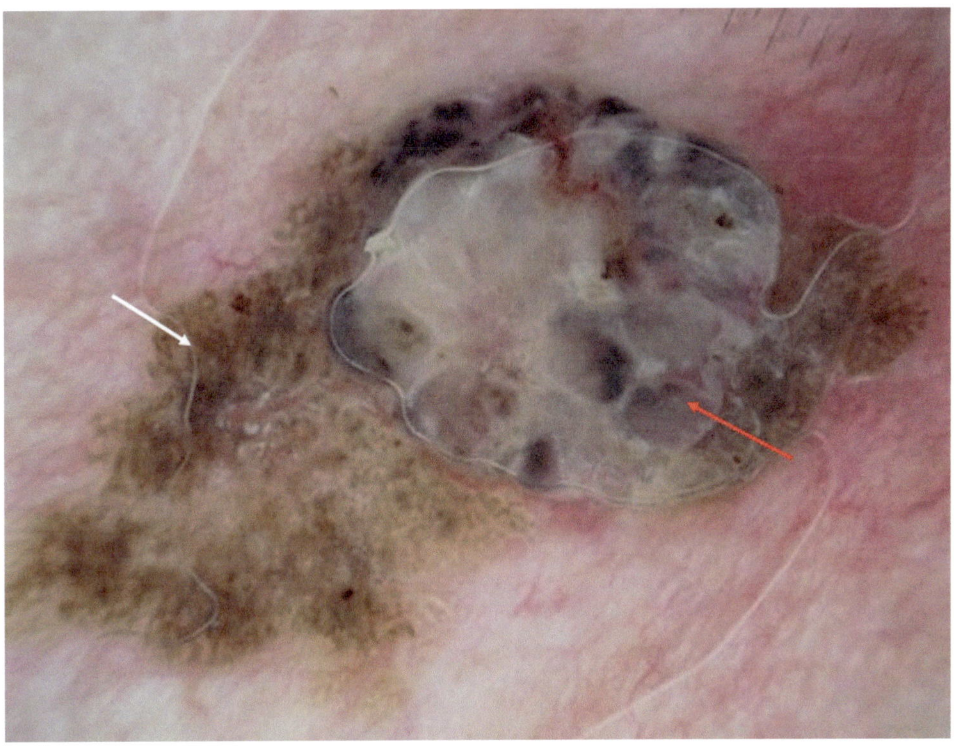

Fig. 3.20 Collision tumors—seborrheic keratosis (white arrow) and basal cell carcinoma (red arrow)—as a melanoma simulator

Nonmelanocytic Melanoma Simulators

Basal cell carcinoma
- Squamous cell carcinoma
- Actinic keratosis
- Ink-spot lentigo
- Seborrheic keratosis
- Dermatofibroma
- Thrombosed hemangioma
- Hematomas
- Pyogenic granuloma
- Eccrine poroma
- Collision tumors

Melanocytic Melanoma Simulators

Atypical nevus (Clark's nevus)
- Recurrent nevus
- Combined nevus
- Blue nevus
- Spitz-Reed nevus
- Melanocytic maculae
- Longitudinal melanonychia

4 Criteria of Non-melanocytic Benign Lesions

Horacio Cabo and Aimilios Lallas

Seborrheic Keratosis (SK)

Dermoscopic criteria of SK are *milia-like cysts, pseudofollicular openings*, and a typical *vascular pattern with hairpin vessels* (Figs. 4.1, 4.2, and 4.3).

Solar lentigo (SL) is nowadays considered as a flat SK. Dermoscopy features of SL are *fingerprint-like structures, moth-eaten border, and jelly sign* (Figs. 4.4 and 4.5).

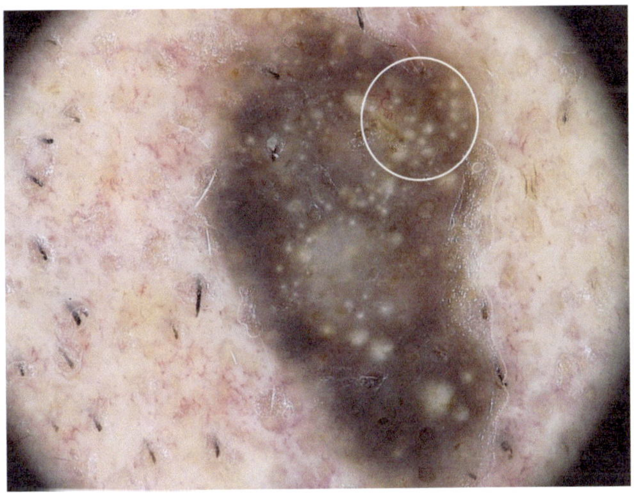

Fig. 4.1 SK with multiple milia-like cysts—circular structures, white-yellow in color and small in size (white circle)

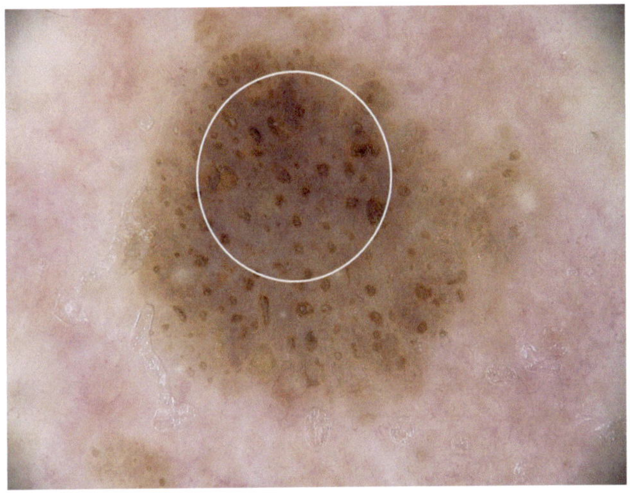

Fig. 4.2 SK with multiple pseudofollicular openings—yellowish, light brown, dark brown, or black, circular in shape, and of small size, presenting the typical appearance of a pore or a comedo (white circle)

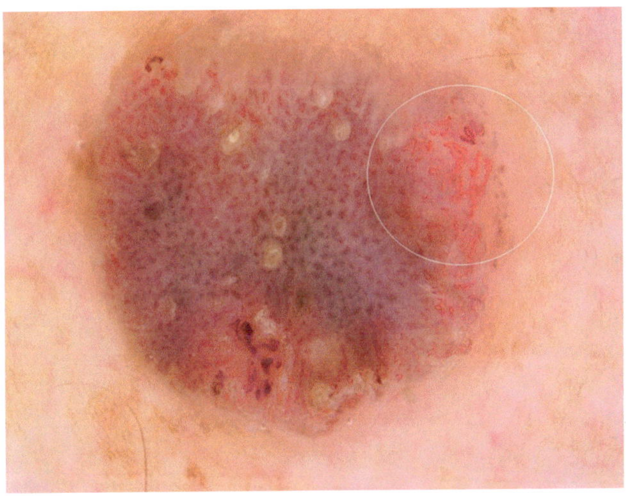

Fig. 4.3 SK with multiple hairpin vessels (white circle)

H. Cabo (✉)
Instituto de Investigaciones Médicas "A. Lanari". Dermatology Section, University of Buenos Aires, Buenos Aires, Argentina

A. Lallas
First Department of Dermatology, Aristotle University of Thessaloniki, Thessaloniki, Greece

H. Cabo, A. Lallas (eds.), *Comprehensive Atlas of Dermatoscopy Cases*, https://doi.org/10.1007/978-3-319-76932-5_4

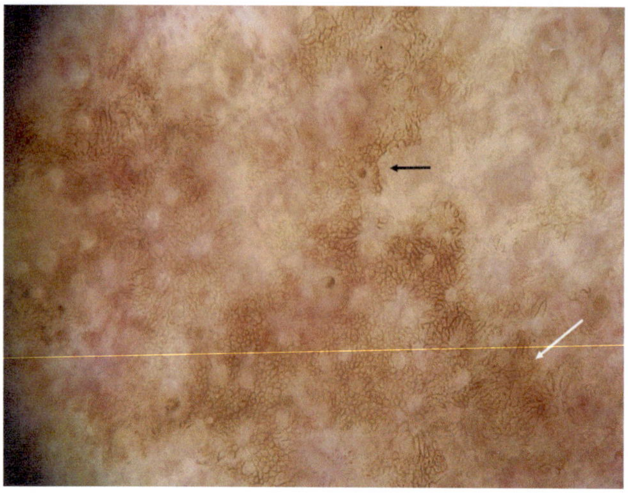

Fig. 4.4 SL (fingerprint-like structures) brown structures, made up of fine parallel lines in fingerprint fashion (white arrow) and moth-eaten border—concave edge of the lesion resembling the bite of a moth (black arrow)

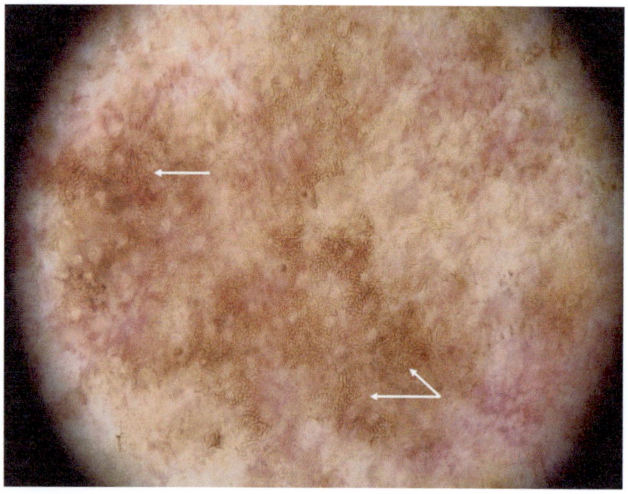

Fig. 4.5 SL—fingerprint-like structures (white arrows)

Angiomas (A)

The dermoscopic hallmark of angiomas are the so-called lacunae, which are *well-demarcated areas of red or blue-red, blue-black, or black color.* Notably, each lacuna should be a perfectly homogeneous roundish structure without any structures (vessels) seen within it. Lacunae are typically multiple and they may vary in size and color within the same lesion (Figs. 4.6 and 4.7).

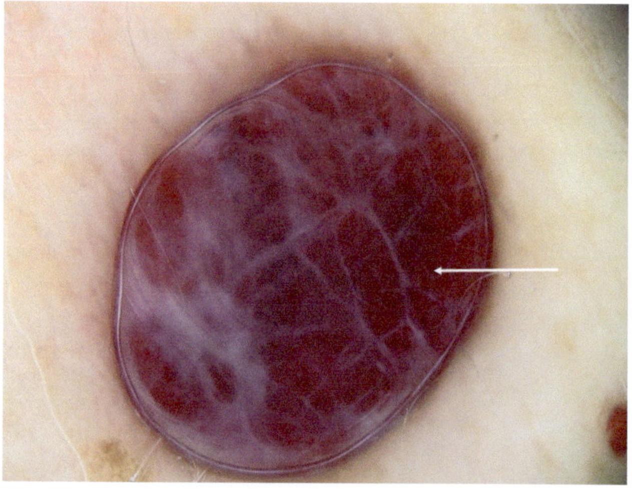

Fig. 4.6 Angioma—well-demarcated lacunae on a blue-red pigment background without any dermatoscopic structures within (white arrow)

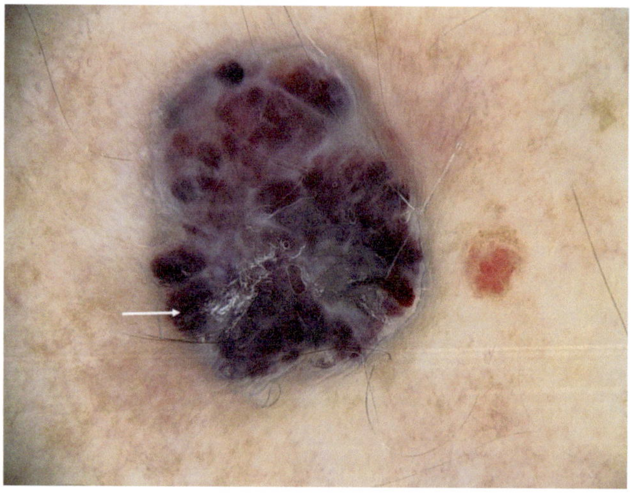

Fig. 4.7 Angioma—well-demarcated blue-red lacunae (white arrow)

Dermatofibroma (D)

Dermoscopy patterns of D are *delicate peripheral pigment network, central white patch or area with a scar-like appearance, and white shiny lines* (Figs. 4.8 and 4.9).

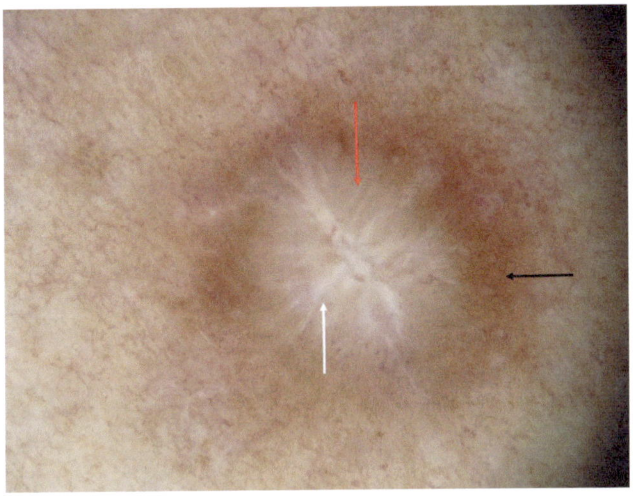

Fig. 4.8 Dermatofibroma delicate pigment network (black arrow), central white patch (red arrow), and white shine lines (white arrow)

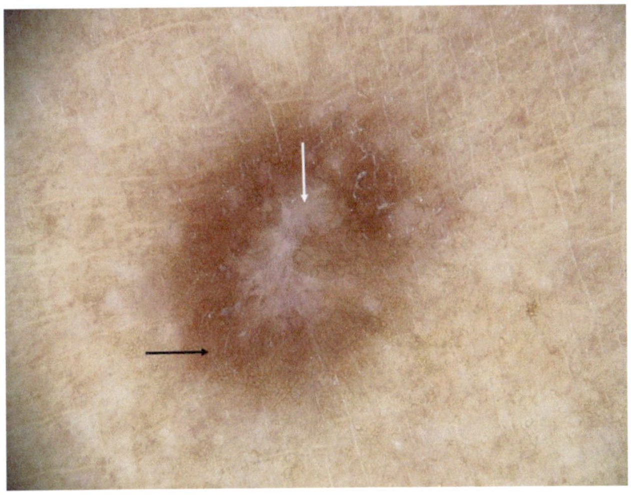

Fig. 4.9 Dermatofibroma delicate pigment network (black arrow), central white patch (white arrow)

5 Criteria of Non-melanocytic Malignant Lesions

Horacio Cabo and Aimilios Lallas

Basal Cell Carcinoma (BCC)

BCC is dermoscopically typified by its characteristic vascular pattern (arborizing vessels), the presence of pigmented structures, and ulceration. White shiny strands and blotches are an additional criterion seen only with polarized light (Figs. 5.1, 5.2, 5.3, 5.4, 5.5, and 5.6).

Vascular pattern: arborizing vessels (thick vessels with multiple branches) and superficial fine telangiectasia

Pigmented structures: there are two main subcategories, depending on the depth of pigment

- Brown-colored structures:
  - *Maple leaflike areas*
  - *Spoke-wheel areas*
  - *Concentric structures*
- Blue-gray-colored structures:
  - *Multiple blue-gray dots or small globules*
  - *Blue-gray ovoid nests*

Ulcerations: single or multiple and in different sizes and colors

White shiny blotches and strands

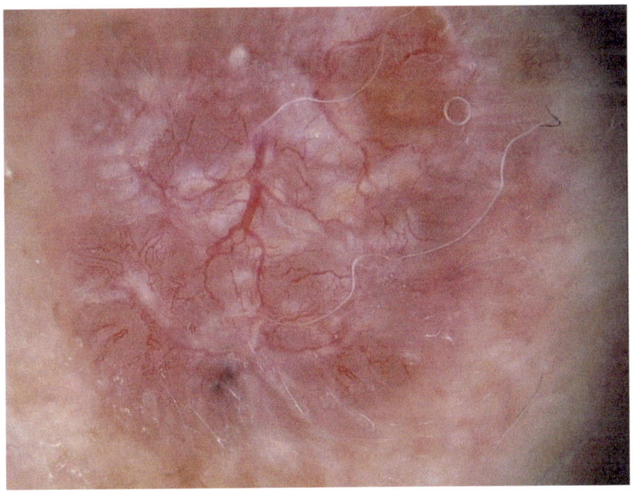

Fig. 5.1 BCC with arborizing vessels

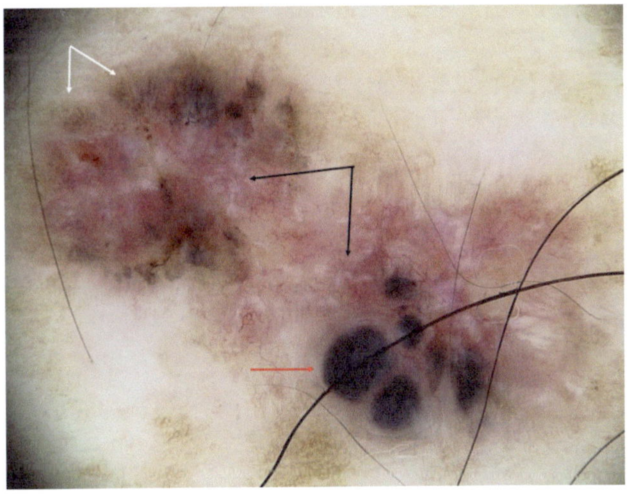

Fig. 5.2 BCC notice leaflike structures (white arrows), large blue-gray areas or globules (red arrow), and white shiny lines or crystalline structures (black arrows)

H. Cabo (✉)
Instituto de Investigaciones Médicas "A. Lanari". Dermatology Section, University of Buenos Aires, Buenos Aires, Argentina

A. Lallas
First Department of Dermatology, Aristotle University of Thessaloniki, Thessaloniki, Greece

H. Cabo, A. Lallas (eds.), *Comprehensive Atlas of Dermatoscopy Cases*, https://doi.org/10.1007/978-3-319-76932-5_5

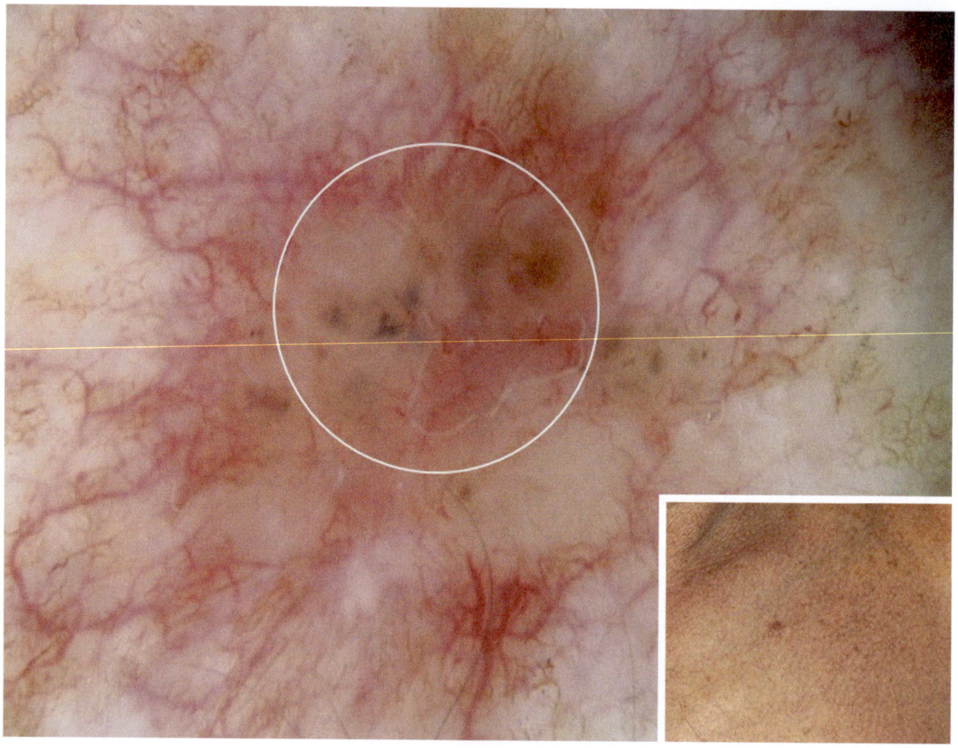

Fig. 5.3 BCC with the presence of blue-gray dots (white circle)

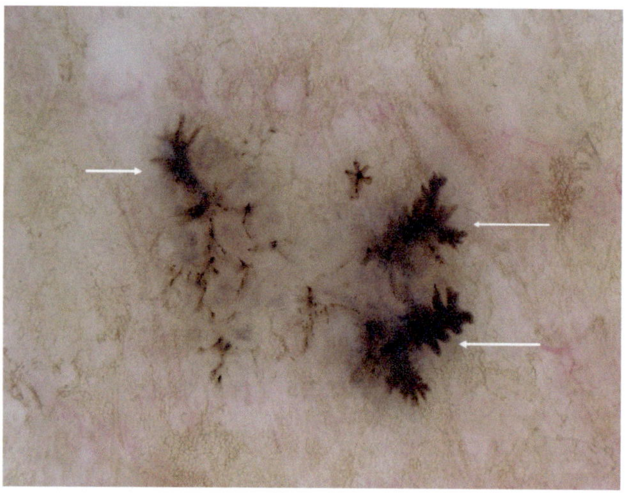

Fig. 5.4 BCC with leaflike structures (white arrows)

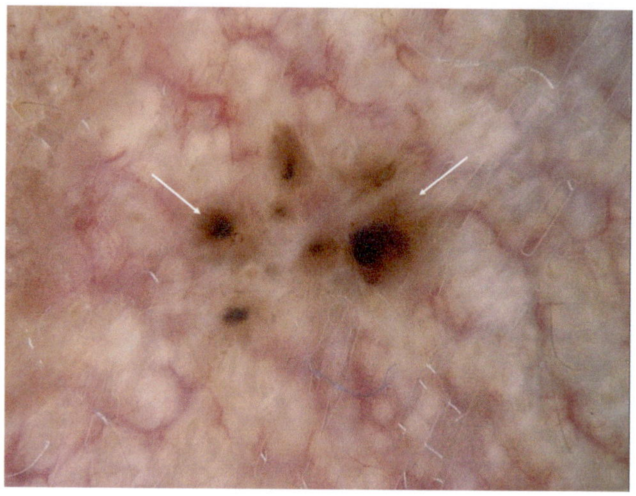

Fig. 5.5 BCC with spoke-wheel areas or radial areas (white arrows)

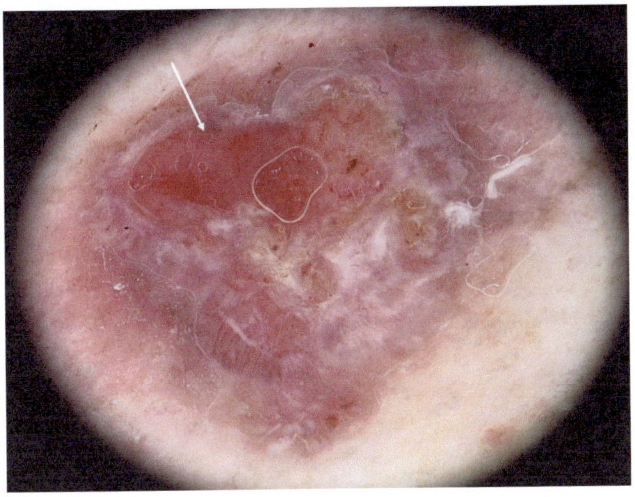

Fig. 5.6 BCC notice the ulceration (white arrow)

Actinic Keratosis (AK) and Squamous Cell Carcinoma (SCC)

AK: dermoscopy criteria are (Figs. 5.7 and 5.8):

Strawberry-like pattern
Vascular pattern with fine undulated vessels surrounding the hair follicle and dotted vessels
Superficial yellowish-white scales
Hyperkeratotic follicles
Rosettes

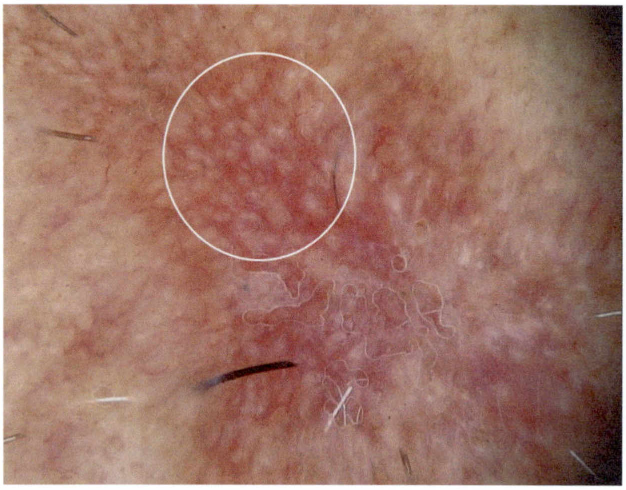

Fig. 5.7 AK: strawberry pattern (white circle)

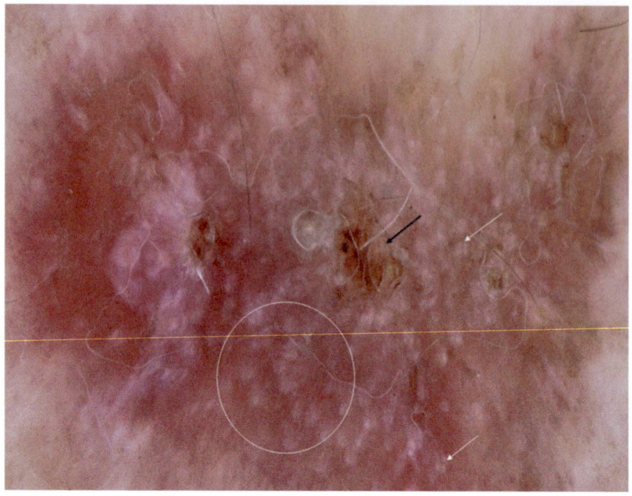

Fig. 5.8 AK: rosette-like structures (white arrows), strawberry pattern (white circle), and superficial yellowish-white scales (black arrow)

SCC Can Be In Situ or Infiltrating

SCC in situ *or Bowen's disease* shows (Figs. 5.9 and 5.10):

In nonpigmented forms, a *vascular pattern with glomerular vessels in focal distribution*

In the pigmented forms, the dermoscopy criteria are:

Linear arrangement of red, brown, or gray dots in the periphery of the lesion
Brown color
Structureless areas
Hypopigmented areas (pink, skin colored, or white)

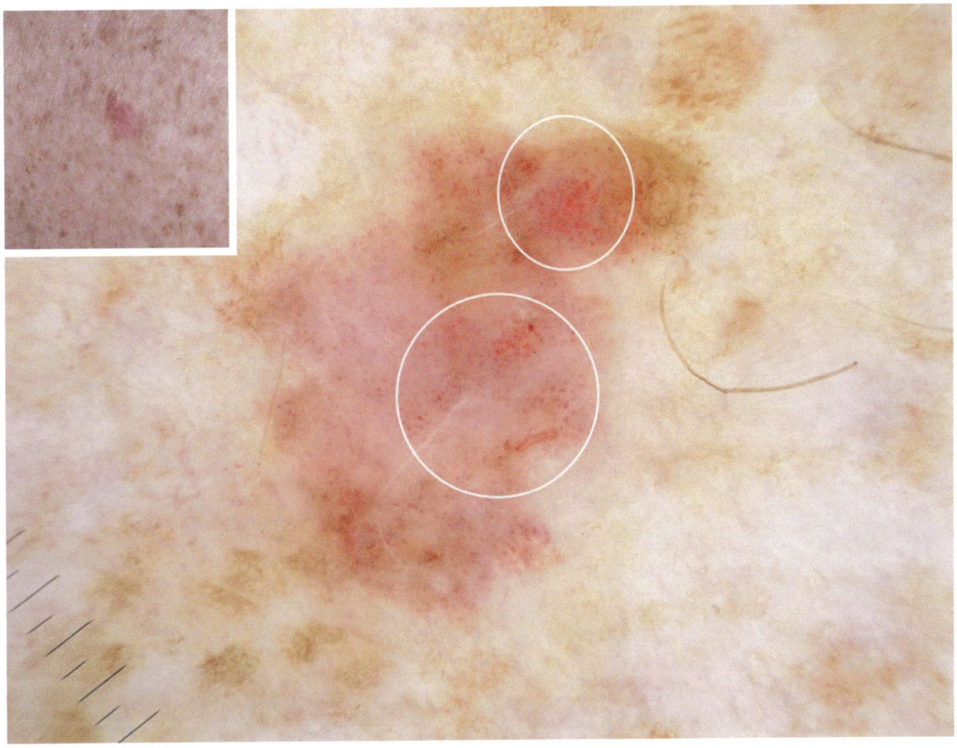

Fig. 5.9 Bowen's disease: vascular pattern with glomerular vessels in focal distribution (white circles)

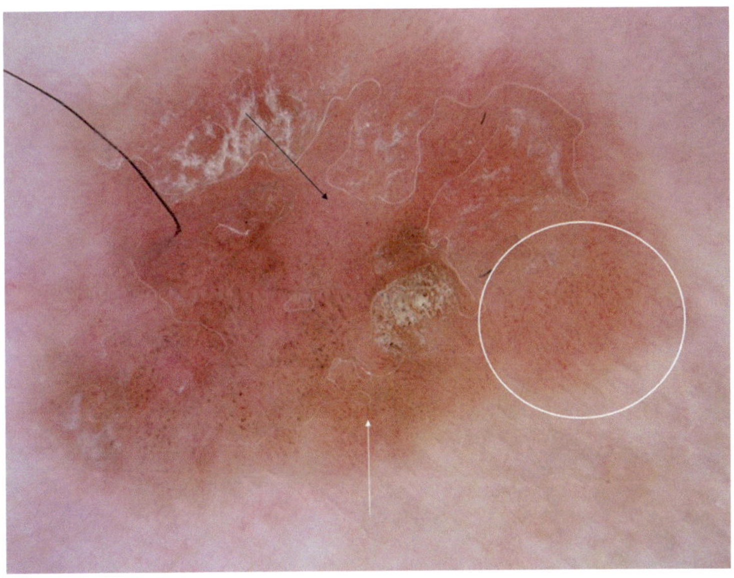

Fig. 5.10 Pigmented SCC: linear arrangement of red dots in the periphery of the lesion (white circle), brown color (white arrow) and structureless hypopigmented red areas (black arrow)

The dermoscopic pattern of invasive SCC depends on the grade of histopathologic differentiation (Figs. 5.11 and 5.12).

Well-differentiated SCC is typified by:

Hyperkeratotic areas usually located in the central part of the tumor (surface keratin)
White circles and white areas
Hairpin vessels arranged in the periphery of the lesion or glomerular vessels
Ulceration

Poorly differentiated SCC is typified by:

Red predominant color
Bleeding
Polymorphous vessels
Intense vascularity

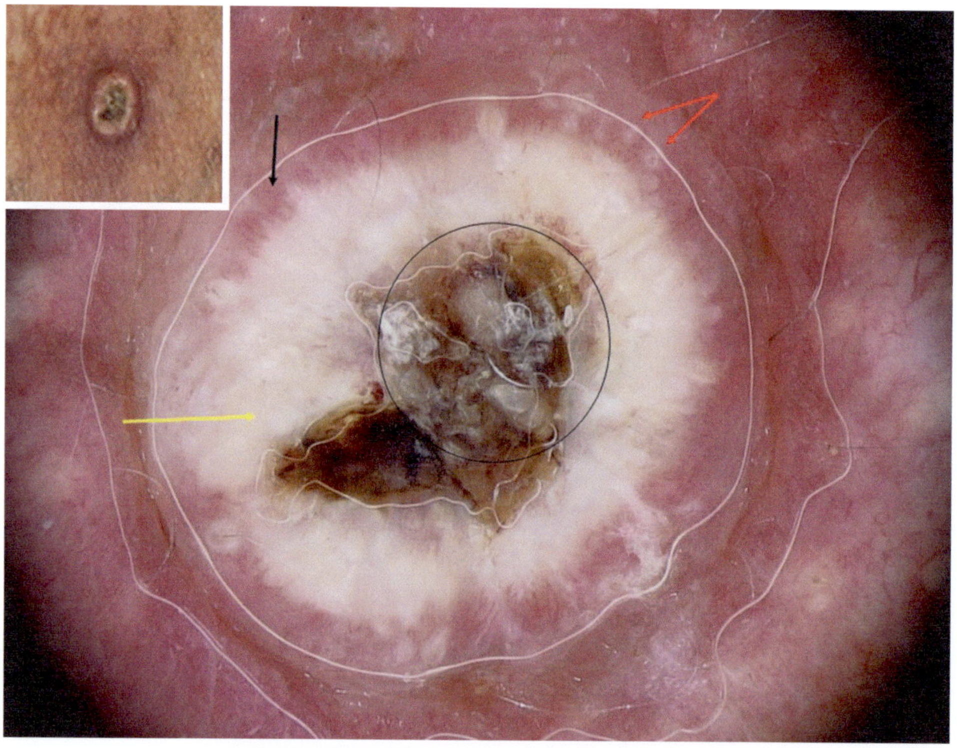

Fig. 5.11 Infiltrating SCC with hyperkeratotic areas in the central part of the lesion (black circle), white circles (red arrows), white areas (yellow arrow), and hairpin vessels arranged in the periphery of the lesion (black arrow)

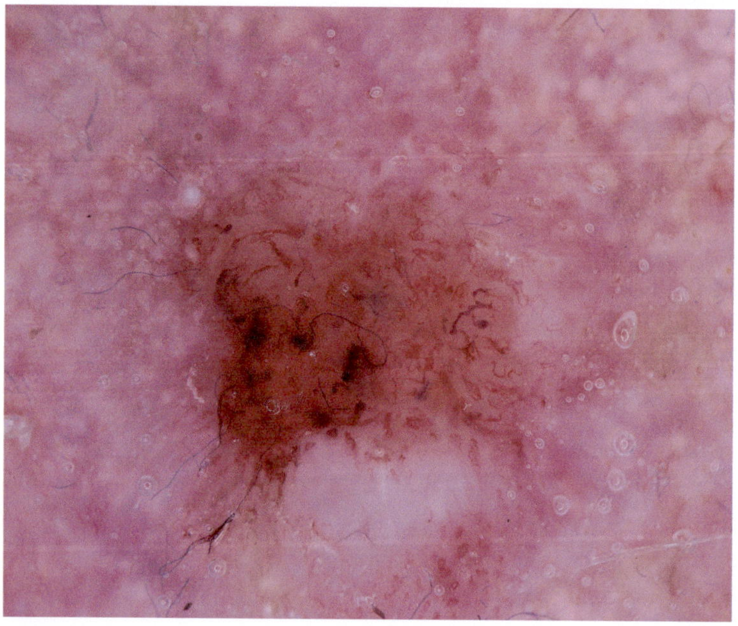

Fig. 5.12 Poorly differentiated SCC is typified by a red predominant color, dense vascularity, and polymorphous vessels

Flat Pigmented Lesion on the Scalp

6

Emilia Noemi Cohen Sabban

Case 1

Sex: male
Age: 67
Surface (flat/palpable/nodular): flat
Maximum diameter: 1 cm
Duration of the lesion: 2 years
History of morphologic changes: yes
Personal history of skin cancer (if yes, please specify): no
Family history of skin cancer (if yes, please specify): no
Skin phototype: III
Total nevus count: (<10, 10–50, 50–100, >100): 10–50
Other clinical findings (optional):

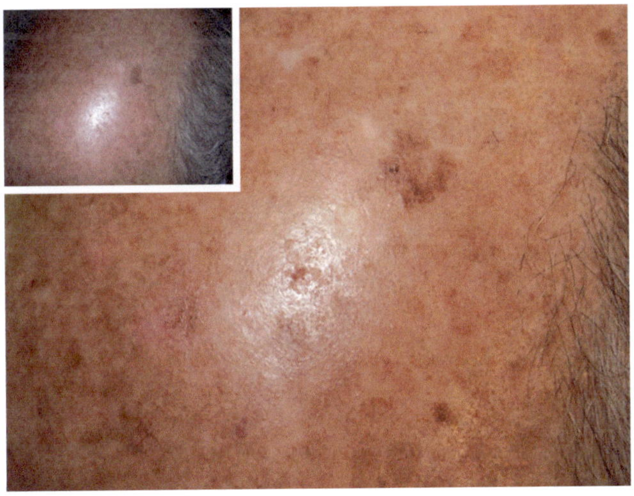

Fig. 6.1 Clinical view: asymmetric pigmented lesion in the scalp

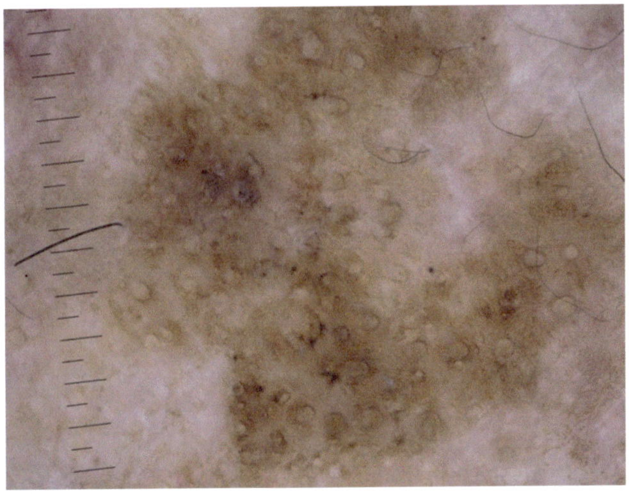

Fig. 6.2 Dermoscopy view: irregular lesion with different colors (different shades of brown and blue-gray colors)

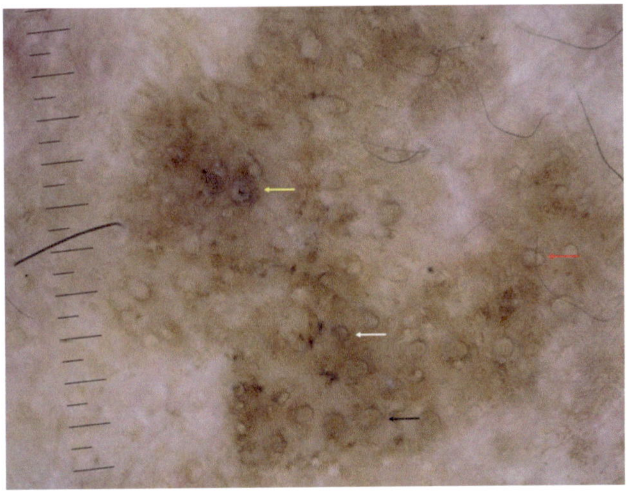

Fig. 6.3 Dermoscopy view: blue-gray color (yellow arrow), pigmentation of follicular openings (red arrow), asymmetric pigmentation of follicular openings (white arrow), two concentric circles (black arrow)

E. N. Cohen Sabban
Instituto de Investigaciones Médicas "A. Lanari". Chief of Dermatology Section, University of Buenos Aires, Buenos Aires, Argentina

H. Cabo, A. Lallas (eds.), *Comprehensive Atlas of Dermatoscopy Cases*, https://doi.org/10.1007/978-3-319-76932-5_6

Key Message

The first dermoscopy manifestations of lentigo maligna on the face appear around and in the hair follicle, with the presence of pigmentation of follicular openings (symmetric, asymmetric, and two concentric circles), so we have to rule out lentigo maligna.

Blue-gray color on the face is suggestive of lentigo maligna as well.

7 Palpable Lesion on the Scalp

Alon Scope, John Paoli, and Zoe Apalla

Case 1: A.S.

Sex: female
Age: 60
Surface (flat/palpable/nodular): palpable
Maximum diameter: 10 mm
Duration of the lesion: unknown (spouse noted the scalp lesion in the past month)
History of morphologic changes: unknown
Personal history of skin cancer (if yes, please specify): history of multiple in situ melanomas on the upper extremities and torso
Family history of skin cancer (if yes, please specify): negative
Skin phototype: II
Total nevus count (<10, 10–50, 50–100, >100): 10–50
Other clinical findings (optional):

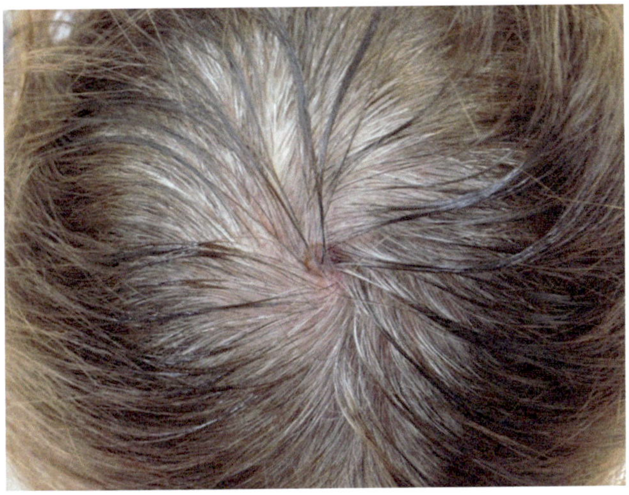

Fig. 7.1 Clinical image of a 10-mm plaque, with asymmetrically distributed brown-pink colors, in the mid-parietal scalp

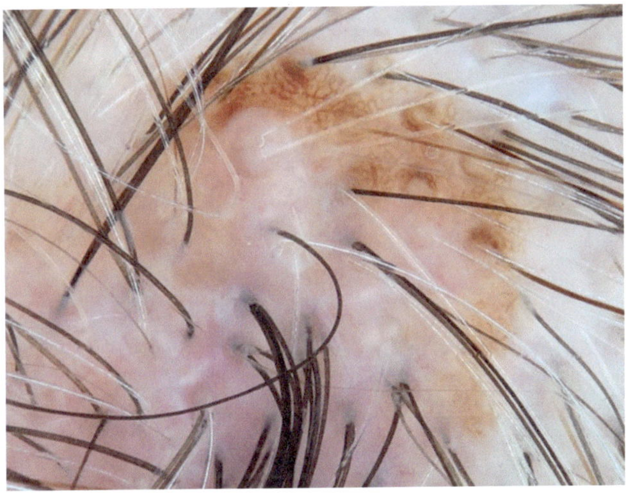

Fig. 7.2 Dermoscopy view

A. Scope (✉)
Melanoma and Pigmented Lesion Clinic,
Chaim Sheba Medical Center, Ramat-Gan, Israel

Faculty of Medicine, Tel Aviv University, Tel Aviv, Israel

J. Paoli
University of Gothenburg, Gothenburg, Sweden

Z. Apalla
First Department of Dermatology, Aristotle University of Thessaloniki, Thessaloniki, Greece

H. Cabo, A. Lallas (eds.), *Comprehensive Atlas of Dermatoscopy Cases*, https://doi.org/10.1007/978-3-319-76932-5_7

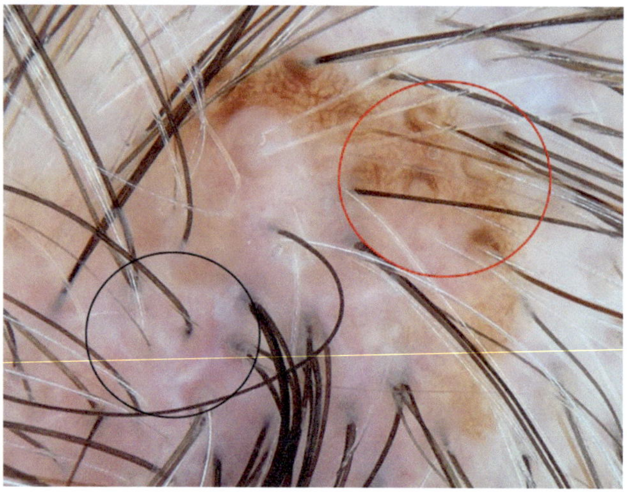

Fig. 7.3 Dermoscopy image of the lesion. The flat brown pole shows a reticular pattern and asymmetrically pigmented follicular openings (creating incomplete brown circles) (red circle). The palpable pink pole shows a homogenous pattern with vascular blush and chrysalis (shiny white lines), as well as relative scarcity of hair follicles (black circle). Irregular vessels were observed during in vivo examination

Key Message

Histopathology reports a melanoma 0.7 mm in thickness. The dermoscopic findings in the pigmented area suggest a melanoma arising in association with sun-damaged skin. Women often part their hair in the mid-parietal scalp and cumulative sun damage may occur. This case also highlights the need to carefully look and palpate the scalp during periodic examination, as melanoma can occur within the hairy scalp. Patients should encourage their hairdresser to bring to their attention any scalp lesions noted during hair salon visit.

Case 2: J.P.

Sex: male
Age: 81 years
Surface (flat/palpable/nodular): slightly raised, ulcerated
Maximum diameter: 18 mm
Duration of the lesion: 6 months
History of morphologic changes: patient had noted ulceration during the past weeks.
Personal history of skin cancer (if yes, please specify): multiple actinic keratoses and basal cell carcinomas
Family history of skin cancer (if yes, please specify): unknown
Skin phototype: I
Total nevus count (<10, 10–50, 50–100, >100): <10
Other clinical findings (optional):

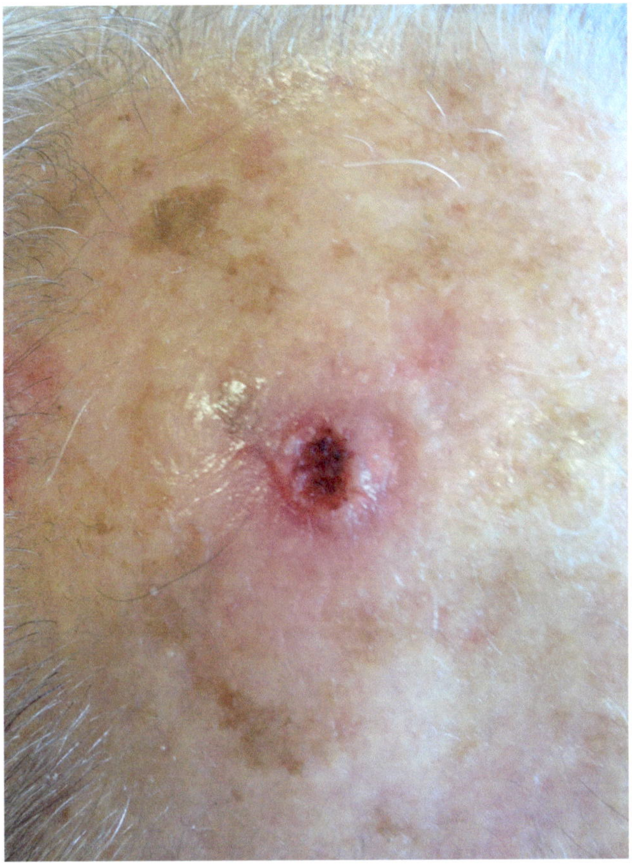

Fig. 7.4 Clinically, a pinkish-white, slightly raised nodule with central ulceration is observed in UV-damaged skin on the bald scalp of this elderly man

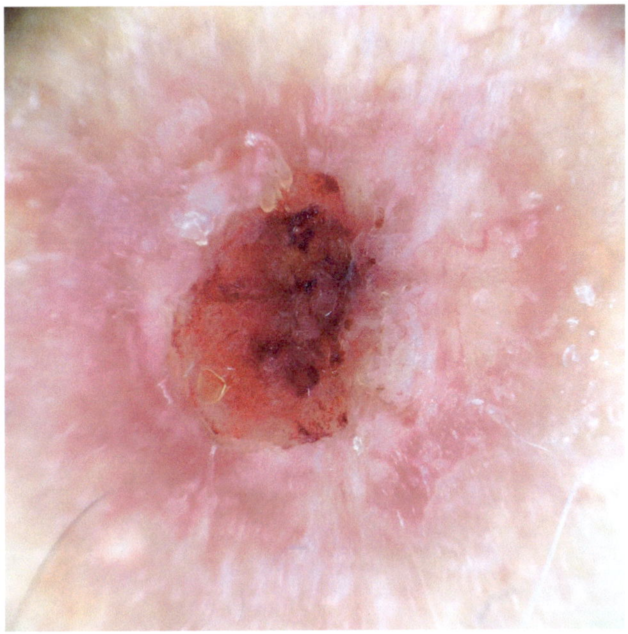

Fig. 7.5 Dermoscopy view

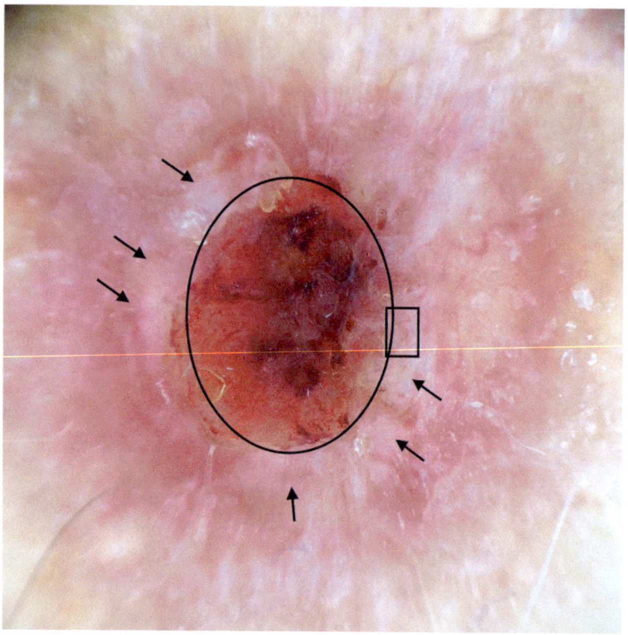

Fig. 7.6 Peripheral white structureless areas (black narrows) are noted surrounding a central yellow-orange keratin mass with a very large number of blood spots and irregular vessels (black circle). At 3 o'clock, a multilobular hairpin vessel with radial distribution is observed (black square)

Key Message

Histopathology confirmed the diagnosis of an invasive squamous cell carcinoma with poor differentiation. The central keratin mass combined with blood spots surrounded by white structureless areas and with or without hairpin vessels are typical for squamous cell carcinoma. The fact that the red color is predominant and the irregular vessels are indicative of poor differentiation and can help guide the surgeon to choose a larger surgical margin when carrying out the excision to ensure complete removal.

Case 3: Z.A.

Sex: male
Age: 75
Surface (flat/palpable/nodular): flat
Maximum diameter: 1.5 cm
Duration of the lesion: 3.5 months
History of morphologic changes: gradually enlarging, bleeding
Personal history of skin cancer (if yes, please specify): actinic keratoses
Family history of skin cancer (if yes, please specify): no
Skin phototype: III
Total nevus count (<10, 10–50, 50–100, >100): <10
Other clinical findings (optional):

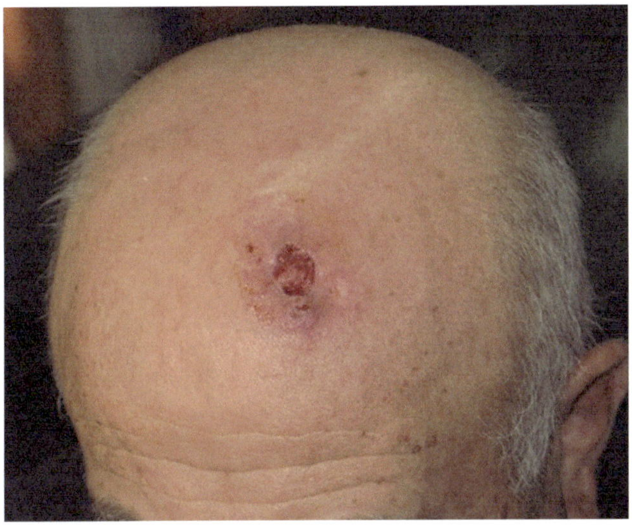

Fig. 7.7 Ulcerated reddish plaque involving the frontal-parietal area of the scalp

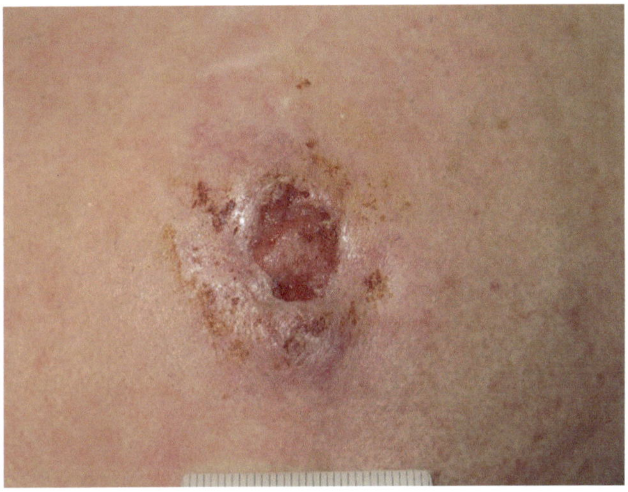

Fig. 7.8 In a closer view, we can observe the abrupt borders of the lesion and the bleeding base of the ulcer

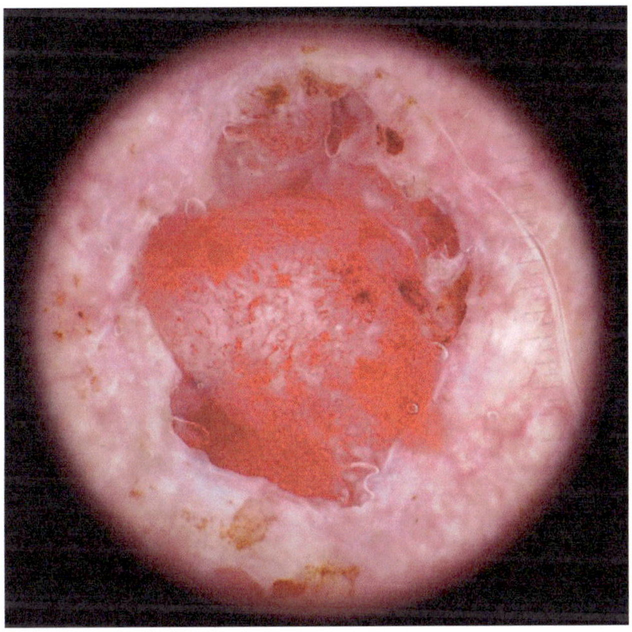

Fig. 7.9 Dermoscopy view

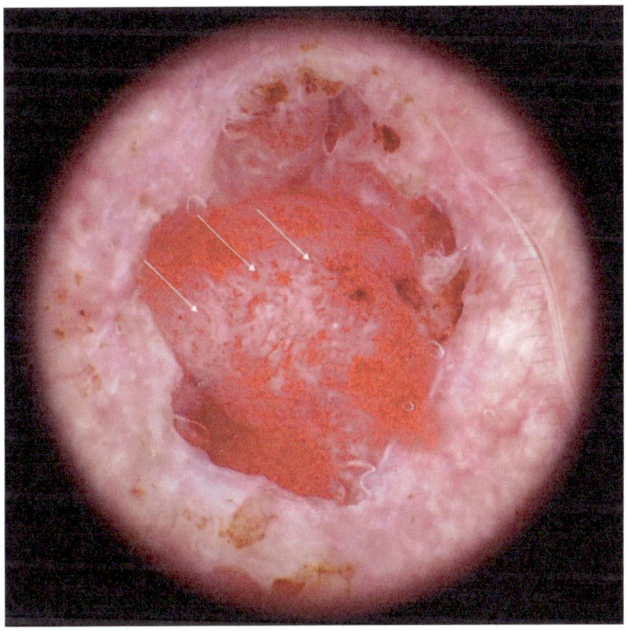

Fig. 7.10 Dermatoscopy highlights the abrupt border of the ulcer and the presence of many atypical vessels in the ulcerated area, resulting in a homogenous red coloration (white arrows). Dermatoscopic structures as white scales, white halos, or white circles are not seen in this lesion

Key Message

Red color as the result of intense tumor vascularization in dermatoscopy is suggestive of malignancy. In this case, the diagnosis was poorly differentiated squamous cell carcinoma. The presence of vessels in more than 50% of the tumor's surface and a diffuse distribution of vessels and bleeding are significantly associated with poor differentiation.

8 Flat Pigmented Lesions on the Face

Aimilios Lallas, Chryssoula Papageorgiou, and Elvira Moscarella

Case 1 A.L.

Sex: female
Age: 50
Surface (flat/palpable/nodular): flat
Maximum diameter: 5 mm
Duration of the lesion: 1 year
History of morphologic changes: no
Personal history of skin cancer (if yes, please specify): no
Family history of skin cancer (if yes, please specify): no
Skin phototype: II
Total nevus count: (<10, 10–50, 50–100, >100): 10–50
Other clinical findings (optional): few solar lentigos mainly on the face

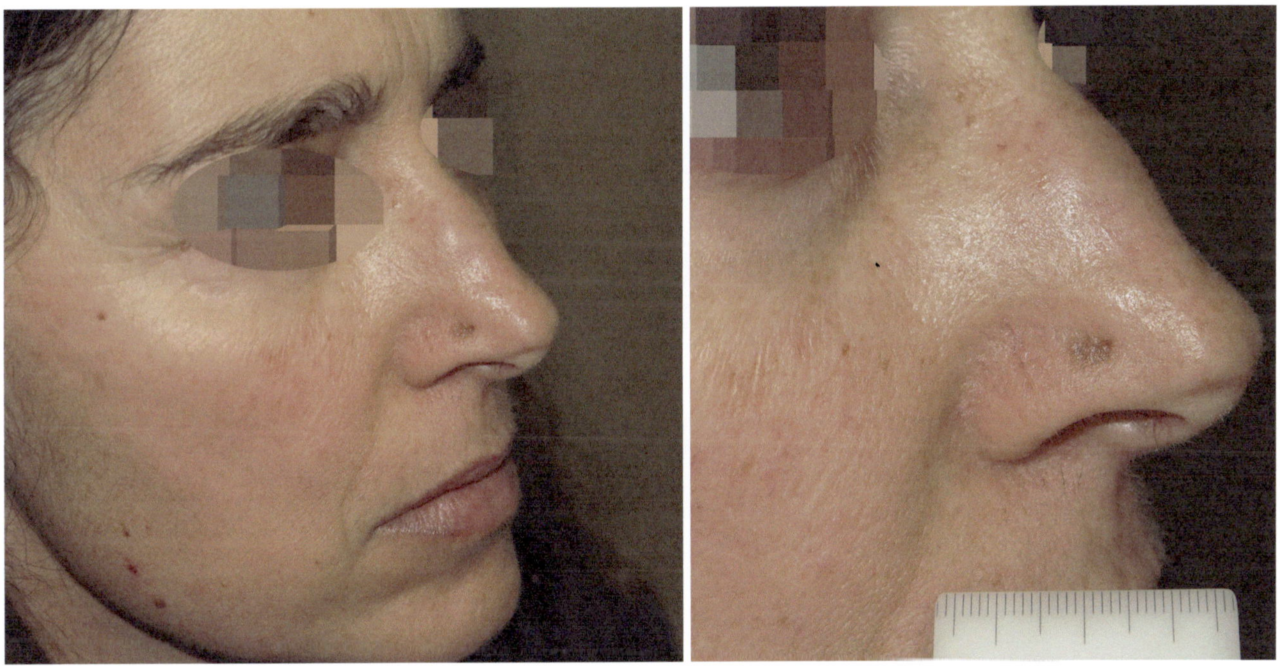

Fig. 8.1 and 8.2 On clinical examination, there is flat, pigmented lesion with irregular borders located on the right side of the nose

A. Lallas (✉) · C. Papageorgiou
First Department of Dermatology, Aristotle University of Thessaloniki, Thessaloniki, Greece

E. Moscarella
Dermatology and Skin Cancer Unit, Arcispedale S Maria Nuova, IRCCS, Reggio Emilia, Modena, Italy

H. Cabo, A. Lallas (eds.), *Comprehensive Atlas of Dermatoscopy Cases*, https://doi.org/10.1007/978-3-319-76932-5_8

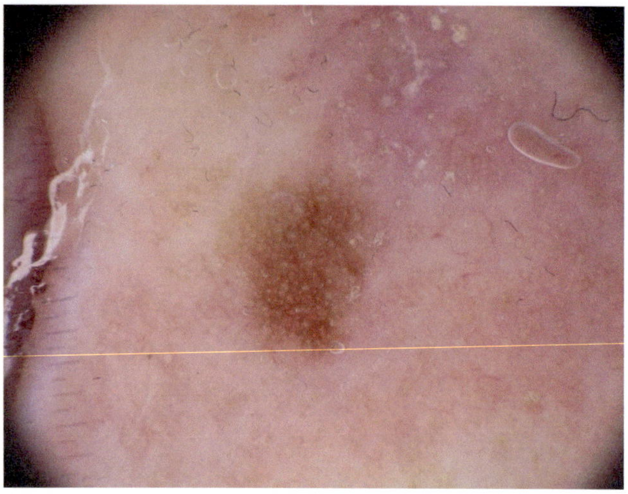

Fig. 8.3 Dermoscopy view

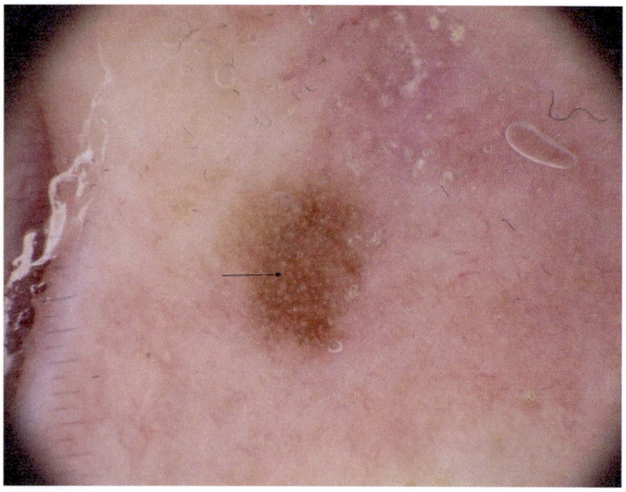

Fig. 8.4 Dermoscopically, the lesion exhibits a peudonetwork (black arrow), namely, diffuse, brown color interrupted by white follicular openings. No other criteria suggestive of melanoma or any other diagnosis can be seen. However, this was a melanoma in situ

Key Message

The differential diagnosis of lentigo maligna melanoma from solar lentigo and pigmented actinic keratosis can be highly challenging, because these tumors are characterized by a significant overlap of dermoscopic criteria. The only safe strategy to diagnose early melanomas like this one is to biopsy any flat facial lesion that cannot be safely diagnosed as a pigmented actinic keratosis or a solar lentigo/seborrhea keratosis.

Case 2 E.M.

Sex: male
Age: 40
Surface (flat/palpable/nodular): flat
Maximum diameter: 0.7 cm
Duration of the lesion: unknown
History of morphologic changes: no
Personal history of skin cancer (if yes, please specify): no
Family history of skin cancer (if yes, please specify): no
Skin phototype: III
Total nevus count: (<10, 10–50, 50–100, >100): 10–50
Other clinical findings (optional): seborrheic keratosis on the trunk

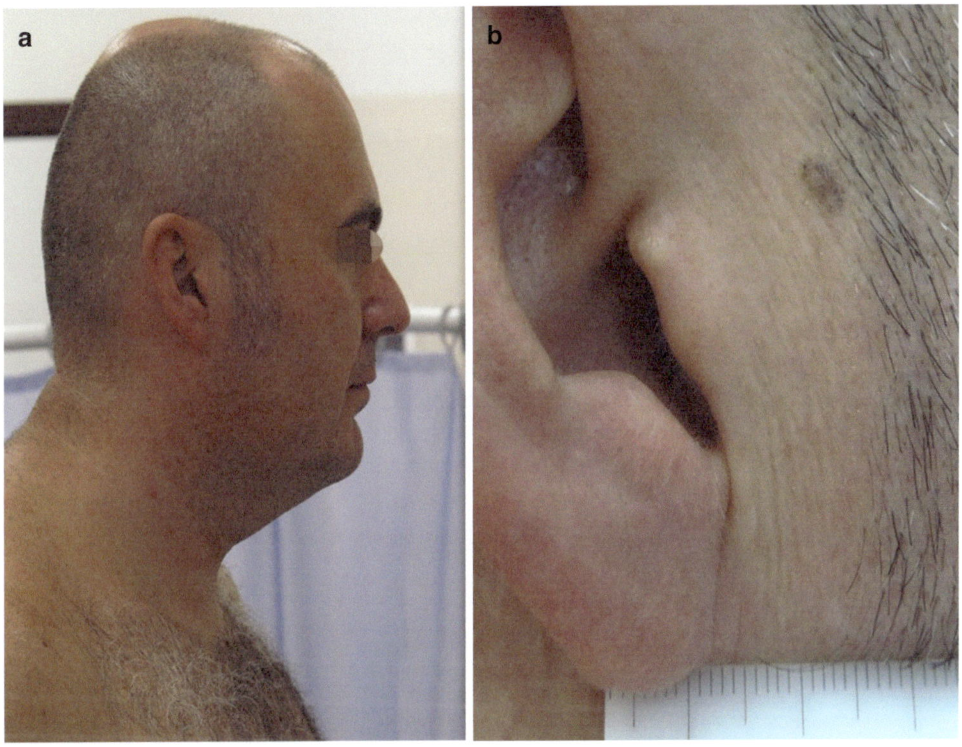

Fig. 8.5 (**a**) Pigmented lesion located on the right preauricular area. (**b**) Close-up showing a well-demarcated border. Color variegation from light brown to grey is visible

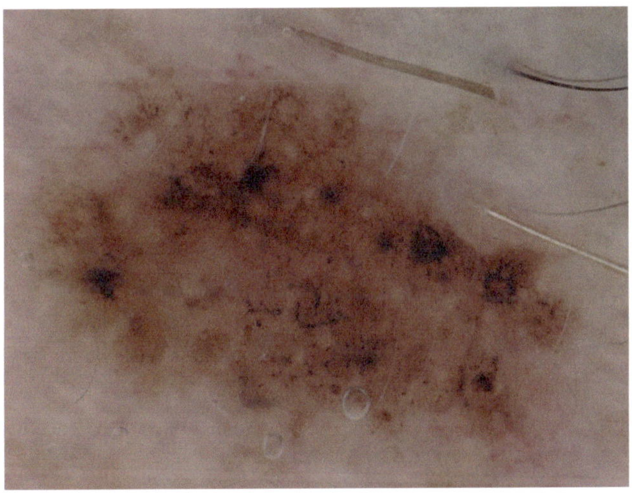

Fig. 8.6 Dermoscopy view

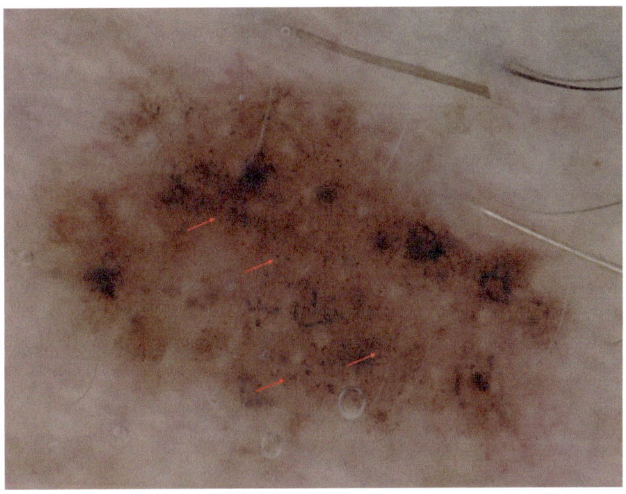

Fig. 8.7 In dermoscopy, multiple loosely arranged brown to grey globules and dots in focus are visible (red arrows)

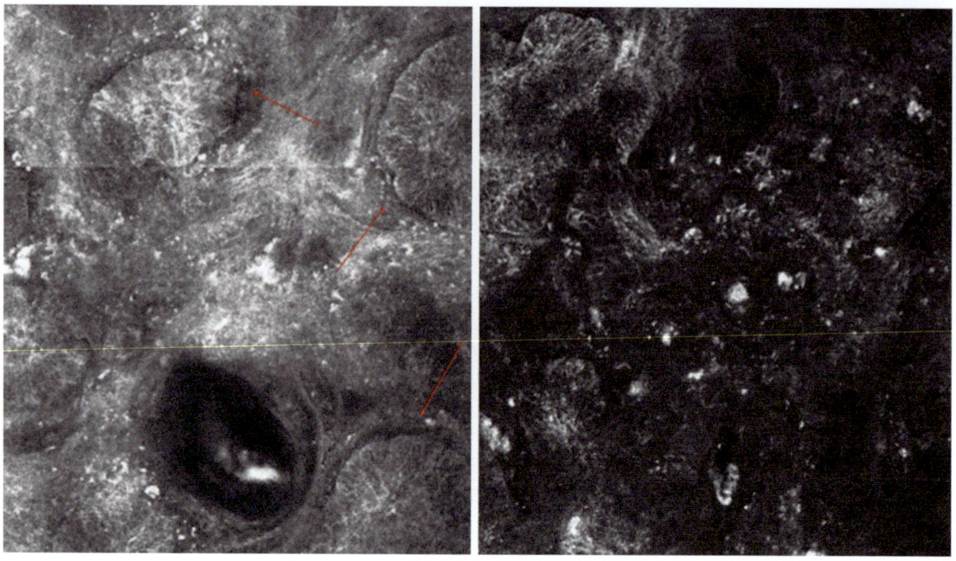

Fig. 8.8 In reflectance confocal microscopy, basaloid islands composed of highly refractile dendritic cells are visible; these islands are well demarcated with visible peripheral clefting

Key Message

The multiple loosely arranged brown to gray globules and dots "in focus" correspond in histology to pigmented basaloid nests. This is a relatively recently described feature of basal cell carcinoma (BCC) that allows the correct diagnosis in early BCC cases. The color, brown to gray, suggests a location in the epidermis and upper dermis. In histology, this was a superficial-type basal cell carcinoma.

Case 3 M.K., R.P.B.

Sex: male
Age: 89
Surface (flat/palpable/nodular): flat
Maximum diameter: 3 × 3 cm
Duration of the lesion: 3 months
History of morphologic changes: persistent pigmentation on the left forehead following radiotherapy (60Gy) of a lentigo maligna 3 months ago
Personal history of skin cancer (if yes, please specify): multiple squamous cell carcinomas
Family history of skin cancer (if yes, please specify): no
Skin phototype: II
Total nevus count: (<10, 10–50, 50–100, >100): 10–50
Other clinical findings (optional):

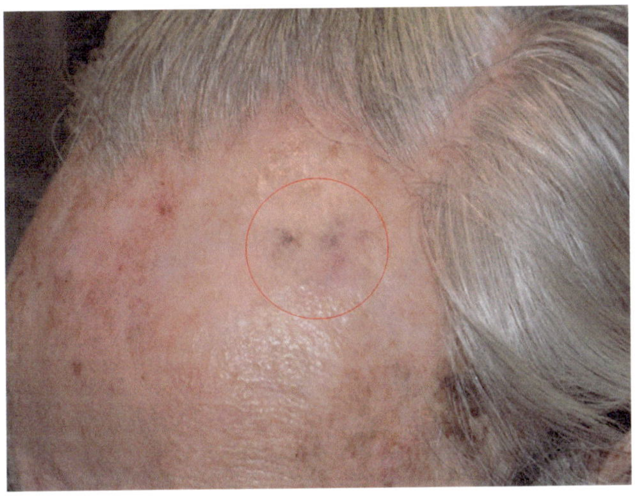

Fig. 8.9 Clinical picture of a grayish lesion with scattered pigment and unclear borders on the left forehead (red circle)

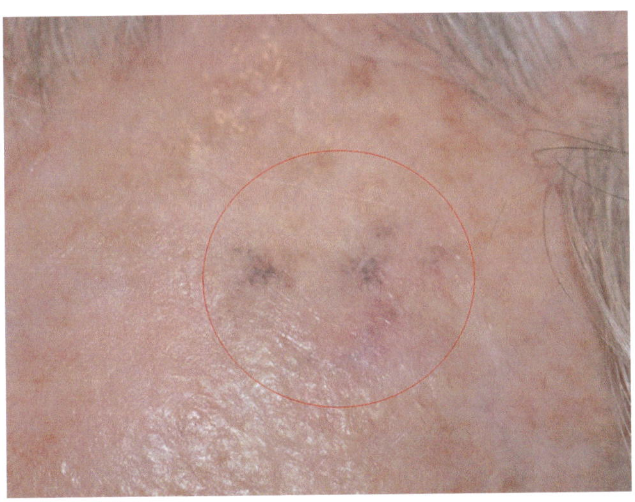

Fig. 8.10 Close-up clinical picture of the pigmented lesion on the left forehead revealing multiple islands of grayish pigment and a slight perifocal erythema (red circle)

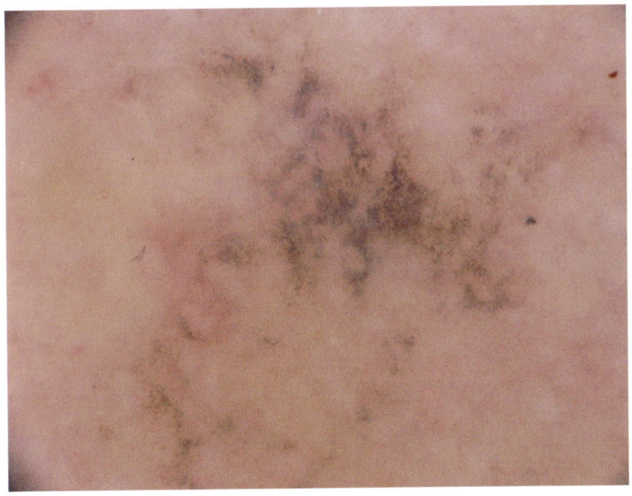

Fig. 8.11 Dermoscopy view

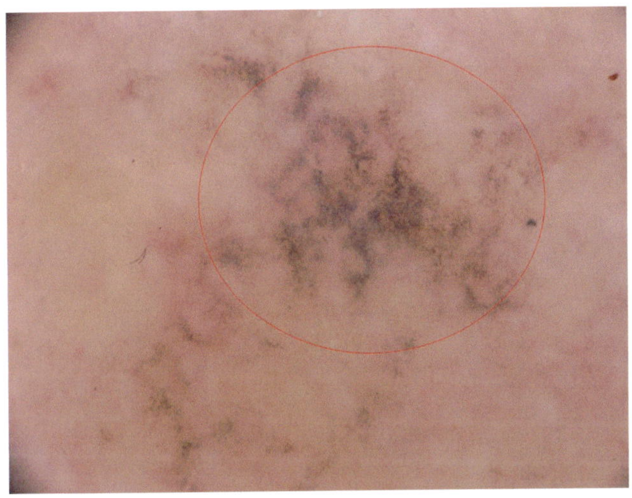

Fig. 8.12 Dermoscopy picture with diffuse and asymmetric, partly polygonal and perifollicular, grayish peppering and parts with a discrete whitish veil (red circle)

Key Message
Unspecific dermoscopic picture with regression, which points to a melanocytic lesion. Because of the polygonal and asymmetric perifollicular arrangement, the lesion was biopsied to rule out relapsing lentigo maligna or melanoma. No melanocytes have been found, and a histological diagnosis of radiodermatitis with pigment incontinence has been made.

9 Flat Nonpigmented Lesions on the Face

Aimilios Lallas

Case No: 1

Sex: female
Age: 59
Surface (flat/palpable/nodular): flat
Maximum diameter: 6 mm
Duration of the lesion: 7 months
History of morphologic changes: yes, slowly enlarging
Personal history of skin cancer (if yes, please specify): no
Family history of skin cancer (if yes, please specify): no
Skin phototype: II
Total nevus count: (<10, 10–50, 50–100, >100): 10–50
Other clinical findings (optional):

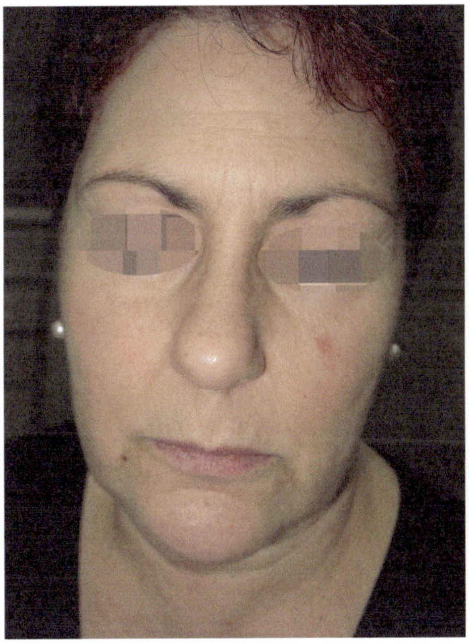

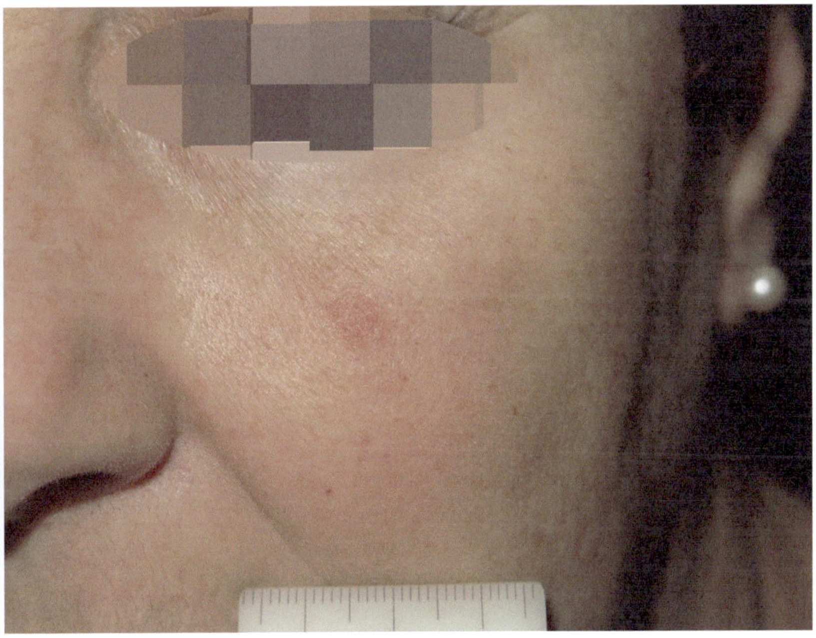

Fig. 9.1and 9.2 On clinical examination, there is an erythematous, scaly plaque on the left cheek

A. Lallas
First Department of Dermatology, Aristotle University of Thessaloniki, Thessaloniki, Greece

H. Cabo, A. Lallas (eds.), *Comprehensive Atlas of Dermatoscopy Cases*, https://doi.org/10.1007/978-3-319-76932-5_9

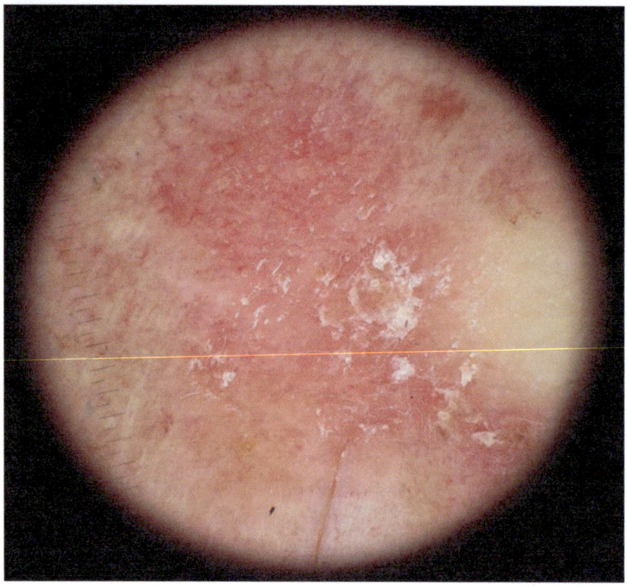

Fig. 9.3 Dermoscopy view

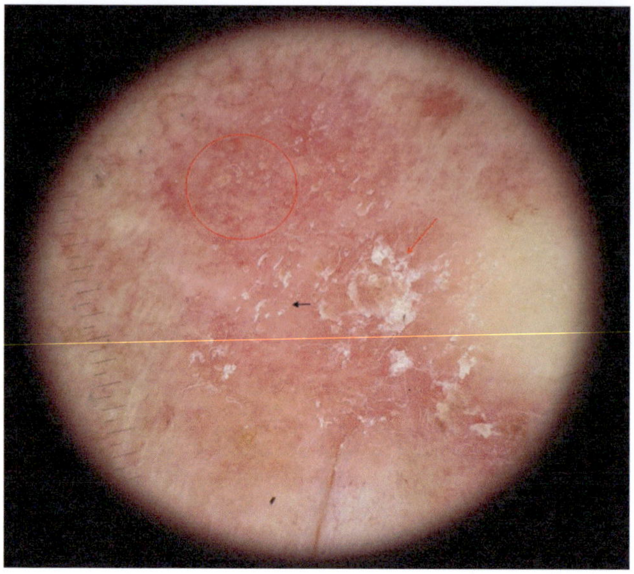

Fig. 9.4 Dermoscopy reveals a red pseudonetwork pattern and an erythematous background along with white to yellow, keratotic, and enlarged follicular openings (known as "strawberry pattern") mainly in the upper side of the lesion (red circle). Moreover, white to yellow scales are also seen (red arrow). White circles are also visible around few hair follicles (black arrow)

Key Message

The white color and in this case the white circles around the hair follicles are indicative of a keratinocytic tumor. The clinical and dermoscopic images with the characteristic strawberry pattern allow a safe diagnosis of actinic keratosis.

Palpable Pigmented Lesions on the Face

10

Horacio Cabo, Aimilios Lallas, Wilhem Stolz, Zoe Apalla, Michael Kunz, and Ralph P. Braun

Case 1: H.C.

Sex: female
Age: 74
Surface (flat/palpable/nodular): palpable
Maximum diameter: 6 mm
Duration of the lesion: >1 year
History of morphologic changes: no
Personal history of skin cancer (if yes, please specify): no
Family history of skin cancer (if yes, please specify): no
Skin phototype: II
Total nevus count (<10, 10–50, 50–100, >100): 10–50
Other clinical findings (optional):

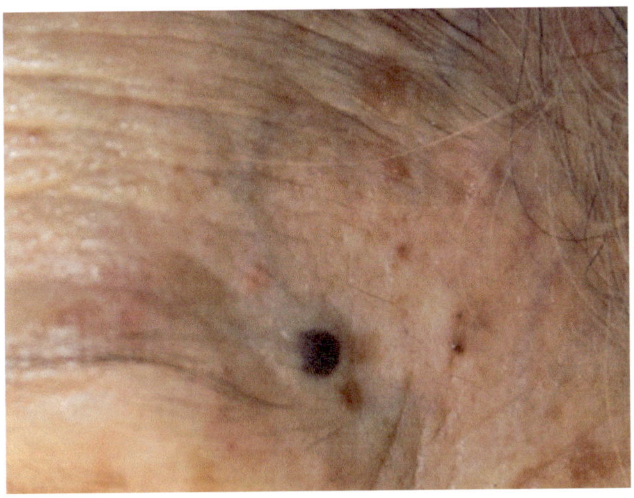

Fig. 10.1 Clinical view: blue elevated symmetric small lesion on the forehead

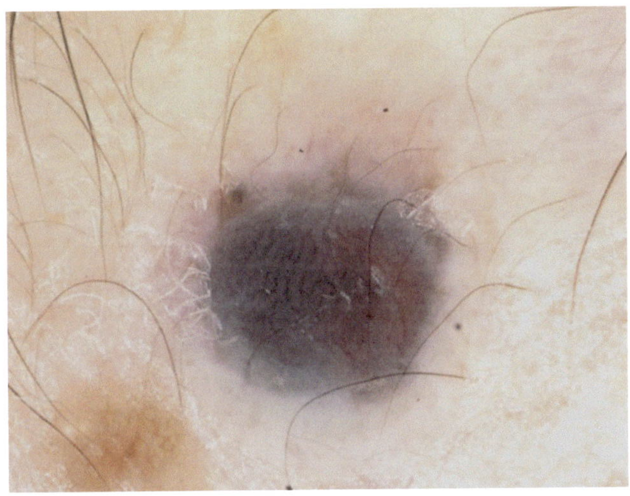

Fig. 10.2 Dermoscopy view

H. Cabo (✉)
Instituto de Investigaciones Médicas "A. Lanari". Dermatology Section, University of Buenos Aires, Buenos Aires, Argentina

A. Lallas · Z. Apalla
First Department of Dermatology, Aristotle University of Thessaloniki, Thessaloniki, Greece

W. Stolz
Dermatology Department, Klinikum Schwabing, Munich, Germany

M. Kunz · R. P. Braun
Department of Dermatology, University of Zürich, Zürich, Switzerland

H. Cabo, A. Lallas (eds.), *Comprehensive Atlas of Dermatoscopy Cases*, https://doi.org/10.1007/978-3-319-76932-5_10

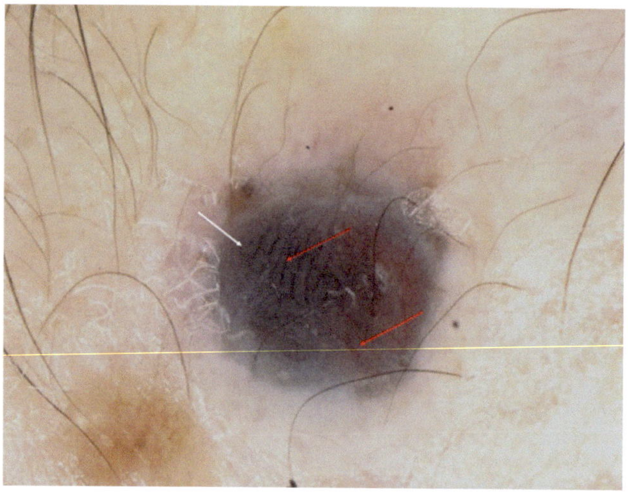

Fig. 10.3 Dermoscopy view: large areas with blue-gray pigmentation (white arrow); arborizing vessels (red arrows)

Key Message

Diagnosis: Basal cell carcinoma

The three major criteria of this tumor are the following:

- Blue-gray pigmentation (depending on the configuration, we will see different structures, and this case has large blue-gray areas)
- Arborizing vessels
- Ulceration (It is not present in this case)

Case 2: A.L.

Sex: male
Age: 52
Surface (flat/palpable/nodular): palpable
Maximum diameter: 4 mm
Duration of the lesion: 6 months
History of morphologic changes: yes, gradually enlarging
Personal history of skin cancer (if yes, please specify): yes, melanoma
Family history of skin cancer (if yes, please specify): no
Skin phototype: III
Total nevus count (<10, 10–50, 50–100, >100): 50–100
Other clinical findings (optional):

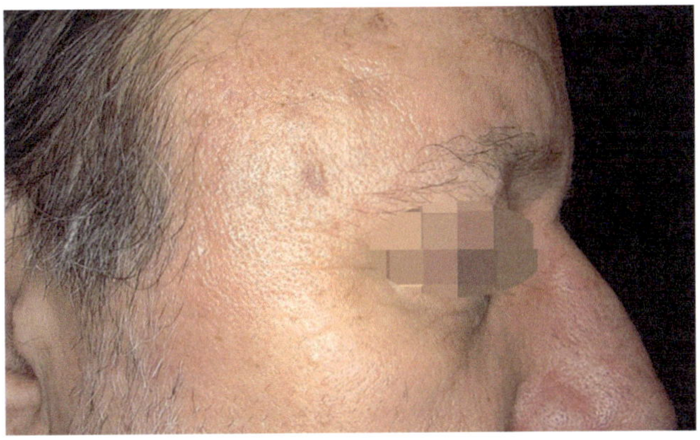

Fig. 10.4 On clinical examination, there is a solitary reddish plaque involving the frontal-temporal area of the scalp

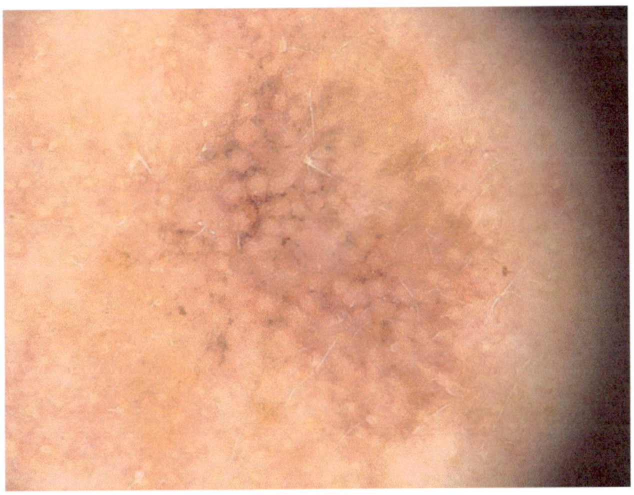

Fig. 10.5 Dermoscopy view

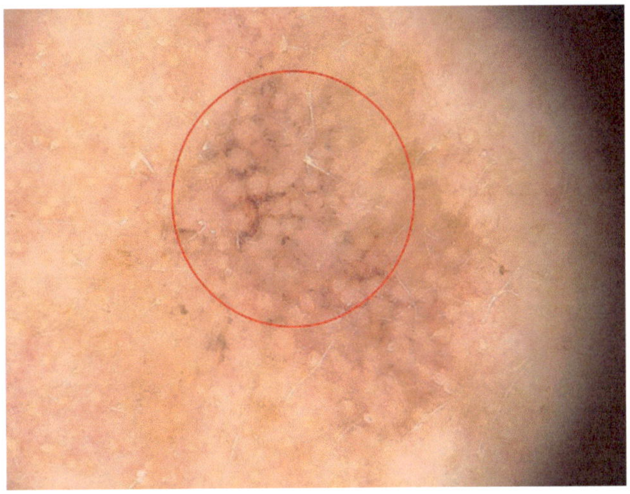

Fig. 10.6 Background erythema, brown to gray rhomboidal lines and gray dots around the follicular openings can be dermoscopically seen (red circle). Notably, the pigmentation tends not to obliterate the follicular openings but is limited to the interfollicular space allowing the follicular openings to be visible and evident

Key Message

Gray color (either as dots/globules or rhomboidal structures) can be confounding when dealing with facial pigmented lesions as it can be present in both lentigo maligna melanoma and pigmented actinic keratosis. However, in this case, the red color and mainly the distribution of pigmentation that let the follicles large and evident suggest the diagnosis of pigmented actinic keratosis.

Case 3: W.S.

Sex: female
Age: 47
Surface (flat/palpable/nodular): palpable
Maximum diameter: 2 mm
Duration of the lesion: unknown
History of morphologic changes: yes
Personal history of skin cancer (if yes, please specify): no
Family history of skin cancer (if yes, please specify): no
Skin phototype: III
Total nevus count (<10, 10–50, 50–100, >100): 10–50
Other clinical findings (optional):

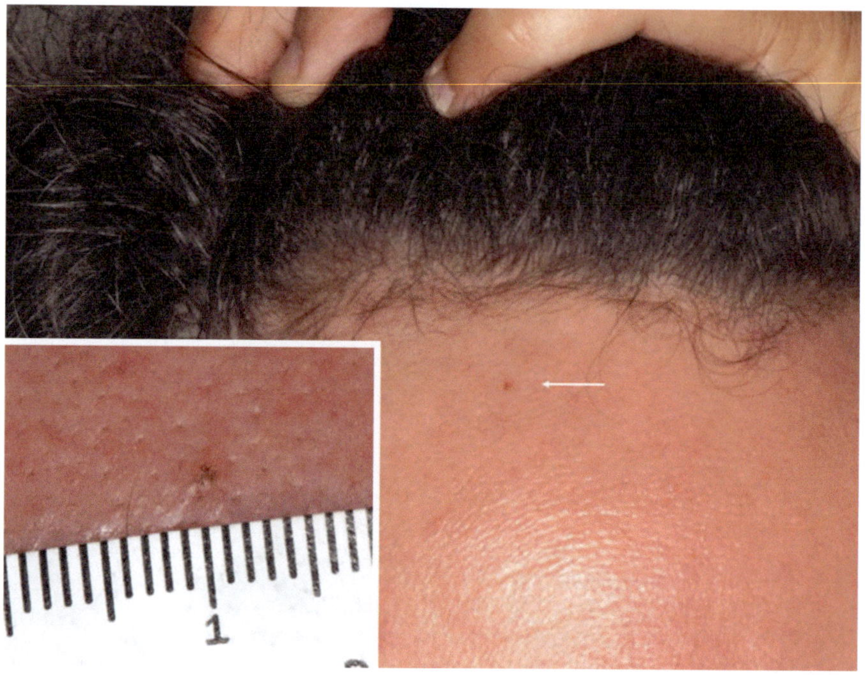

Fig. 10.7 Clinical view of a forehead lesion (white arrow); close-up (inset)

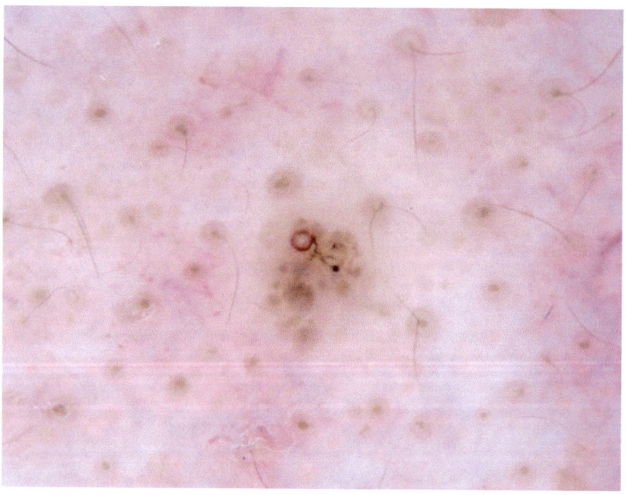

Fig. 10.8 Dermoscopy view

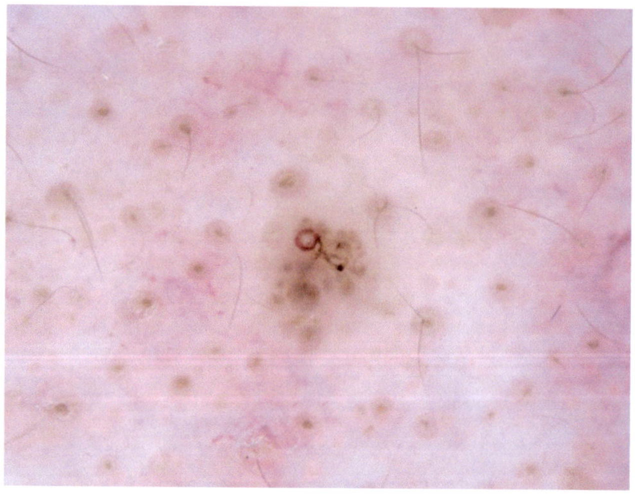

Fig. 10.9 Dermoscopy view: superficial erosion (blue arrow); blue-gray globules (white arrows); thick vessels (red arrow); leaf-like structures (black arrow); brown peripheral areas (yellow arrow)

Key Message
Diagnosis: Pigmented basal cell carcinoma
Dermoscopy clues:

- Superficial erosion
- Blue-gray globules
- Thick vessels
- Leaf-like structures
- Brown peripheral areas

Case 4: Z.A.

Sex: male
Age: 62
Surface (flat/palpable/nodular): palpable
Maximum diameter: 4 mm
Duration of the lesion: 2 months
History of morphologic changes: gradually growing
Personal history of skin cancer (if yes, please specify): yes, actinic keratosis
Family history of skin cancer (if yes, please specify): yes, NMSCs
Skin phototype: III
Total nevus count (<10, 10–50, 50–100, >100): <10
Other clinical findings (optional): asymptomatic

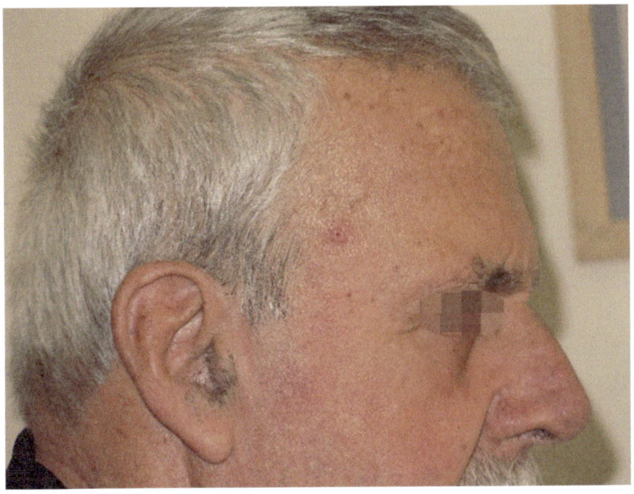

Fig. 10.10 A small asymptomatic pinkish papule, located in the left temple area

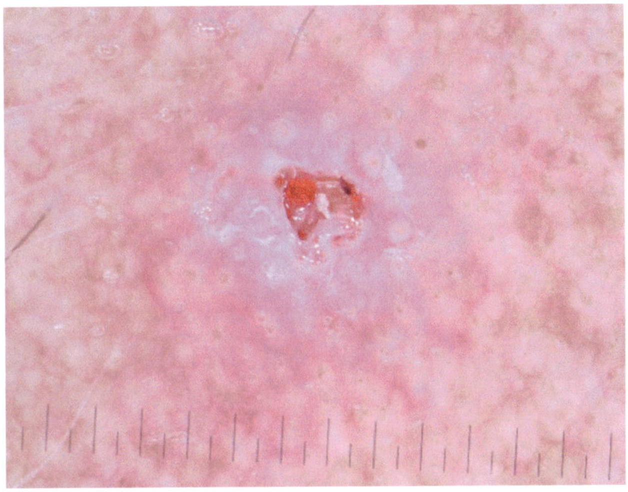

Fig. 10.12 Dermoscopy view

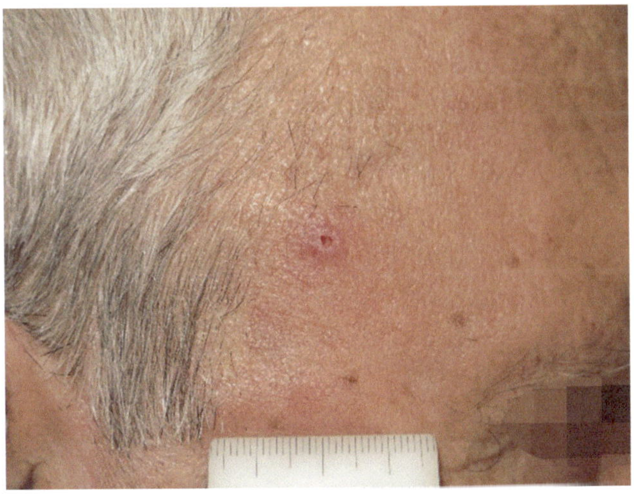

Fig. 10.11 In a closer view, we can observe the central ulceration, resulting in a crateriform morphology

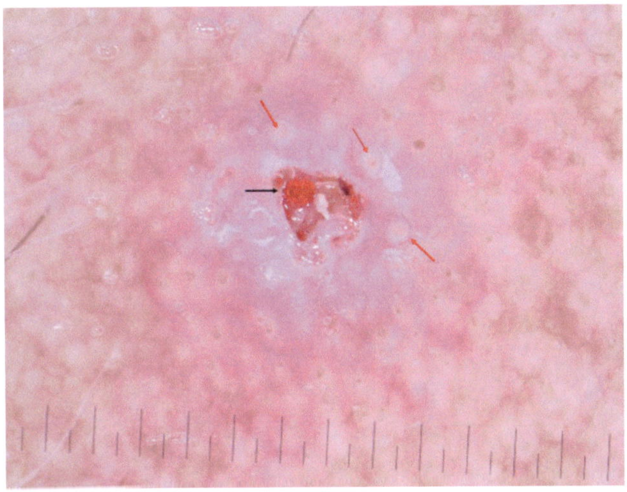

Fig. 10.13 In dermoscopy view we recognize the central ulceration (black arrow), as well as the presence of white circles around dilated follicular openings (red arrows), a finding strongly suggestive of a well-differentiated squamous cell carcinoma

Key Message

It is well known that the clinical and dermatoscopic features of invasive cutaneous squamous cell carcinoma depend on the histopathological grade of differentiation. If the clinical scenario is consistent, the presence of white circles and central ulceration in dermatoscopy strongly indicate a well-differentiated squamous cell carcinoma.

Case 5: M.K., R.P.B.

Sex: male
Age: 89
Surface (flat/palpable/nodular): palpable
Maximum diameter: 1 cm
Duration of the lesion: 1 month
History of morphologic changes: rapidly growing painless papule on the right forehead
Personal history of skin cancer (if yes, please specify): multiple squamous cell carcinomas
Family history of skin cancer (if yes, please specify): no
Skin phototype: II
Total nevus count (<10, 10–50, 50–100, >100): 10–50
Other clinical findings (optional): –

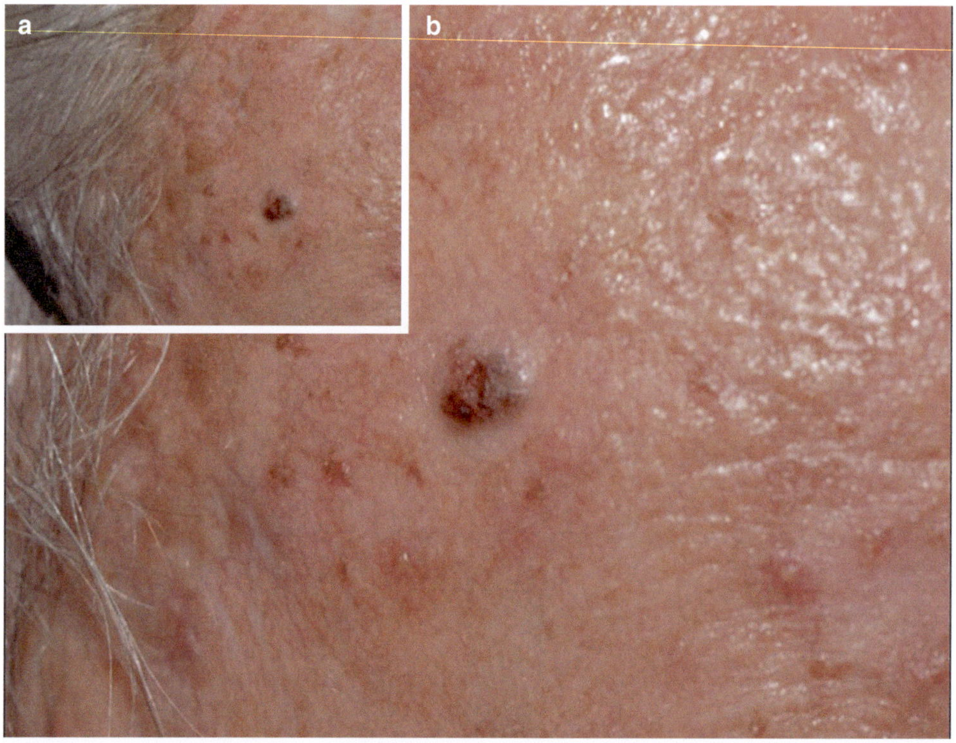

Fig. 10.14 (**a**) Clinical picture of a well-demarcated brown eroded papule on the left forehead; (**b**) close-up clinical picture of the brown papule on the left forehead revealing a verrucous surface and erosions

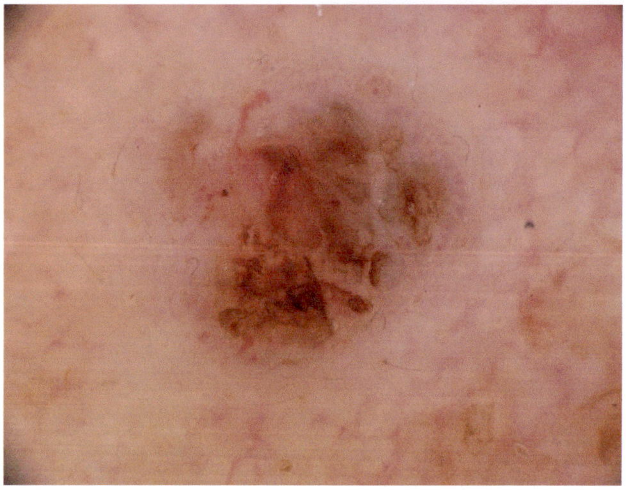

Fig. 10.15 Dermoscopy view

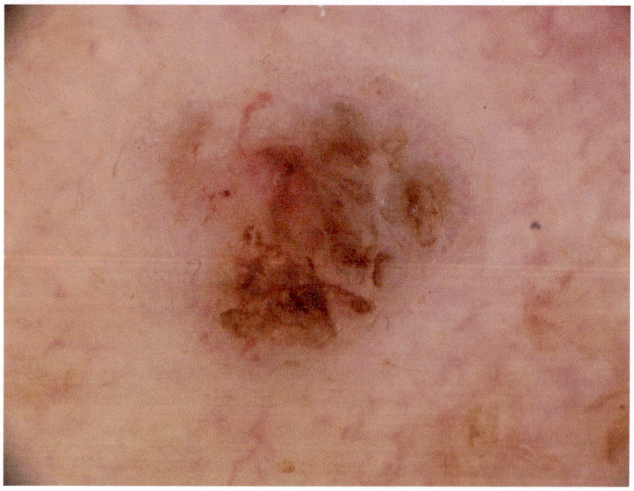

Fig. 10.16 Dermoscopic picture of a non-melanotic lesion with central yellowish scale, ulceration (multiple hairs stuck to lesion are a clue to ulceration), and peripheral focal glomerular and hairpin vessels surrounded by a whitish halo

Key Message

The dermoscopic picture shows multiple clues to a keratinizing tumor such as squamous cell carcinoma. The tumor was resected, and histology showed a poorly differentiated squamous cell carcinoma of 1 cm thickness.

Palpable Nonpigmented Lesion on the Face

11

Chryssoula Papageorgiou and Aimilios Lallas

Case 1: A.L.

Sex: male
Age: 56
Surface (flat/palpable/nodular): palpable
Maximum diameter: 4 mm
Duration of the lesion: unknown
History of morphologic changes: yes
Personal history of skin cancer (if yes, please specify): no
Family history of skin cancer (if yes, please specify): no
Skin phototype: III
Total nevus count (<10, 10–50, 50–100, >100): 10–50
Other clinical findings (optional): photodamaged skin and numerous actinic keratosis on the scalp

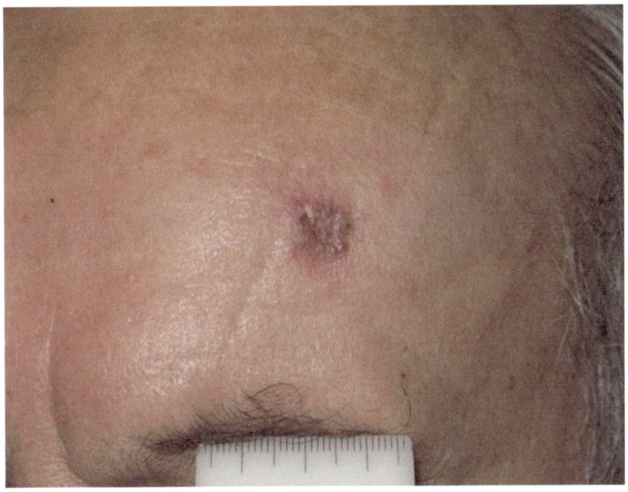

Fig. 11.1 Asymptomatic erythematous plaque on the forehead

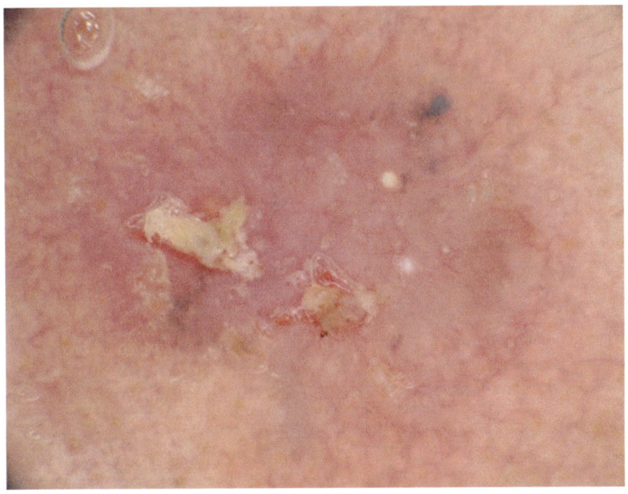

Fig. 11.2 Dermoscopy view

C. Papageorgiou (✉) · A. Lallas
First Department of Dermatology, Aristotle University of Thessaloniki, Thessaloniki, Greece

H. Cabo, A. Lallas (eds.), *Comprehensive Atlas of Dermatoscopy Cases*, https://doi.org/10.1007/978-3-319-76932-5_11

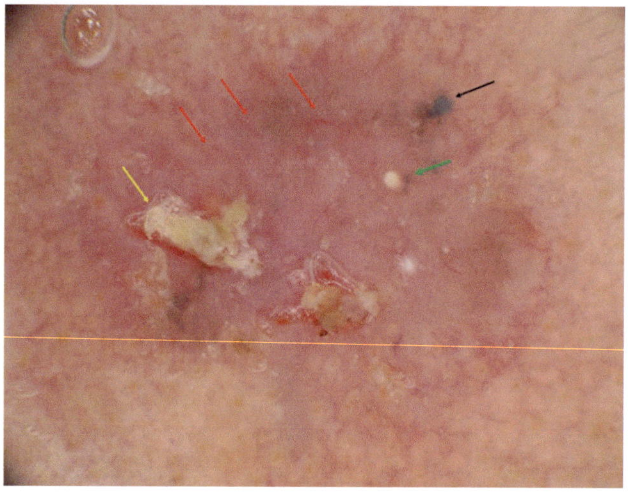

Fig. 11.3 Dermoscopy reveals linear and branching vessels (red arrows), hyperkeratosis (yellow arrow), a few milia-like cysts (green arrow), and a blue-gray roundish area (black arrow)

Key Message

The dermoscopic characteristics are indicative of basal cell carcinoma of nodular type. The presence of a blue-gray nest leaves no diagnostic doubt, since blue-gray globules/nests represent a highly specific criterion for BCC. In contrast, linear branching vessels represent a frequent BCC criterion but not so specific, since they can be seen in other tumors, like those of adnexal origin.

12 Nodular Pigmented Lesions on the Face

Caterina Longo

Case 1

Sex: F
Age: 75
Surface (flat/palpable/nodular): nodular
Maximum diameter: 1 cm
Duration of the lesion: unknown
History of morphologic changes: yes
Personal history of skin cancer (if yes, please specify): previous BCC and multiple AKs
Family history of skin cancer (if yes, please specify): no
Skin phototype: II
Total nevus count (<10, 10–50, 50–100, >100): 10–50
Other clinical findings (optional): no

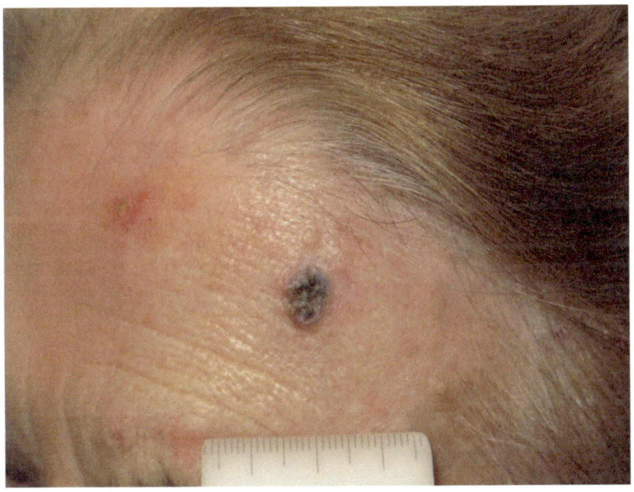

Fig. 12.1 A heavily pigmented lesion located on the forehead, with hyperkeratotic surface and well-demarcated borders

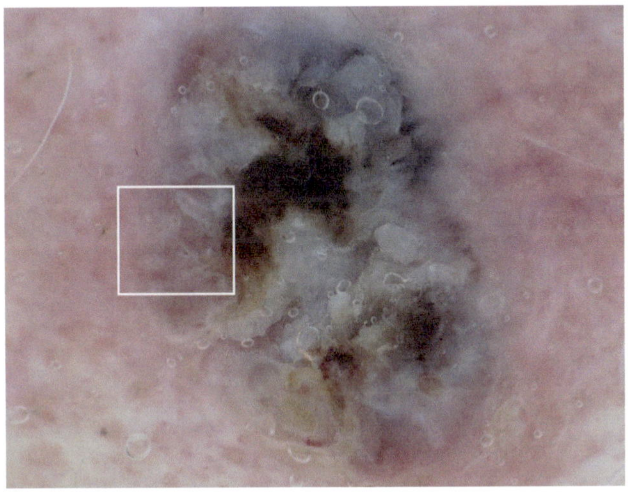

Fig. 12.2 Dermoscopy view

C. Longo
Dermatology Unit, University of Modena and Reggio Emilia, Modena, Italy

H. Cabo, A. Lallas (eds.), *Comprehensive Atlas of Dermatoscopy Cases*, https://doi.org/10.1007/978-3-319-76932-5_12

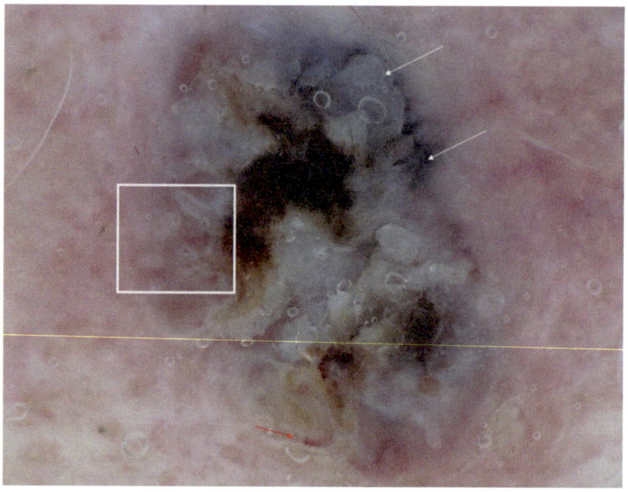

Fig. 12.3 In dermoscopy, black and blue structureless areas are visible over a with structureless area (white arrows). A thick linea vessel is visible at one side of the lesion (red arrow). Multiple white circles are visible (white square)

Key Message

White circles, visible as white annular structures surrounding follicular openings, are a strong clue for the diagnosis of squamous cell carcinoma. In this case, the lesion was pigmented, exhibiting blue and black color, thus entering differential diagnosis with a pigmented basal cell carcinoma. Although rare, pigmentation in SCC can occur. Dermoscopy clues are helpful for the diagnosis.

Nodular Nonpigmented Lesion on the Face

13

Caterina Longo, Giuseppe Argenziano, Gabriella Brancaccio, Aimilios Lallas, Chryssoula Papageorgiou, Daniel Morgado Carrasco, Natalia Espinosa, and Cristina Carrera

Case 1 C.L.

Sex: female
Age: 78 years old
Surface (flat/palpable/nodular): nodular
Maximum diameter: 1 cm
Duration of the lesion: few weeks
History of morphologic changes: rapidly growing
Personal history of skin cancer (if yes, please specify): none
Family history of skin cancer (if yes, please specify): negative
Skin phototype: III
Total nevus count (<10, 10–50, 50–100, >100): <10
Other clinical findings (optional):

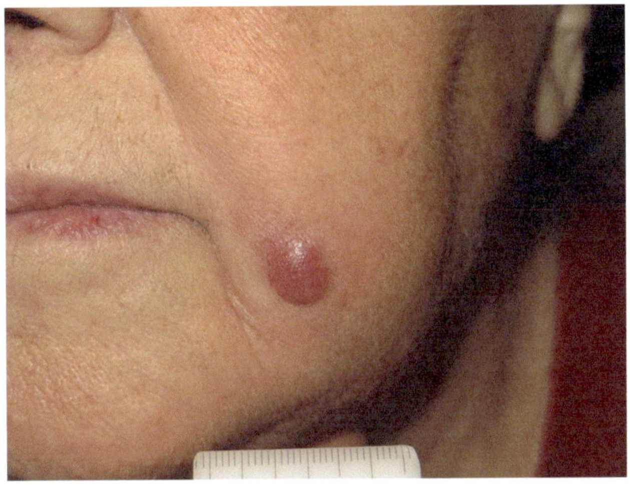

Fig. 13.1 A woman in her 78s showed the presence of a solitary cherry red nodule on her right cheek

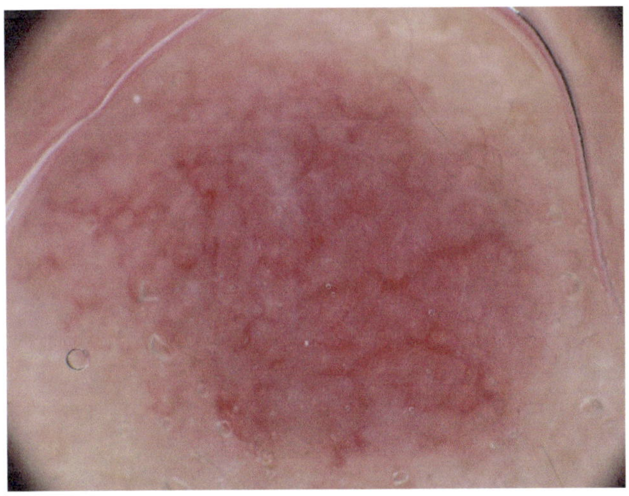

Fig. 13.2 Dermoscopy view

C. Longo (✉)
Dermatology Unit, University of Modena and Reggio Emilia, Modena, Italy

G. Argenziano · G. Brancaccio
Dermatology Unit, University of Campania, Naples, Italy
e-mail: gabri.brancaccio@gmail.com

A. Lallas · C. Papageorgiou
First Department of Dermatology,
Aristotle University of Thessaloniki, Thessaloniki, Greece

D. M. Carrasco · N. Espinosa · C. Carrera
Dermatology Department, University of Barcelona, Hospital Clínic de Barcelona, Villarroel 170, 08036 Barcelona, Spain
e-mail: ccarrera@clinic.cat

H. Cabo, A. Lallas (eds.), *Comprehensive Atlas of Dermatoscopy Cases*, https://doi.org/10.1007/978-3-319-76932-5_13

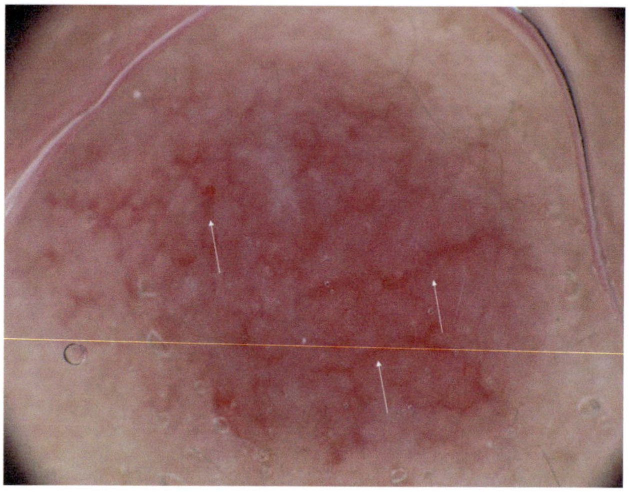

Fig. 13.3 Dermoscopically, the lesion was typified by the presence of pinkish structureless areas and serpentine not in focus vessels (white arrows). The lesion was excised, and the histologic diagnosis was Merkel cell carcinoma

Key Message

Merkel cell carcinoma (MCC) is a rare primary cutaneous carcinoma with neuroendocrine differentiation.

MCC typically arises on the head and neck of elderly people, and it is more common in men. Clinically, it presents as an asymptomatic, rapidly growing, red nodule. The acronym AEIOU has been recently proposed to summarize its most common clinical features: *A* asymptomatic, *E* expanding rapidly, *I* immune suppression, *O* older than 50 years, *U* ultraviolet-exposed site on fair skin. Dermoscopically, MCC is typified by the presence of polymorphic vascular pattern, composed of milky-red clods/areas in association with one or more additional vascular structures. These findings are not specific for MCC as they can be found also in other locally aggressive tumors.

The golden rule not to miss a MCC is to excise any given solitary growing nodule occurring in elderly, especially on limbs and the head. Dermoscopy could be of help although no specific diagnostic criteria permit to make a definite and reliable diagnosis.

Case 2 G.A., G.B.

Sex: male
Age: 54
Surface (flat/palpable/nodular): nodular
Maximum diameter: 1 cm
Duration of the lesion: 2 months
History of morphologic changes: yes, rapid growth
Personal history of skin cancer (if yes, please specify): no
Family history of skin cancer (if yes, please specify): no
Skin phototype: II
Total nevus count (<10, 10–50, 50–100, >100): <10
Other clinical findings (optional): the presence of severe photodamage

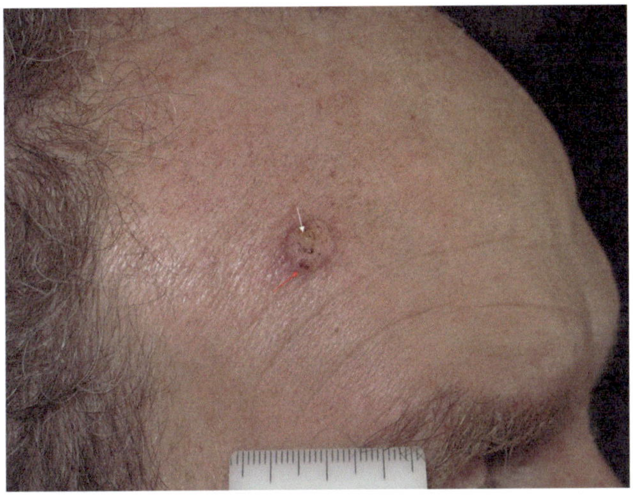

Fig. 13.4 Macroscopically the dome-shaped nodule is characterized by a keratotic central plug (white arrow) and blood crusts (red arrow)

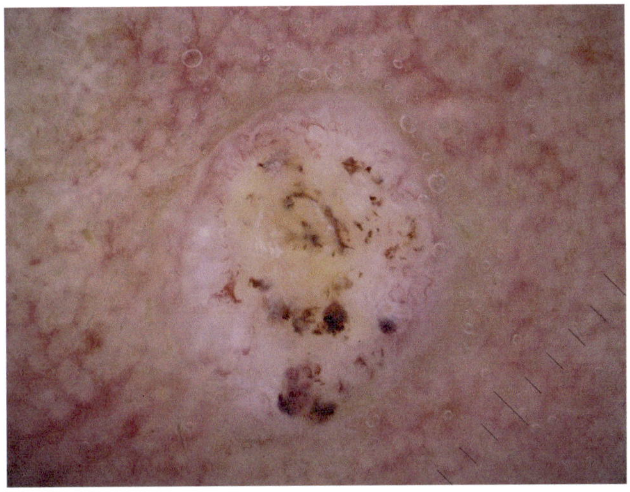

Fig. 13.5 Dermoscopy view

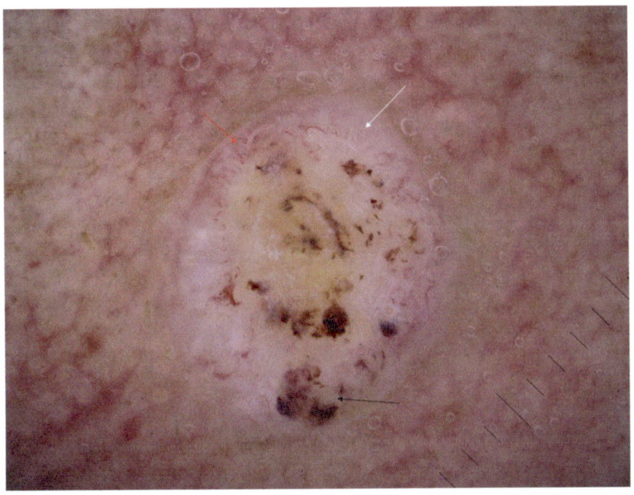

Fig. 13.6 Dermoscopically above the central keratotic plug is clearly visible a diffuse whitish coloration (white arrow), favoring a keratinocytic proliferation. On this whitish background, numerous thin hairpin vessels are visible at the periphery (red arrow). Some crusts and dark red to black areas are signs of ulceration (black arrow)

Key Message

The clinical and dermoscopy images allow a straightforward diagnosis of a keratinocytic tumor. Taking into account the history and the white color, a well-differentiated type of squamous cell carcinoma (keratoacanthoma-like) is clearly recognizable.

Case 3 A.L.

Sex: female
Age: 56
Surface (flat/palpable/nodular): nodular
Maximum diameter: 1.4 cm
Duration of the lesion: 11 months
History of morphologic changes: yes, gradually growing
Personal history of skin cancer (if yes, please specify): yes, actinic keratosis
Family history of skin cancer (if yes, please specify): no
Skin phototype: II
Total nevus count (<10, 10–50, 50–100, >100): <10
Other clinical findings (optional):

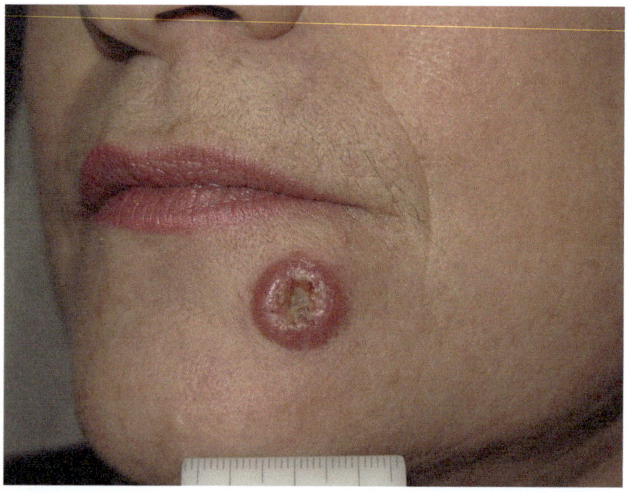

Fig. 13.7 Macroscopically, there is a well-demarcated and indurated hyperkeratotic nodule presenting with a central ulceration

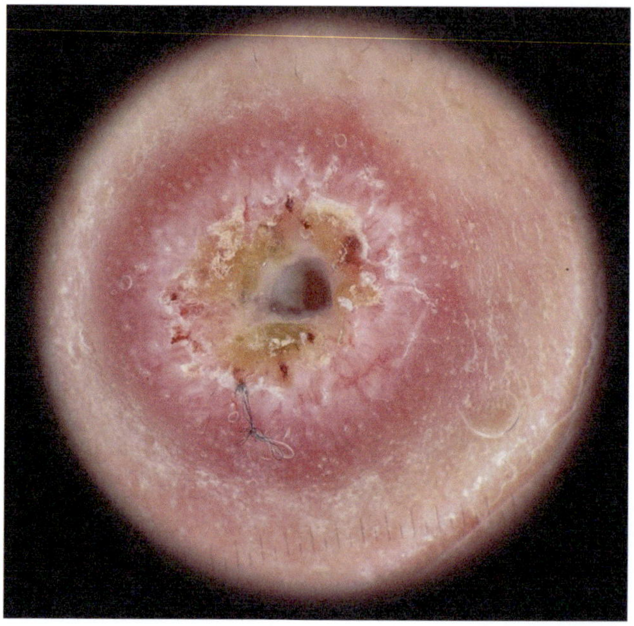

Fig. 13.8 Dermoscopy view

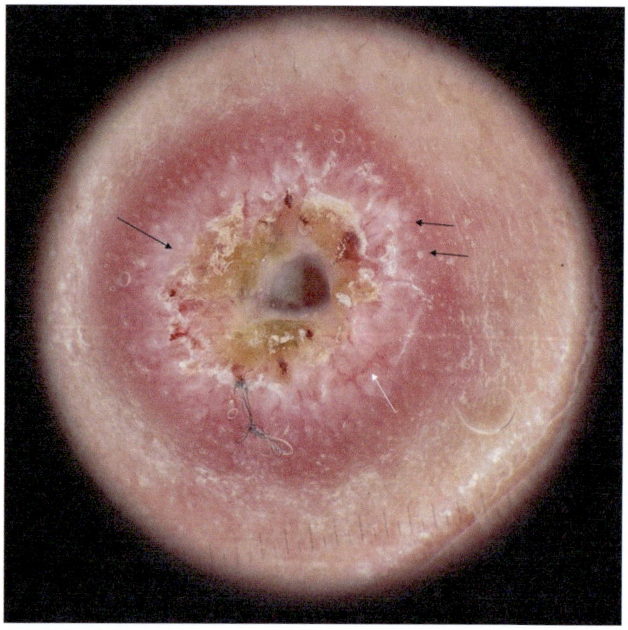

Fig. 13.9 Dermoscopically, we can observe the central ulcer surrounded by white and yellow amorphous masses of keratin and blood crusts. Additionally, white structureless areas and white circles are seen (black arrows). Numerous linear irregular vessels are also recognized by dermoscopy (white arrow)

Key Message

White color is a marker of keratinocytic proliferation and is the predominant color (either as white structureless areas or white circles or white halos or white masses of keratin) when referring to a well-differentiated type of squamous cell carcinoma. On the other hand, red is the predominant color when referring to a poorly differentiated type of squamous cell carcinoma as a result of the presence of bleeding and dense vascularity. In this case, both colors are present as described above. The lesion proved to be a moderately differentiated squamous cell carcinoma after the histopathological examination, a result that explains the presence of both white and red color with characteristics of both well- and poorly differentiated SCC, respectively.

Case 4 D.M.C, N.E, C.C.

Sex: female
Age: 39
Surface (flat/palpable/nodular): nodular
Maximum diameter: 1.5 cm
Duration of the lesion: 6 months

History of morphologic changes: a previously healthy woman presented with a 6-month history of a solitary tender nodule on her left cheek.
Personal history of skin cancer (if yes, please specify): no
Family history of skin cancer (if yes, please specify): no
Skin phototype: II
Total nevus count (<10, 10–50, 50–100, >100): 10–50
Other clinical findings (optional):

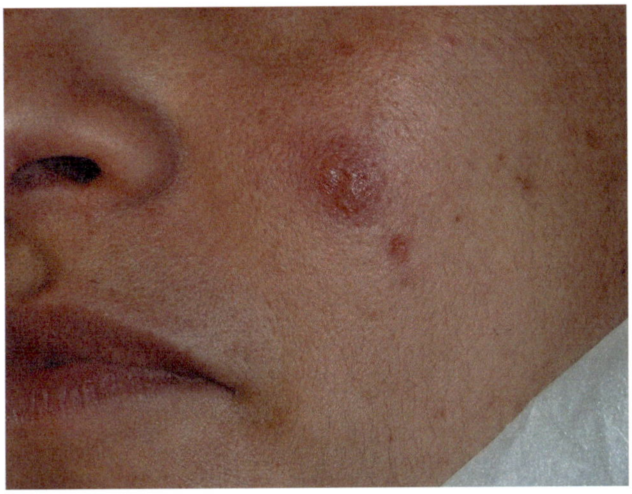

Fig. 13.10 Clinical Image. Tender erythematous nodule on the left cheek developed over the last 6 months

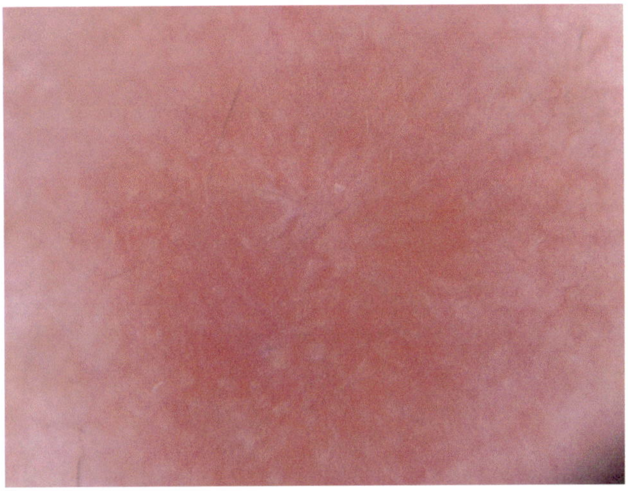

Fig. 13.11 Dermoscopy. Diffuse erythema (white stars), yellow-orange roundish "tear-like" structures (black arrows) and white starburst-like structure (red arrow)

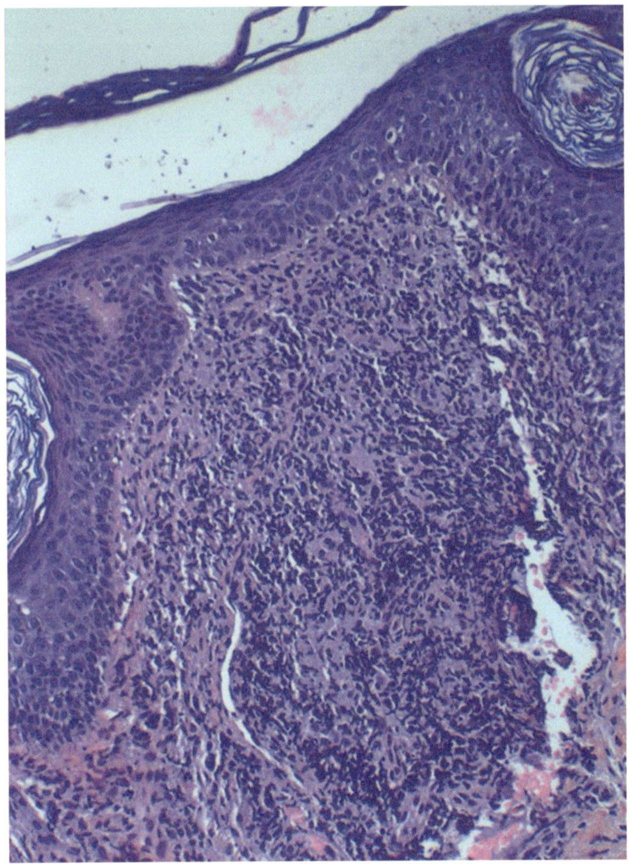

Fig. 13.12 Histology. Dense lymphohistiocytic infiltrate with non-necrotizing granulomas in the dermis (H-E, ×200), Giemsa stain, and microbiologic ancillary studies confirmed the diagnosis of cutaneous leishmaniasis

Key Message

The most frequent dermoscopic findings of cutaneous leishmaniasis are diffuse erythema, yellow-orange roundish structures also called as "yellow tears" and the white starburst-like pattern. Other well-described findings include central erosions or ulcer and crust, diverse vascular patterns and salmon-colored ovoid structures. Dermoscopy helps to establish the differential diagnosis especially from tumoral disorders such as spitzoid tumors or basal cell carcinoma on the face. The yellowish ovoid structures with whitish starburst pattern lead to suspect a granulomatous disease, in addition to the combination with vascular pattern and central erosion make the difference and the correct diagnosis.

Flat Pigmented Lesions on the Trunk

14

Aimilios Lallas, Chryssoula Papageorgiou, Caterina Longo, Horacio Cabo, Renato Marchiori Bakos, Harald Kittler, Giuseppe Argenziano, and Gabriella Brancaccio

Case 1 A.L.

Sex: male
Age: 75
Surface (flat/palpable/nodular): flat
Maximum diameter: 9 mm
Duration of the lesion: unknown
History of morphologic changes: yes
Personal history of skin cancer (if yes, please specify): yes, BCC
Family history of skin cancer (if yes, please specify): no
Skin phototype: III
Total nevus count: (<10, 10–50, 50–100, >100): 10–50
Other clinical findings (optional): Presence of numerous seborrheic keratosis and severe photodamage.

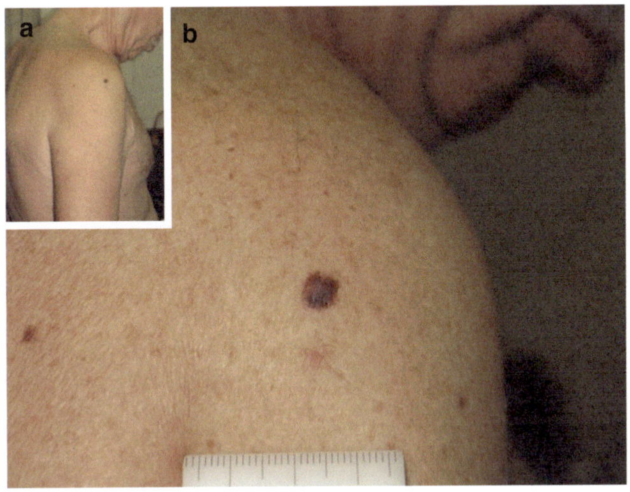

Fig. 14.1 (**a**) Macroscopically, there is a heavily pigmented lesion located on the right shoulder that stands out from the rest of the lesions. (**b**) In a closer view, the lesion is characterized by asymmetry in color and shape

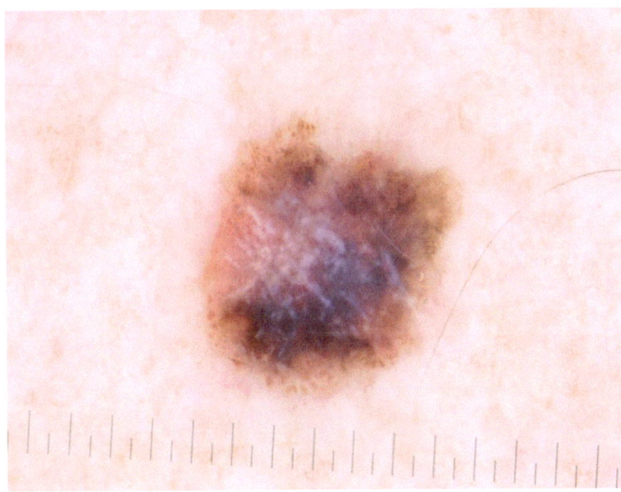

Fig. 14.2 Dermoscopy view

A. Lallas (✉) · C. Papageorgiou
First Department of Dermatology, Aristotle University of Thessaloniki, Thessaloniki, Greece

C. Longo
Dermatology Unit, University of Modena and Reggio Emilia, Modena, Italy

H. Cabo
Instituto de Investigaciones Médicas "A. Lanari". Dermatology Section, University of Buenos Aires, Buenos Aires, Argentina

R. M. Bakos
Universidade Federal do Rio Grande do Sul, Porto Alegre, Brazil

H. Kittler
Department of Dermatology, Medical University of Vienna, Vienna, Austria

G. Argenziano · G. Brancaccio
Dermatology Unit, University of Campania, Naples, Italy

H. Cabo, A. Lallas (eds.), *Comprehensive Atlas of Dermatoscopy Cases*, https://doi.org/10.1007/978-3-319-76932-5_14

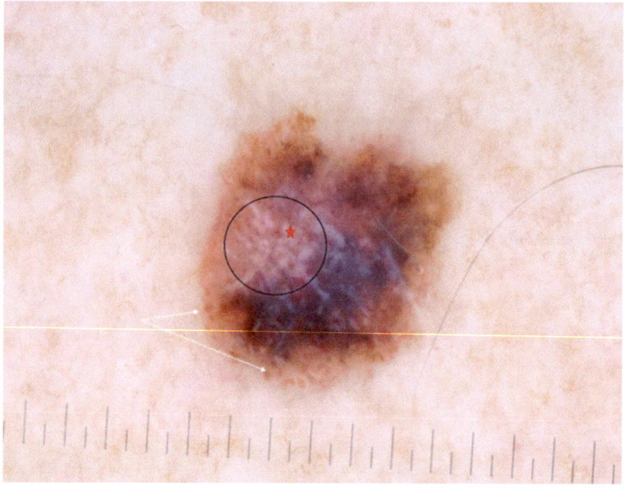

Fig. 14.3 Polarized dermoscopy revealed multiple white shiny streaks (black circle), atypical vessels (red star), and irregularly arranged globules (white arrows)

Key Message

Most of melanomas are easily recognized upon dermoscopic examination, because of the presence of one or more of the so-called melanoma-specific criteria. White shiny streaks represent an additional melanoma-specific criterion, seen only with polarized dermoscopy.

Case 2 A.L.

Sex: male
Age: 60
Surface (flat/palpable/nodular): flat
Maximum diameter: 4 mm
Duration of the lesion: unknown
History of morphologic changes: no
Personal history of skin cancer (if yes, please specify): no
Family history of skin cancer (if yes, please specify): no
Skin phototype: III
Total nevus count: (<10, 10–50, 50–100, >100): 10–50
Other clinical findings (optional): Presence of moderate photodamage and few seborrheic keratosis.

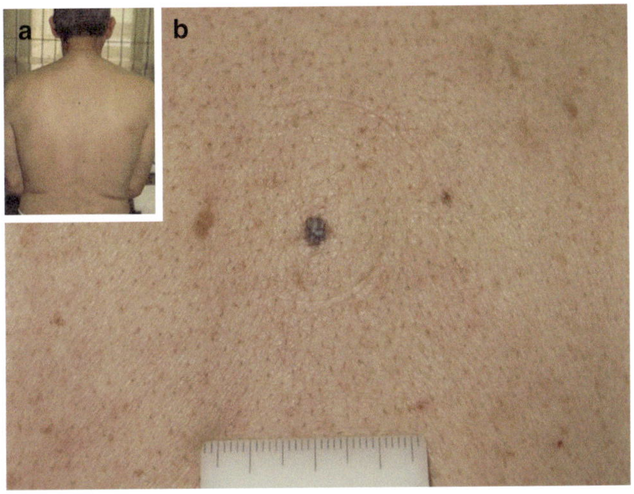

Fig. 14.4 (**a**)Flat pigmented lesion on the center of the upper back; (**b**) close-up of clinical image

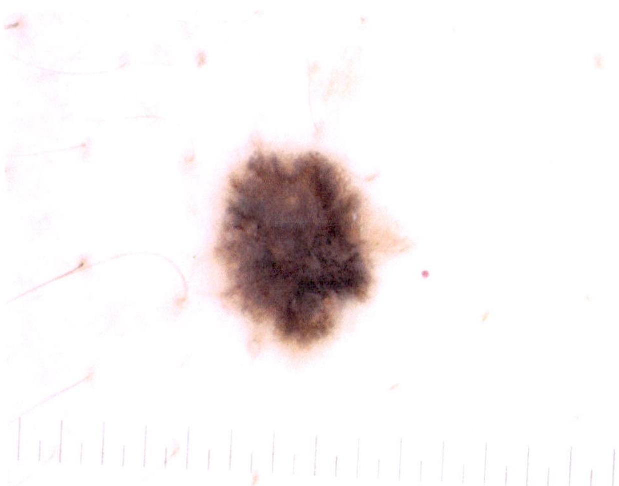

Fig. 14.5 Dermoscopy image

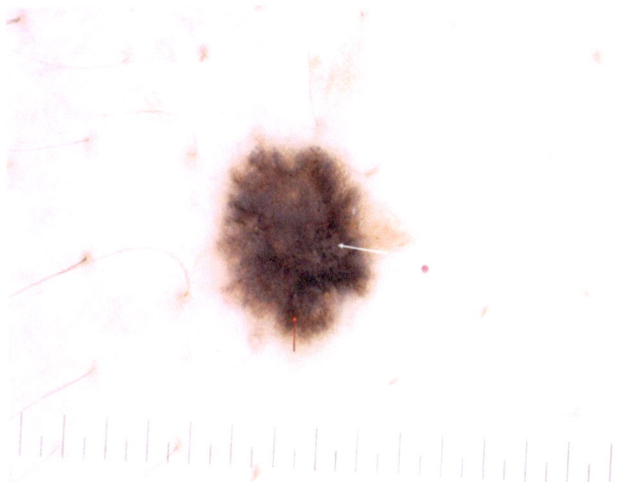

Fig. 14.6 Dermoscopy reveals asymmetry of color, irregular dots (white arrow), and the characteristic irregularly hyperpigmented areas mainly in the lower side of the lesion (red arrow)

Key Message

Irregular dots and blue-white veil are suggestive of melanoma. The presence of irregular hyperpigmented areas represents the most potent dermoscopic predictor of melanoma in situ.

Case 3 C.L.

Sex: male
Age: 73 years old
Surface (flat/palpable/nodular): flat
Maximum diameter: 1.5 cm
Duration of the lesion: unknown
History of morphologic changes: unknown
Personal history of skin cancer (if yes, please specify): basal cell carcinoma
Family history of skin cancer (if yes, please specify): negative
Skin phototype: III
Total nevus count: (<10, 10–50, 50–100, >100): 10–50
Other clinical findings (optional):

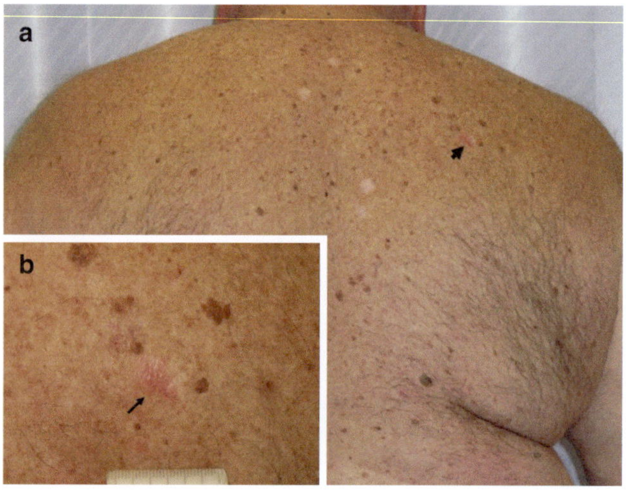

Fig. 14.7 (**a**) A man in his 70s showed the presence of multiple seborrheic keratosis and whitish areas referable to cryotherapy treatment for basal cell carcinomas; (**b**) clinically, an irregularly shaped pinkish patch was noted on his right scapula

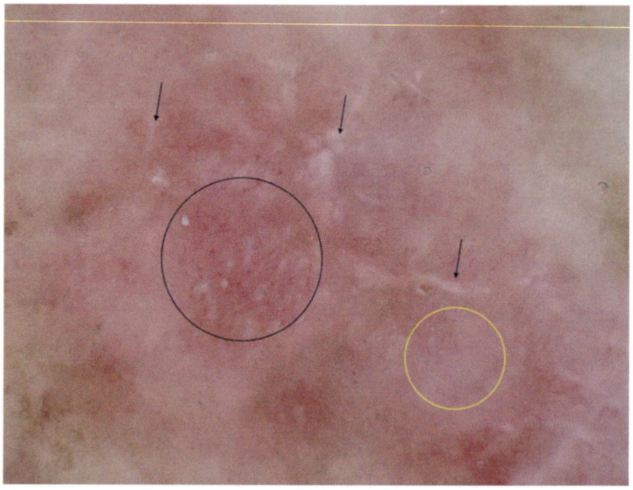

Fig. 14.9 Dermoscopically, the lesion was typified by the presence of pinkish structureless areas (yellow circle), dotted vessels (black circle), and crystalline structures (black arrows)

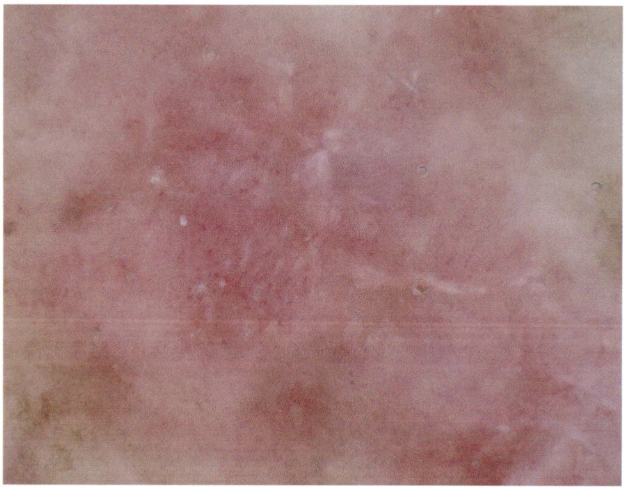

Fig. 14.8 Dermoscopy view

Key Message

The lesion was excised and the histologic diagnosis was invasive melanoma (0.4 mm Breslow thickness).

Amelanotic melanoma is considered the great masquerader since it is difficult to be recognized and differentiated from other benign and malignant lesions. The present case highlights the need to carefully check all lesions despite their clinical appearance. In fact, clinically this melanoma could be diagnosed as basal cell carcinoma because of its unknown growth history and furthermore for the positive history of multiple basal cell carcinomas.

However, dermoscopy revealed the presence of dotted vessels that are typically found in melanocytic lesions, and thus it is considered a positive criterion; additionally, no BCC-specific criteria could be identified, and thus, the diagnosis of melanoma should be considered.

As a general rule, all lesions with no clear-cut diagnostic criteria should be biopsied, and any given lesion with dotted vascular pattern should be regarded as possible melanomas

Case 4 A.L.

Sex: male
Age: 48
Surface (flat/palpable/nodular): flat
Maximum diameter: 6 mm
Duration of the lesion: 1 year
History of morphologic changes: yes
Personal history of skin cancer (if yes, please specify): no
Family history of skin cancer (if yes, please specify): no
Skin phototype: III
Total nevus count: (<10, 10–50, 50–100, >100): 10–50
Other clinical findings (optional): Photodamaged skin.

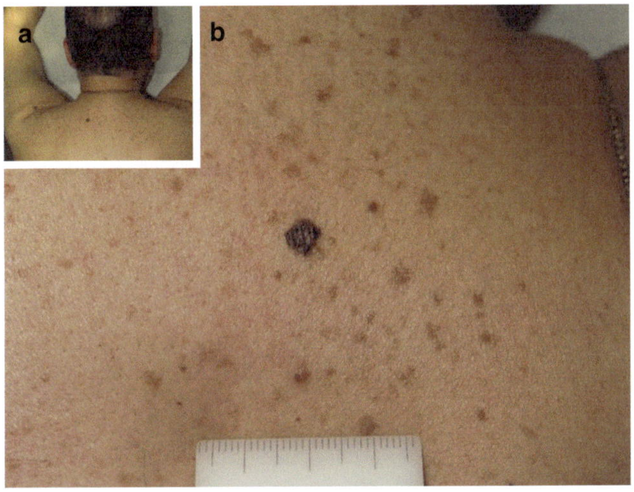

Fig. 14.10 (**a**) Clinical view; (**b**) flat heavily pigmented lesion, surrounded by numerous solar lentigines, on the top of the back

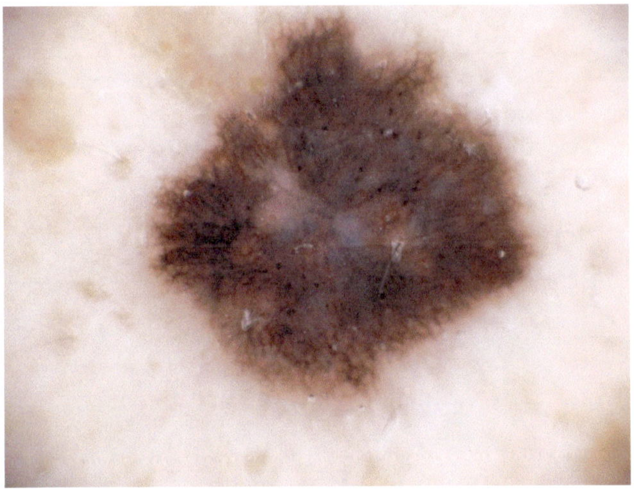

Fig. 14.11 Dermoscopy view

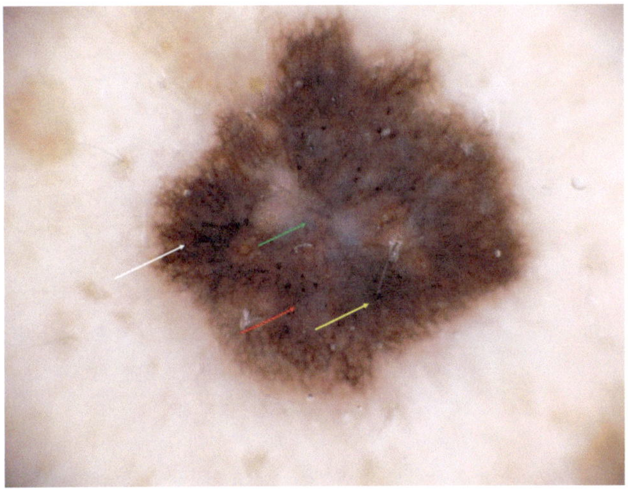

Fig. 14.12 Dermoscopy reveals atypical pigment network (white arrow) and irregular dots and globules (red arrow). Regression structures are also seen in the center of the lesion (green arrow). In the lower side of the lesion, irregular hyperpigmented areas are also apparent (yellow arrow)

Key Message

The combination of atypical network with irregular dots/globules, regression, and irregular hyperpigmented areas is highly suggestive of melanoma.

Case 5 H.C.

Sex: male
Age: 68
Surface (flat/palpable/nodular): flat
Maximum diameter: 10 mm
Duration of the lesion: unknown
History of morphologic changes: yes
Personal history of skin cancer (if yes, please specify): no
Family history of skin cancer (if yes, please specify): no
Skin phototype: III
Total nevus count: (<10, 10–50, 50–100, >100): 10–50
Other clinical findings (optional): the lesion was located in the back and the patient felt itch in this area

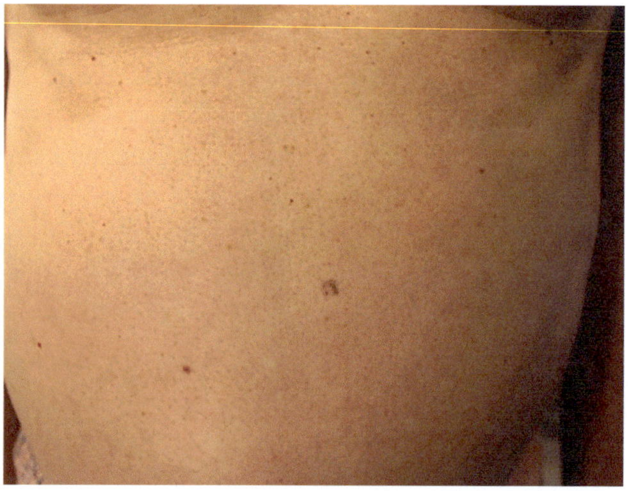

Fig. 14.13 Clinical view: flat irregular lesion on the back with different areas of pigmentation

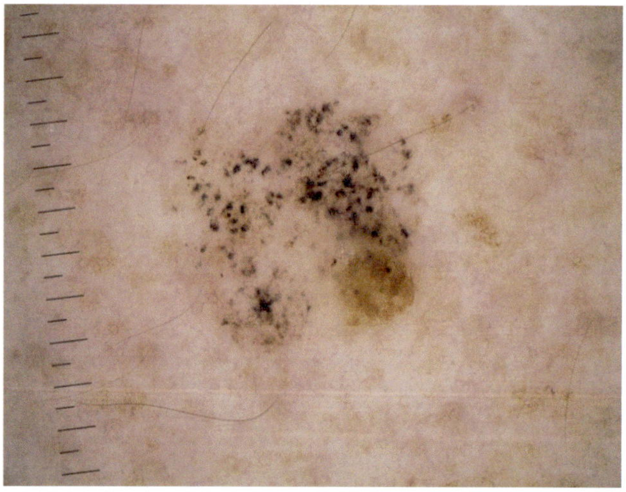

Fig. 14.14 Dermoscopy view

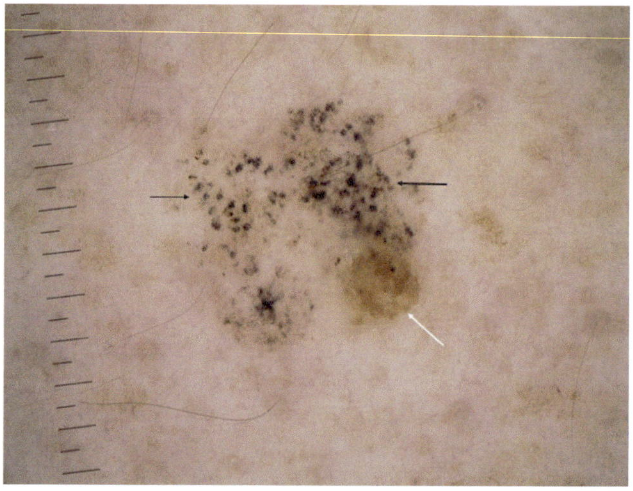

Fig. 14.15 Dermoscopy view: blue-gray round structures, with different size and shape (black arrows); brown area (white arrow)

Key Message

Diagnosis: Seborrheic keratosis with regression

Dermoscopy clue: Seborrheic keratosis may show signs of regression, usually after traumas.

The brown area of the lesion corresponds traces of seborrheic keratosis.

Case 6 A.L.

Sex: male
Age: 60
Surface (flat/palpable/nodular): flat
Maximum diameter: 5 mm
Duration of the lesion: 1 year
History of morphologic changes: yes, slow growth
Personal history of skin cancer (if yes, please specify): no
Family history of skin cancer (if yes, please specify): no
Skin phototype: III
Total nevus count: (<10, 10–50, 50–100, >100): 10–50
Other clinical findings (optional):

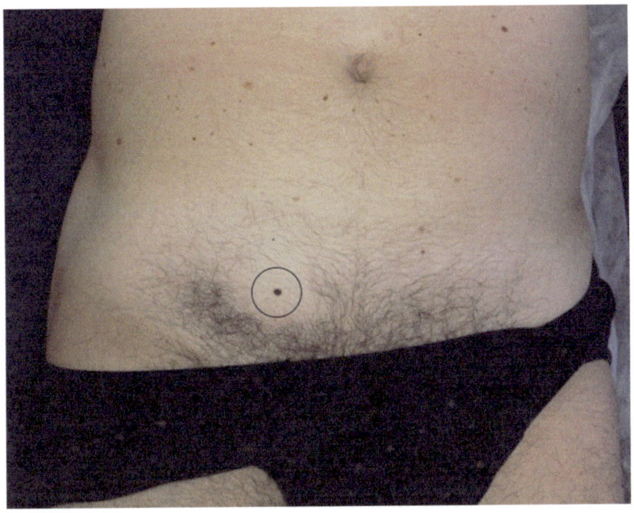

Fig. 14.16 Clinically, there is a symmetric pigmented macule located on the genital area (black circle)

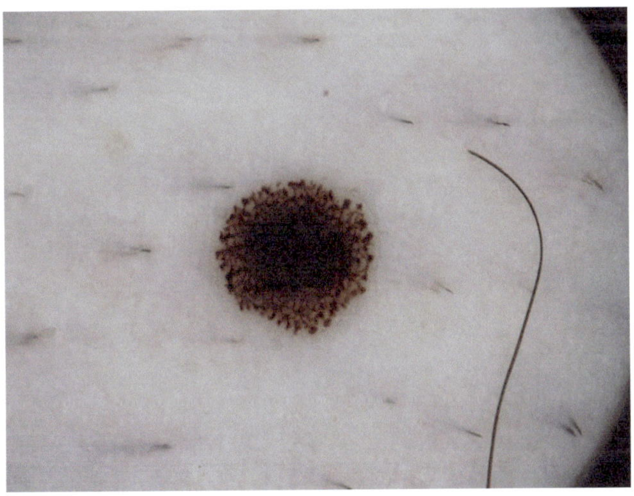

Fig. 14.17 Dermoscopy view

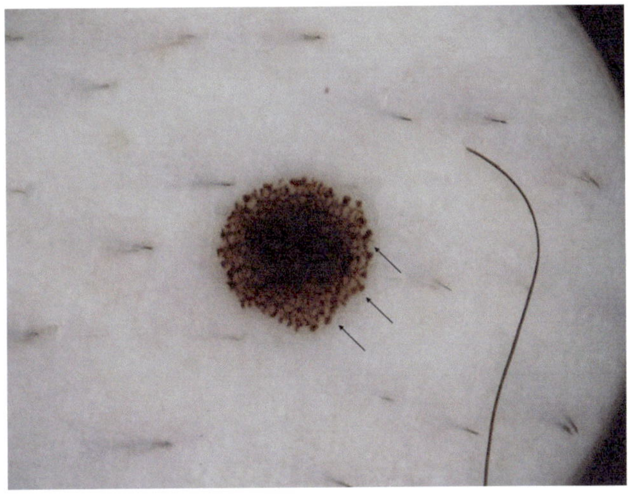

Fig. 14.18 Dermoscopy revealed a symmetric spitzoid-looking lesion characterized by a starburst pattern with a central brown to black pigmented area and asymmetrically distributed peripheral pseudopods (black arrows)

Key Message

The presence of dermoscopic characteristics of a spitzoid lesion along with the age of the patient led to its excision and proved to be a spitzoid melanoma after the histopathological examination. In symmetric flat spitzoid lesions, excision is highly recommended when developing after the age of 12 years, while when developing before this age, the recommended management is follow-up until stabilization.

Case 7 R.M.B.

Sex: male
Age: 50 years old
Surface (flat/palpable/nodular): flat
Maximum diameter: 0.9 cm
Duration of the lesion: unknown
History of morphologic changes: unknown
Personal history of skin cancer (if yes, please specify): yes, basal cell carcinomas
Family history of skin cancer (if yes, please specify): yes, basal cell carcinomas
Skin phototype: III
Total nevus count: (<10, 10–50, 50–100, >100): 10–50
Other clinical findings (optional):

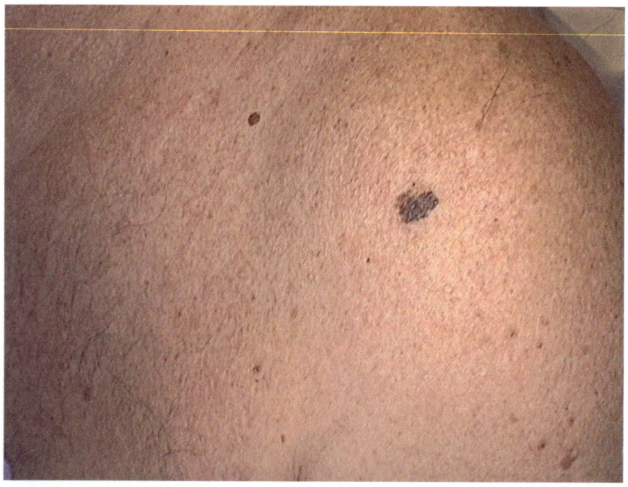

Fig. 14.19 Clinical image of the case showing an asymmetric flat dark brown macule on the anterior aspect of the left shoulder

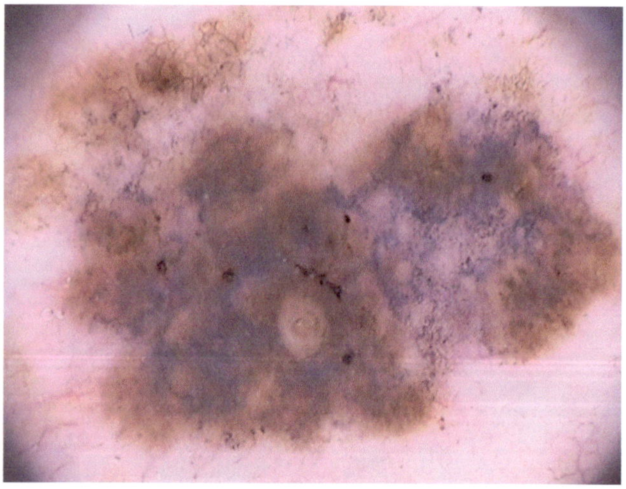

Fig. 14.20 Dermoscopy view

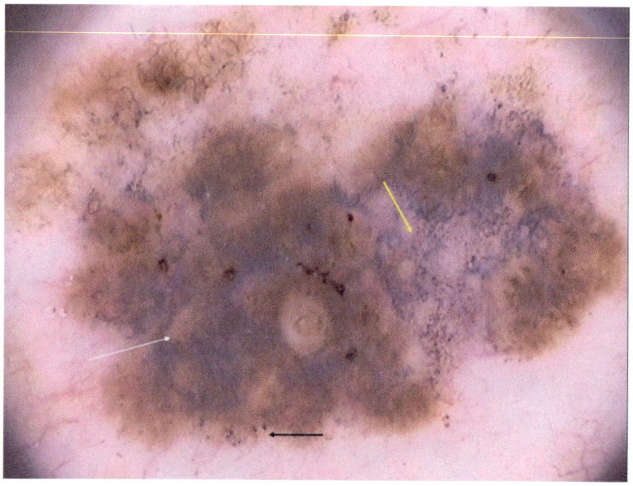

Fig. 14.21 Dermoscopic image showing a multicomponent pattern lesion with multiple colors, asymmetry of dermoscopic structures, atypical network (white arrow); irregular black globules and dots (red arrow) and whitish veil (yellow arrow)

Key Message

Dermoscopy revealed a multicomponent pattern which is mostly associated with malignant melanoma. Asymmetry of structures and multiple colors might also suggest a malignant proliferation. Indeed the major dermoscopic structures (atypical network and irregular globules and dots) corroborate this hypothesis.

Case 8 H.K.

Sex: male
Age: 65
Surface (flat/palpable/nodular): flat
Maximum diameter: 1.5 cm
Duration of the lesion: many years
History of morphologic changes: no
Personal history of skin cancer (if yes, please specify): no
Family history of skin cancer (if yes, please specify): no
Skin phototype: III
Total nevus count: (<10, 10–50, 50–100, >100): 10–50
Other clinical findings (optional):

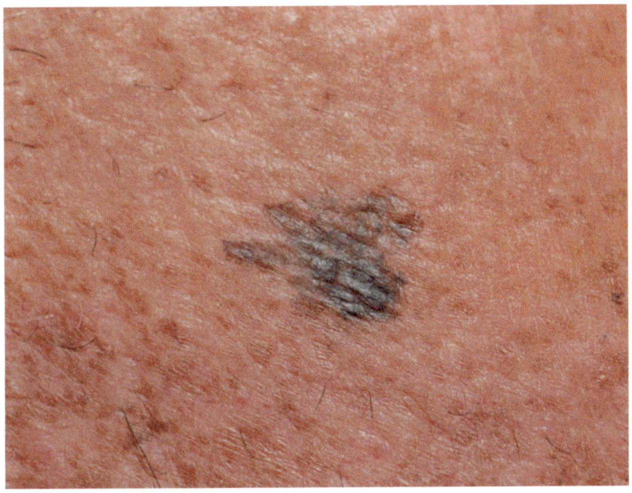

Fig. 14.22 A flat pigmented lesion on chronic sun-damaged skin

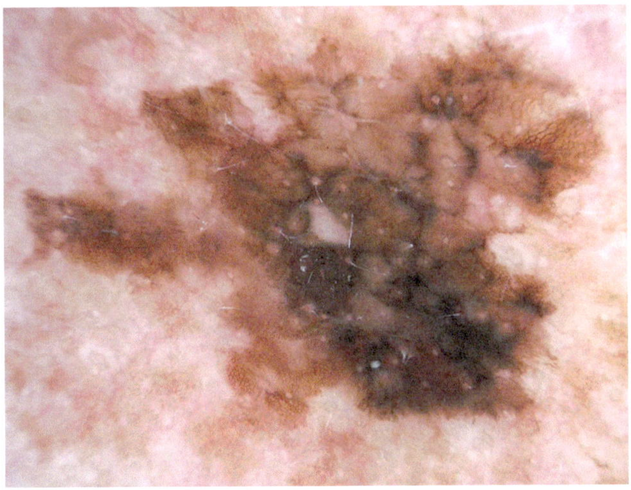

Fig. 14.23 Dermoscopy view

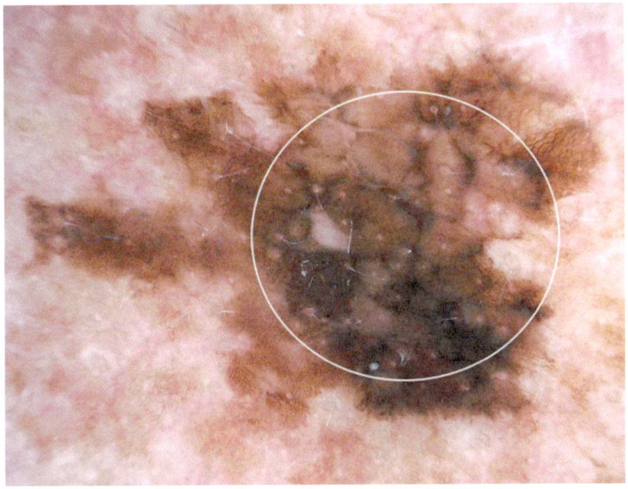

Fig. 14.24 Dermoscopy shows a chaotic lesion with a reticular pattern and polygonal lines (white circle)

Key Message
Polygonal lines are a clue to flat melanoma on chronic sun-damaged skin.

Case 9 P.T.

Sex: male
Age: 45
Surface (flat/palpable/nodular): flat
Maximum diameter: <1 cm
Duration of the lesion:
History of morphologic changes: new appearing lesion
Personal history of skin cancer (if yes, please specify): negative
Family history of skin cancer (if yes, please specify): negative
Skin phototype: II/III
Total nevus count: (<10, 10–50, 50–100, >100): 10–50
Other clinical findings (optional):–

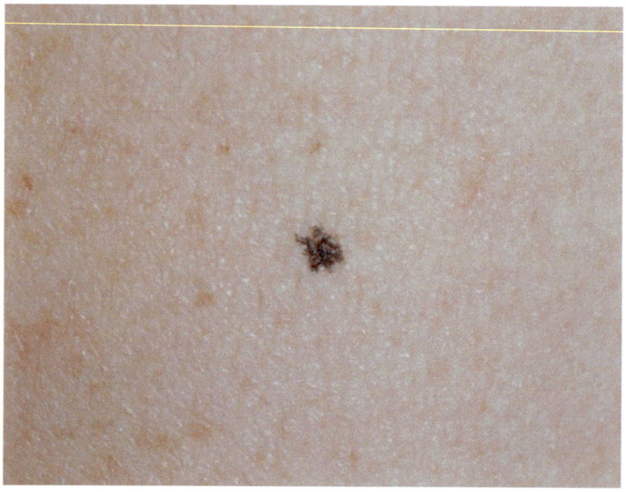

Fig. 14.25 Clinical image of a new appearing spot with dark color and sharp demarcation

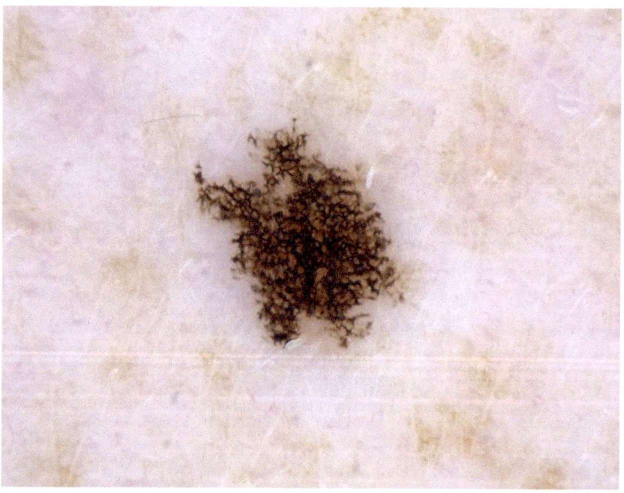

Fig. 14.26 Dermoscopy view

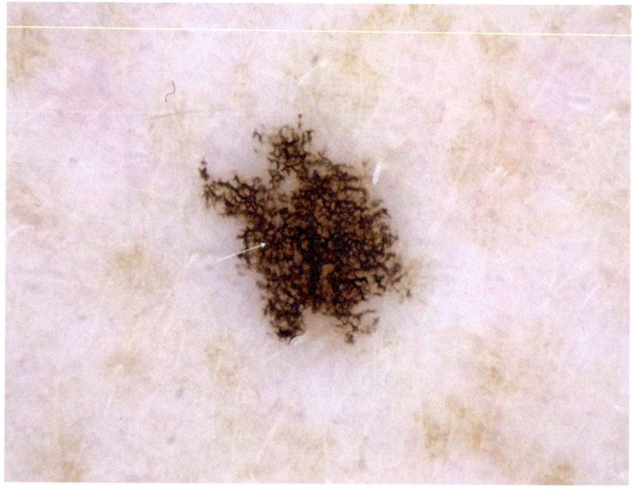

Fig. 14.27 Dermoscopy image of the lesion. One sees reticular lines of dark brown to black color (white arrow). At times, the lines appear thick, in other parts are abruptly interrupted resulting in a "broken-up" network

Key Message

Histology reports a solar lentigo, which in this lesion is in line with an ink-spot lentigo. Ink-spot lentigines are composed of black to dark brown reticular lines that form a "broken" network. Reticular lines are not 100% specific for a melanocytic lesion but can occur, for example, in solar lentigines and seborrheic keratosis. Patients are commonly worried by those lesions because of the dark color but can be reassured by the specific dermoscopic appearance.

Case 10 A.L.

Sex: male
Age: 61
Surface (flat/palpable/nodular): flat
Maximum diameter: 5 mm
Duration of the lesion: unknown

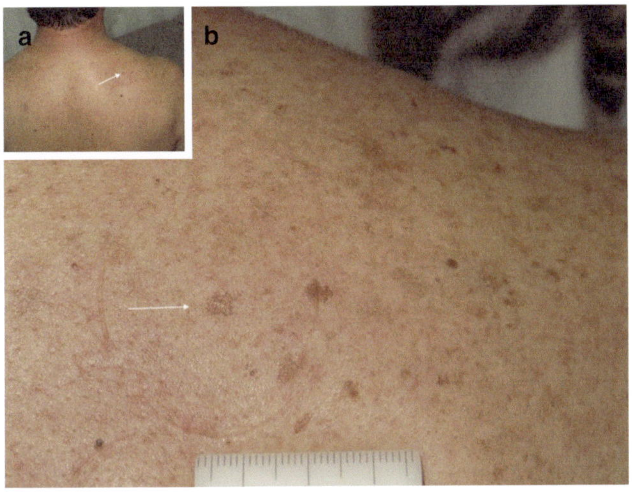

Fig. 14.28 (**a**) Clinical view of the lesion (white arrow); (**b**) clinical close-up: there is a flat pigmented lesion with irregular borders located on the upper side of the back

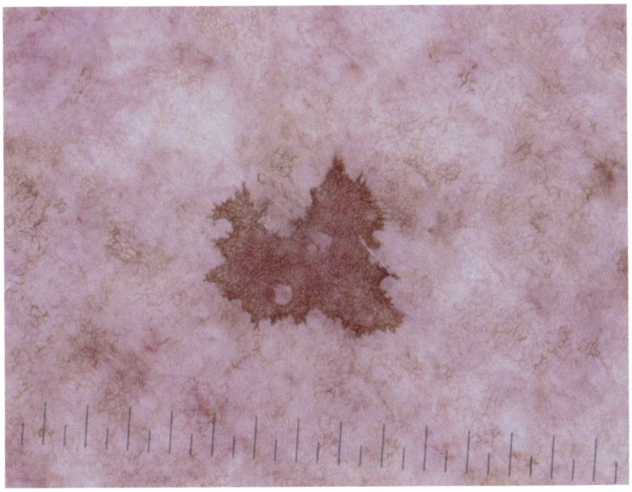

Fig. 14.29 Dermoscopy view

History of morphologic changes: no
Personal history of skin cancer (if yes, please specify): no
Family history of skin cancer (if yes, please specify): no
Skin phototype: III
Total nevus count: (<10, 10–50, 50–100, >100): 10–50
Other clinical findings (optional): Presence of severe photodamage and numerous seborrheic keratosis

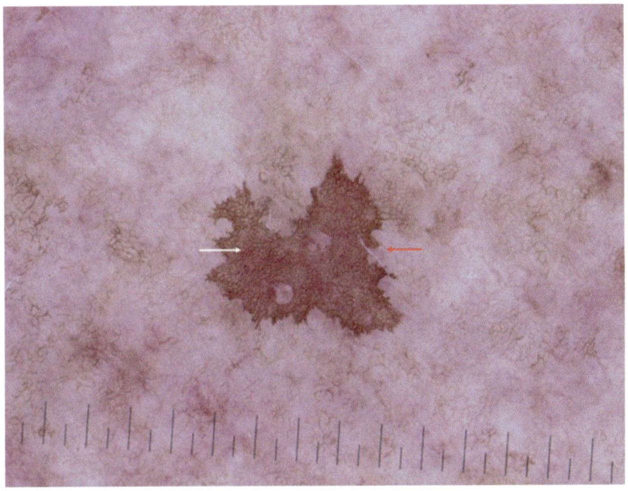

Fig. 14.30 Dermoscopically, the lesion displays densely arranged, roundish to oval brown circles which look like a delicate reticular pattern (white arrow). It is also characterized by sharp concave borders with the pigmentation ending with curved structures ("moth-eaten") (red arrow)

Key Message
The pattern of pigmentation and the "moth-eaten" borders allow a straightforward diagnosis of an extra-facial solar lentigo.

Case 11 G.A., G.B.

Sex: male
Age: **72**
Surface (flat/palpable/nodular): flat
Maximum diameter: 1.2 cm
Duration of the lesion: unknown
History of morphologic changes: yes
Personal history of skin cancer (if yes, please specify): no
Family history of skin cancer (if yes, please specify): no
Skin phototype: III
Total nevus count: (<10, 10–50, 50–100, >100): 50–100
Other clinical findings (optional): Presence of severe photodamage

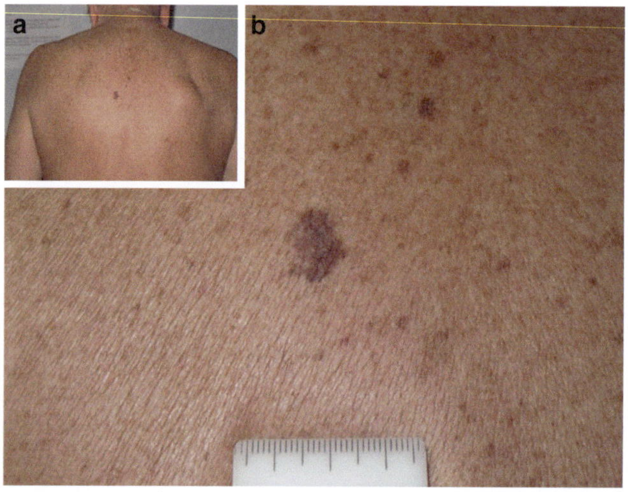

Fig. 14.31 (**a**) Clinical image; (**b**) the lesion, surrounded by signs of photodamage, is clinically asymmetric in color and shape and with irregular borders

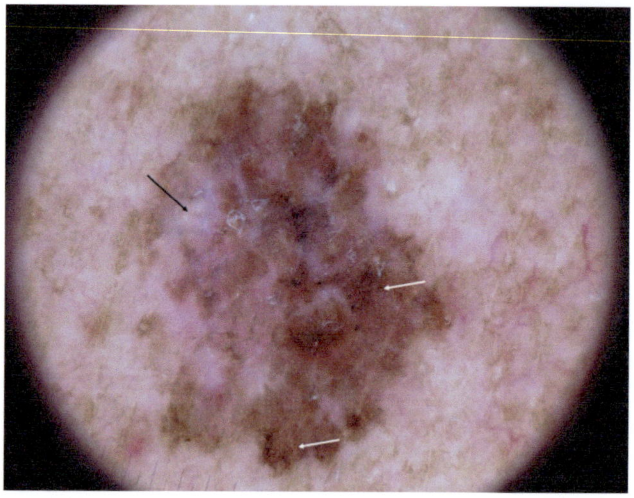

Fig. 14.33 Large amount of regressive features are seen on the left side of the lesion (scar-like areas and gray granules) (black arrow). In the lower-right side is still visible a hint of irregular pigmented network that reveals the melanocytic nature of the lesion (white arrows)

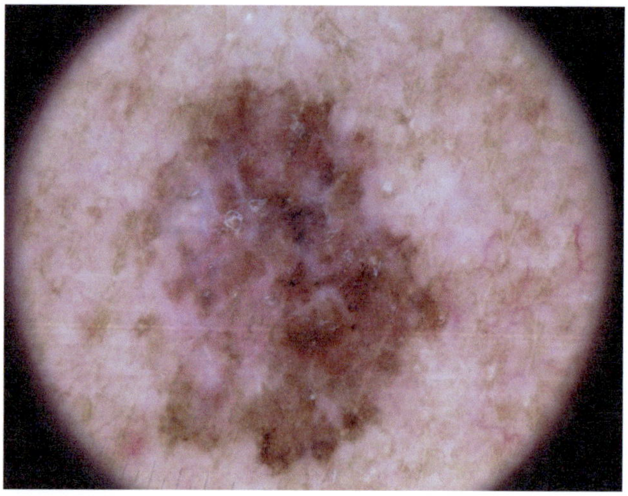

Fig. 14.32 Dermoscopy view

Key Message

In this lesion, the presence of a combination of regressive features and atypical network is the key to diagnose a slow-growing type of superficial melanoma

Case 12 A.L.

Sex: female
Age: 15
Surface (flat/palpable/nodular): flat
Maximum diameter: 2 mm
Duration of the lesion: 1 year
History of morphologic changes: no

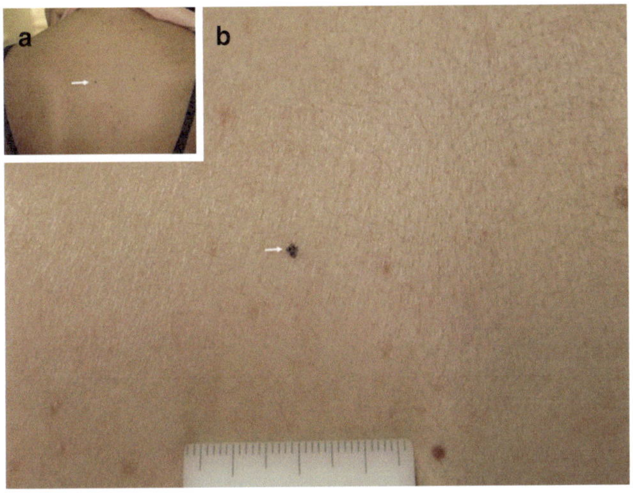

Fig. 14.34 (**a**) Macroscopically, there is a striking, heavily pigmented lesion located on the back (white arrow); (**b**) in a closer view, there is a bizarrely outlined, black macule with irregular shape (white arrow)

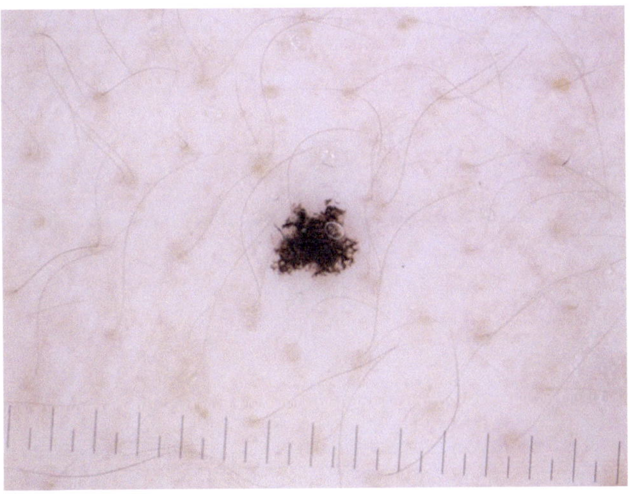

Fig. 14.35 Dermoscopy view

Personal history of skin cancer (if yes, please specify): no
Family history of skin cancer (if yes, please specify): no
Skin phototype: II
Total nevus count: (<10, 10–50, 50–100, >100): 10–50
Other clinical findings (optional): Presence of numerous brown freckles and history of severe sunburn

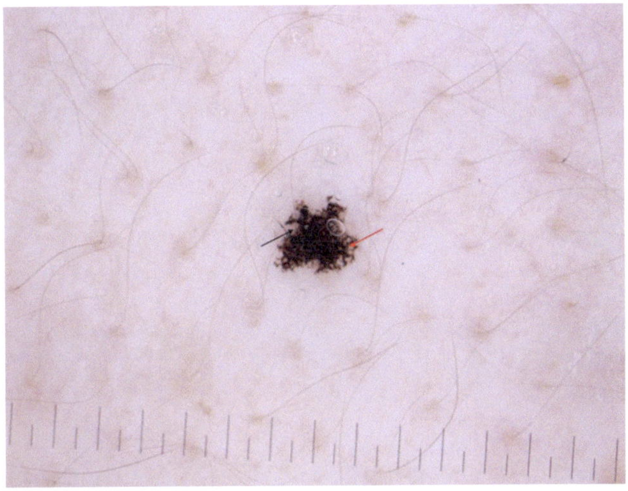

Fig. 14.36 Dermoscopy highlights the dark brown to black and interrupted (broken-up) pigment network consisting of thick lines and wide meshes (red arrow). A sharp concave demarcation is also observed ("moth-eaten" borders) (black arrow)

Key Message

The clinical and dermoscopy images along with the age of the patient and the history of sunburn allow the diagnosis of an ink-spot solar lentigo.

15 Flat Nonpigmented Lesions on the Trunk

Aimilios Lallas, Horacio Cabo, and Gabriel Salerni

Case 1 A. L.

Sex: male
Age: 77
Surface (flat/palpable/nodular): flat
Maximum diameter: 4 mm
Duration of the lesion: unknown
History of morphologic changes: no
Personal history of skin cancer (if yes, please specify): yes, previous BCC
Family history of skin cancer (if yes, please specify): no
Skin phototype: III
Total nevus count: (<10, 10–50, 50–100, >100): <10
Other clinical findings (optional): presence of severe photodamage and actinic keratosis

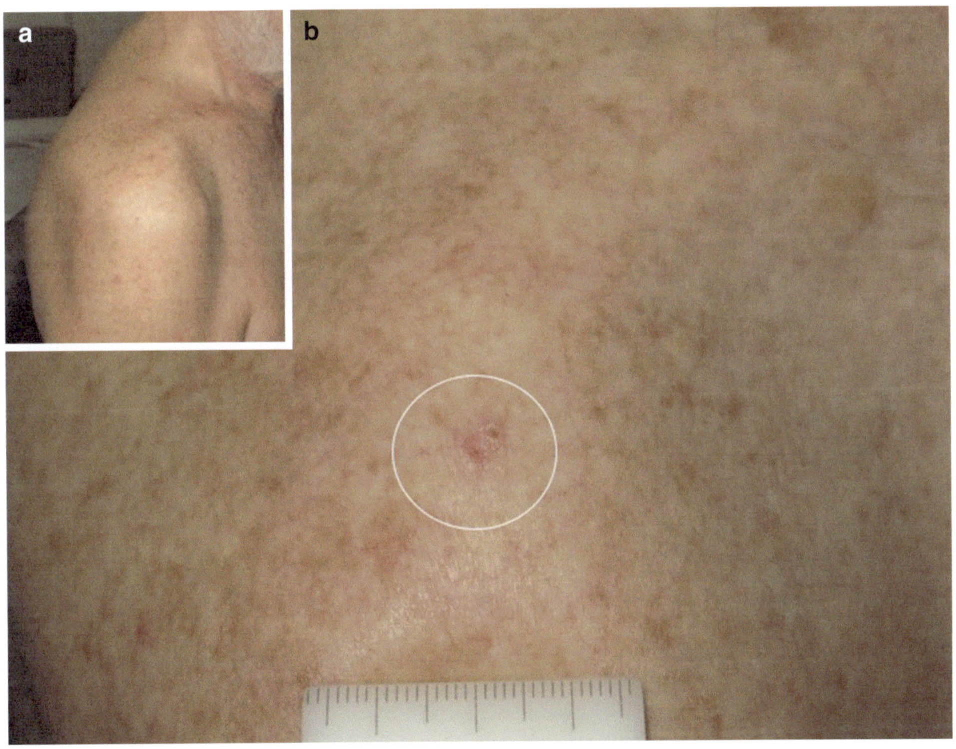

Fig. 15.1 (**a**) Clinical image. (**b**) Close-up: there is a scaly reddish plaque located on the right shoulder (white circle)

A. Lallas (✉)
First Department of Dermatology, Aristotle University of Thessaloniki, Thessaloniki, Greece

H. Cabo
Instituto de Investigaciones Médicas "A. Lanari". Dermatology Section, University of Buenos Aires, Buenos Aires, Argentina

G. Salerni
Dermatologist Doctor in Medicine Universidad Nacional de Rosario and Hospital Provincial del Centenario de Rosario Santa Fe, Santa Fe, Argentina

H. Cabo, A. Lallas (eds.), *Comprehensive Atlas of Dermatoscopy Cases*, https://doi.org/10.1007/978-3-319-76932-5_15

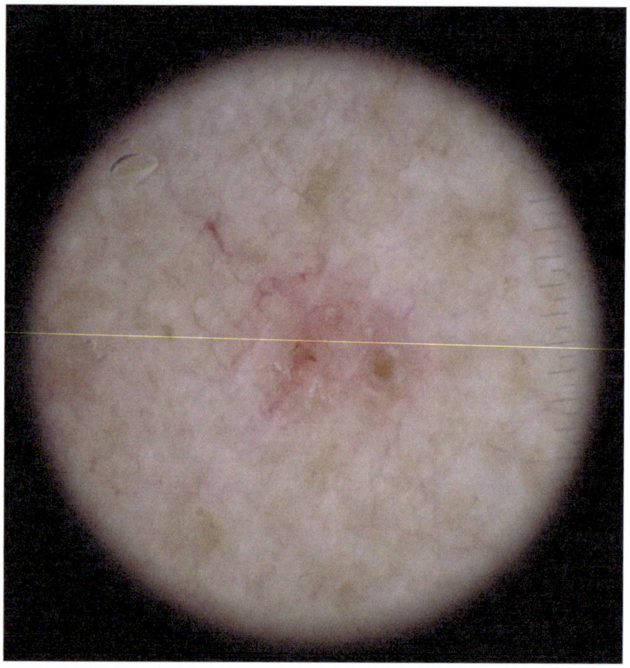

Fig. 15.2 Dermoscopy view

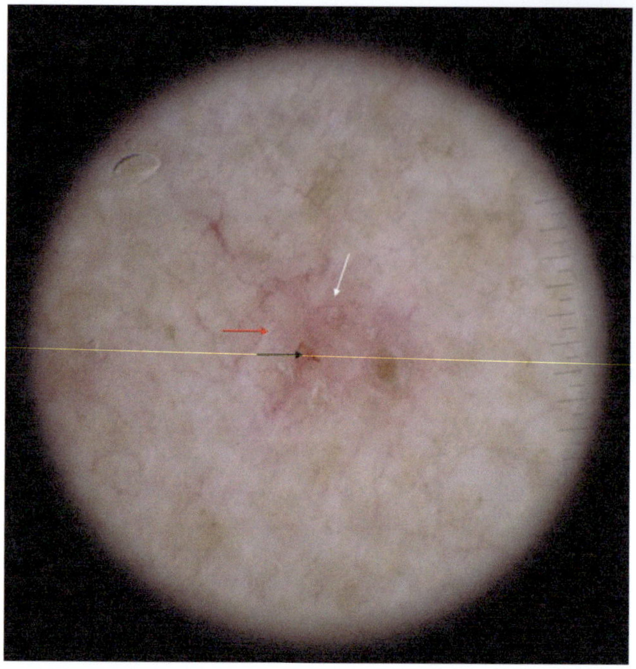

Fig. 15.3 Dermoscopy revealed superficial fine telangiectasia (white arrow), multiple small erosions (black arrow), and shiny white-red structureless areas (red arrow)

Key Message

The clinical and dermoscopic images along with the personal history and the presence of severe photodamage allow the straightforward diagnosis of a superficial basal cell carcinoma. As the histopathologic subtype is the most important factor when deciding on the treatment choice for BCC, nonablative treatments such as imiquimod or cryosurgery are the most effective ones in this sBCC.

Case 2 H.C.

Sex: male
Age: 56
Surface (flat/palpable/nodular): flat
Maximum diameter: 16 mm
Duration of the lesion: > 1 year
History of morphologic changes: yes
Personal history of skin cancer (if yes, please specify): no
Family history of skin cancer (if yes, please specify): no
Skin phototype: II
Total nevus count: (<10, 10–50, 50–100, >100): 50–100
Other clinical findings (optional): very sun-damaged skin

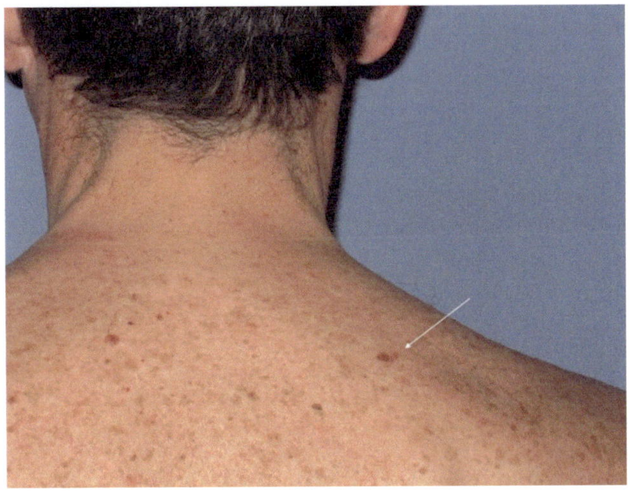

Fig. 15.4 Clinical view: hypopigmented lesion with irregular shape

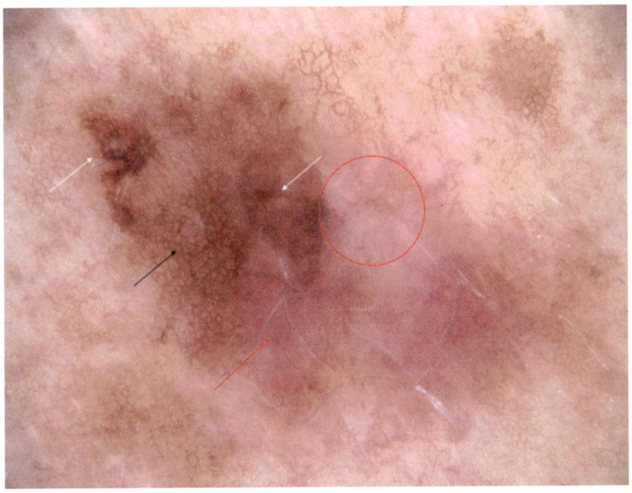

Fig. 15.5 Dermoscopy view

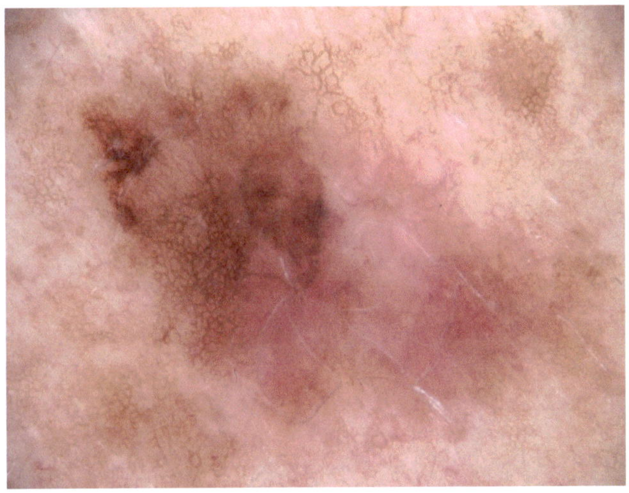

Fig. 15.6 Dermoscopy image: pigmented network (black arrow), atypical pigment network (white arrows), milky red areas (red arrow), and hypopigmented area with irregular and polymorphic vessels (red circle)

Key Message
Diagnosis: Hypomelanotic melanoma
Dermoscopy clues:

- Criteria of melanocytic lesion or traces of pigmentation
- Milky red areas
- Irregular linear and dotted vessels with random and polymorphic pattern

Case 3 G.S.

Sex: female
Age: 19
Surface (flat/palpable/nodular): flat
Maximum diameter: 9 mm
Duration of the lesion: 6 months
History of morphologic changes: shaving excision of dome-shaped lesion 6 months ago
Personal history of skin cancer (if yes, please specify): no
Family history of skin cancer (if yes, please specify): no
Skin phototype: III
Total nevus count: (<10, 10–50, 50–100, >100): 10–50
Other clinical findings (optional):

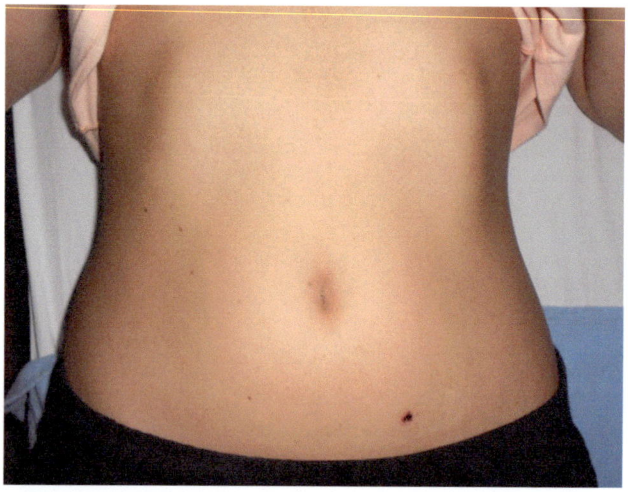

Fig. 15.7 Lesion located on the abdomen, predominantly pink with a symmetric whitish halo and central brown pigmentation

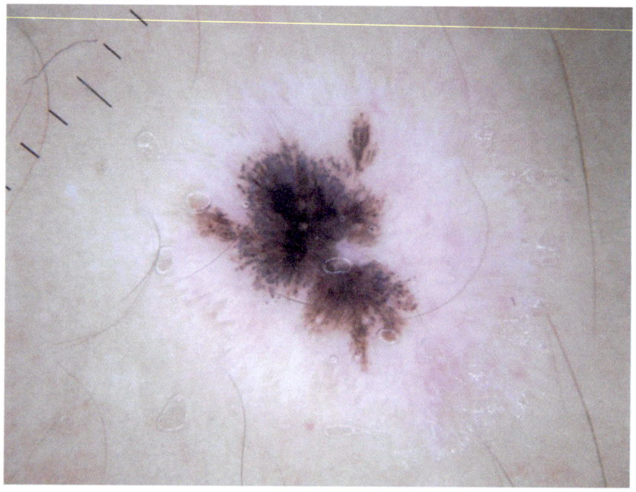

Fig. 15.8 Dermoscopy view

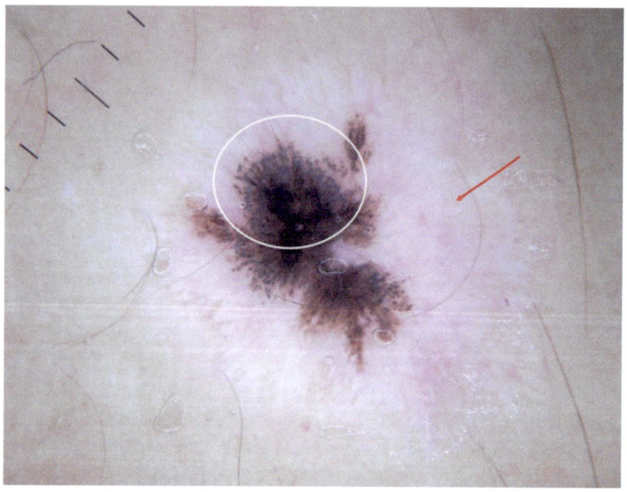

Fig. 15.9 Dermoscopy view: presence of white structureless area with brown radial lines and dots (white circle) and a whitish/pinkish halo (red arrow)

Key Message

The presence of radial lines, symmetry, and centrifugal growth pattern is associated to recurrent nevi, while the presence of circles (especially in facial lesions), eccentric hyperpigmentation at the periphery, chaotic and noncontinuous growth pattern, and the presence of pigmentation beyond the scar's edge are seen in recurrent melanoma.

Clue to the diagnosis: Note that the pigmentation doesn't extend beyond the scar limits.

Palpable Pigmented Lesions on the Trunk

16

Aimilios Lallas, Horacio Cabo, Emilia Noemi Cohen Sabban, Rosario Peralta, Virginia Mariana Gonzalez, Natalia Espinosa, Daniel Morgado, Josep Malvehy, Cristina Carrera, Giovanni Pellacani, Francesca Farnetani, Harald Kittler, Susana Puig, Sonia Rodriguez Saa, and Philipp Tschandl

Case 1: A.L.

Sex: female
Age: 35
Surface (flat/palpable/nodular): palpable
Maximum diameter: 4 mm
Duration of the lesion: unknown
History of morphologic changes: no
Personal history of skin cancer (if yes please specify): no
Family history of skin cancer (if yes please specify): no
Skin phototype: III
Total nevus count: (<10, 10–50, 50–100, >100): 50–100

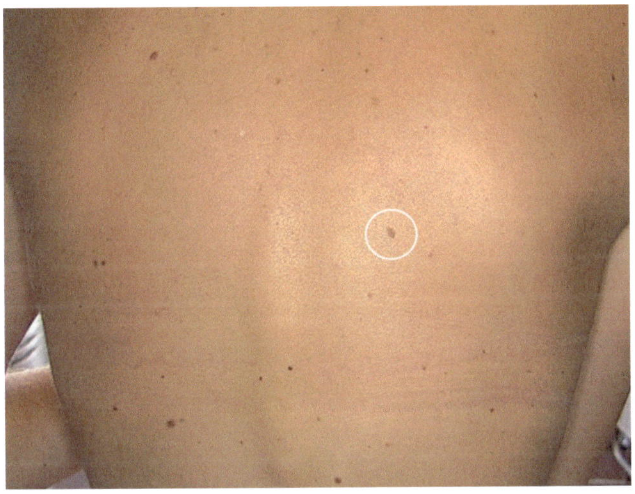

Fig. 16.1 Clinical examination revealed a symmetric, warty, pigmented lesion located on the center of the back, stuck on the skin surface (white circle)

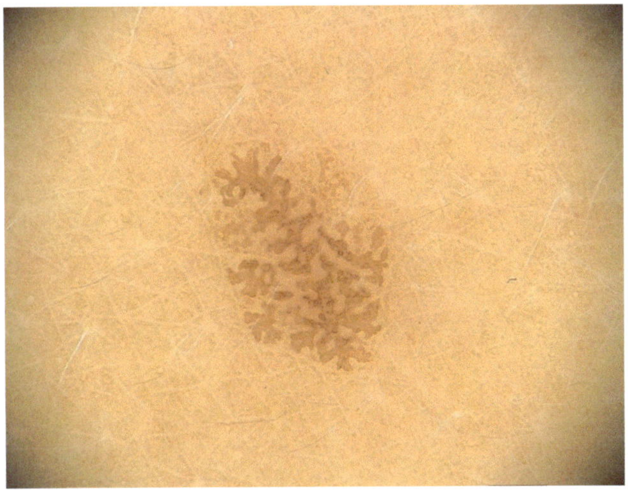

Fig. 16.2 Dermoscopy image

A. Lallas
First Department of Dermatology, Aristotle University of Thessaloniki, Thessaloniki, Greece

H. Cabo · R. Peralta
Instituto de Investigaciones Medicas "A. Lanari". Dermatology Section, University of Buenos Aires, Buenos Aires, Argentina

E. N. Cohen Sabban
Instituto de Investigaciones Médicas "A. Lanari". Chief of Dermatology Section, University of Buenos Aires, Buenos Aires, Argentina

V. M. Gonzalez
Hospital Alemán, Buenos Aires, Argentina

N. Espinosa · D. Morgado · C. Carrera (✉)
Dermatology Department, University of Barcelona, Hospital Clínic de Barcelona, Barcelona, Spain
e-mail: ccarrera@clinic.cat

J. Malvehy · S. Puig
Dermatology Department, Barcelona, Spain

G. Pellacani · F. Farnetani
Department of Dermatology, University of Modena and Reggio Emilia, Modena, Italy

H. Kittler · P. Tschandl
Department of Dermatology, Medical University of Vienna, Vienna, Austria

S. R. Saa
University of Mendoza, Mendoza, Argentina

H. Cabo, A. Lallas (eds.), *Comprehensive Atlas of Dermatoscopy Cases*, https://doi.org/10.1007/978-3-319-76932-5_16

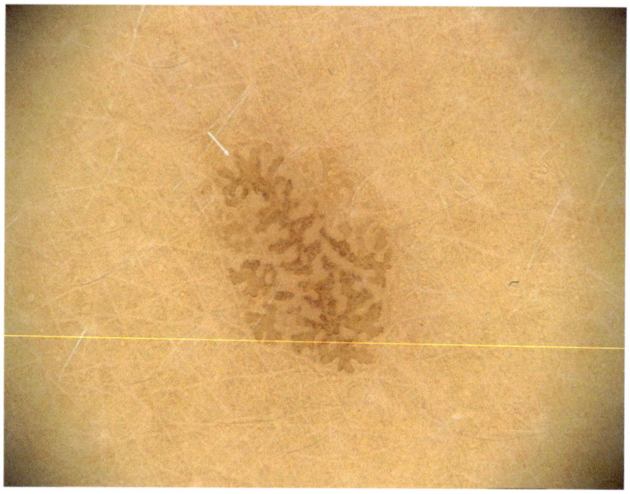

Fig. 16.3 Dermoscopy revealed a cerebriform appearance composed of brown-colored thick linear structures (fat fingers) and a sharply demarcated border at the periphery (white arrow). There are no other structures of seborrheic keratosis like milia-like cysts, comedo-like openings, fingerprint-like structures, or hairpin blood vessels

Key Message

Clinical examination is usually adequate to diagnose a seborrheic keratosis. In equivocal cases such as in this young woman with multiple moles, dermoscopy confirmed our diagnosis with fat fingers being a pathognomonic feature of seborrheic keratosis.

Case 2: A.L.

Sex: female
Age: 49
Surface (flat/palpable/nodular): palpable
Maximum diameter: 1.7 cm
Duration of the lesion: unknown
History of morphologic changes: yes, growth
Personal history of skin cancer (if yes please specify): no
Family history of skin cancer (if yes please specify): no
Skin phototype: III
Total nevus count: **(<10, 10–50, 50–100, >100)**: 50–100
Other clinical findings (optional): Presence of severe photodamage

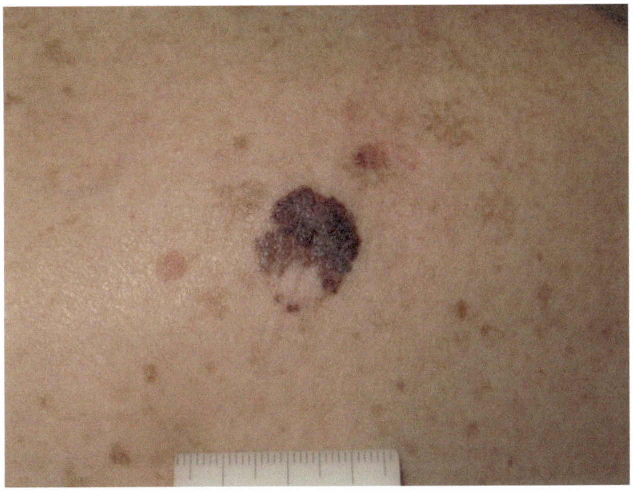

Fig. 16.4 The lesion, located on the right shoulder and surrounded by signs of photodamage, is clinically asymmetric in color with a lack of pigmentation to be seen on the lower side of the lesion

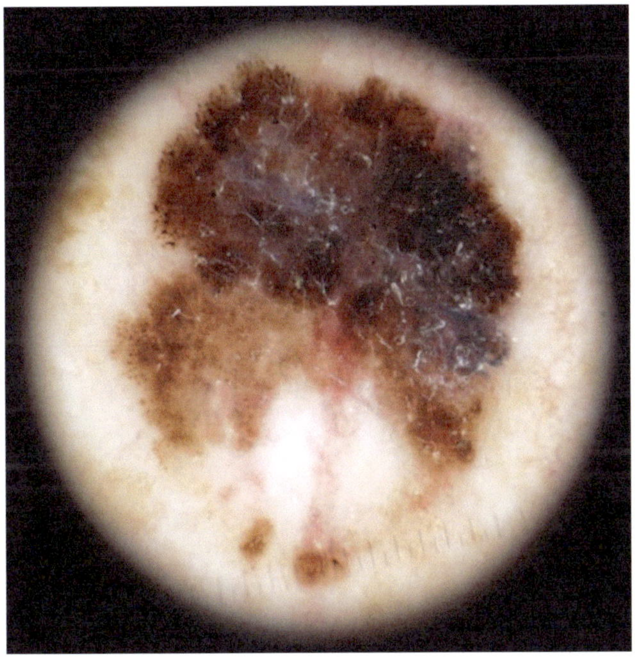

Fig. 16.5 Dermoscopy view

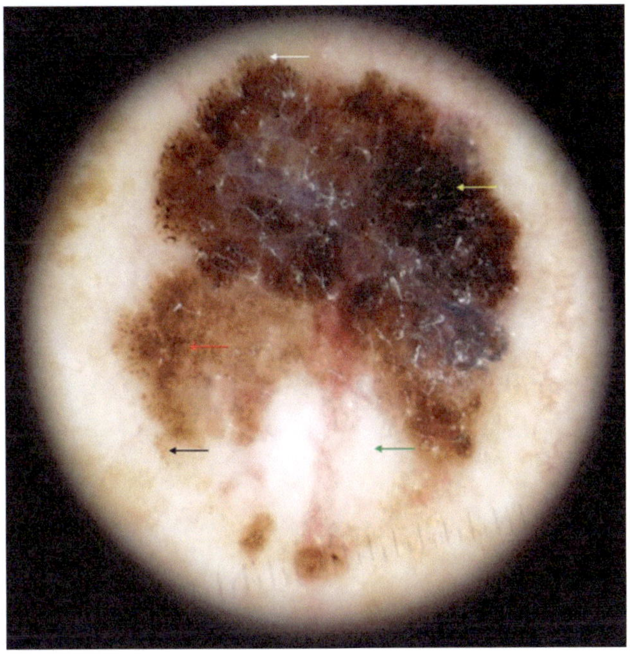

Fig. 16.6 Dermoscopically, the lesion is characterized by a multicomponent pattern. Several dermoscopic features are observed such as atypical pigment network (red arrow), irregular blotches (yellow arrow), and regression structures (both white and blue-gray areas) (green arrow). Moreover, in the lower left side we can see irregular dots (black arrow). Finally, in the upper left side of the lesion, at the periphery, irregular streaks are also visible (white arrow)

Key Message

Atypical network, regression, irregular streaks at the periphery, and irregular globules/dots are main dermoscopic features of superficial spreading melanoma.

Case 3: A.L.

Sex: male
Age: 39
Surface (flat/palpable/nodular): palpable
Maximum diameter: 7 mm
Duration of the lesion: unknown
History of morphologic changes: no
Personal history of skin cancer (if yes please specify): yes, melanoma
Family history of skin cancer (if yes please specify): no
Skin phototype: III
Total nevus count: **(<10, 10–50, 50-100, >100)**: 10–50
Other clinical findings (optional):

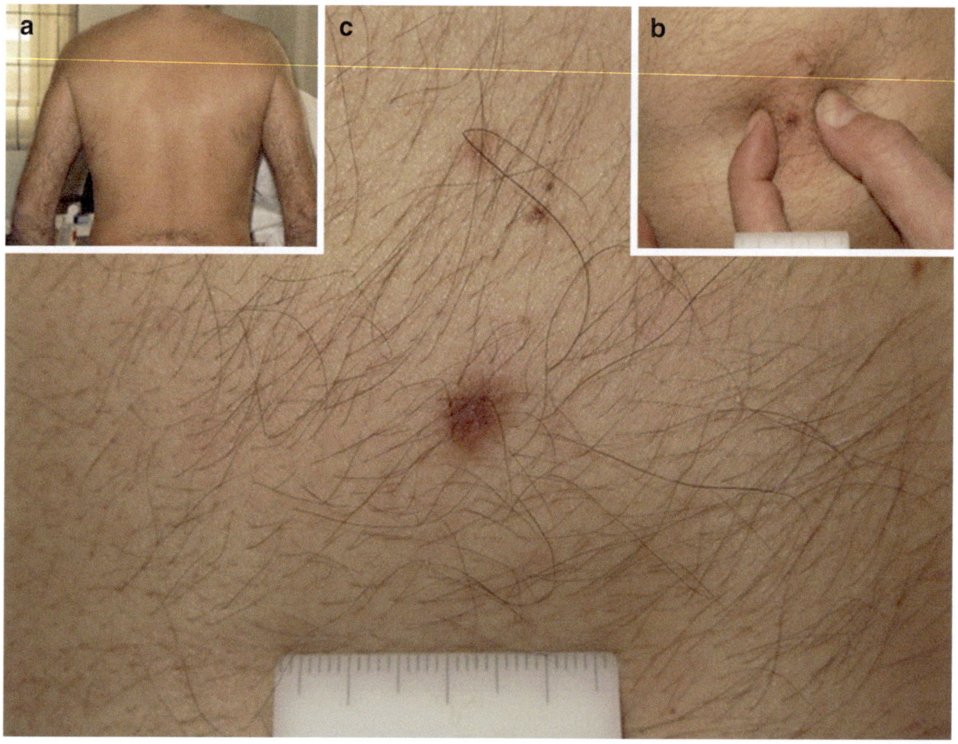

Fig. 16.7 (**a**, **b**) Clinically, there is a firm plaque with a light-brown and red color located on the back. (**c**) A dimple-like depression following lateral compression is also apparent

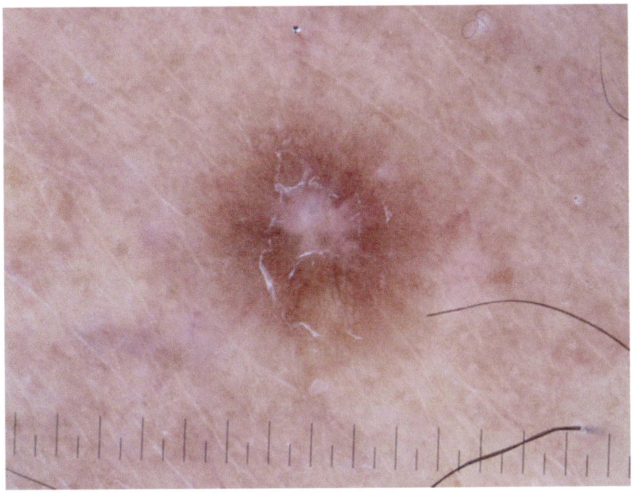

Fig. 16.8 Dermoscopy image

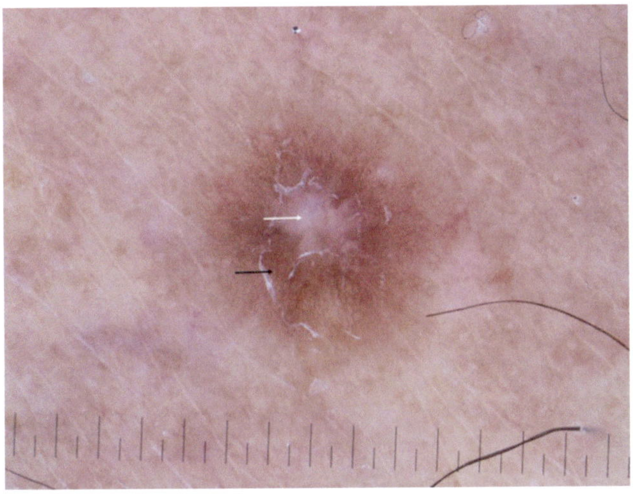

Fig. 16.9 Dermoscopy revealed a sharply demarcated central white (scar-like) patch (white arrow); surrounded by a delicate, regular, light-brown pigment network (black arrow)

Key Message

Clinical examination with the characteristic clinical sign of the dimple-like depression is usually enough to recognize a dermatofibroma. However, the central scar-like patch highlighted by dermoscopy is an additional useful clue verifying the diagnosis.

Case 4: A.L.

Sex: male
Age: 48
Surface (flat/palpable/nodular): palpable
Maximum diameter: 1.1 cm
Duration of the lesion: 1 year
History of morphologic changes: yes, gradually enlarging
Personal history of skin cancer (if yes please specify): no
Family history of skin cancer (if yes please specify): no
Skin phototype: III
Total nevus count: **(<10, 10–50, 50–100, >100)**: 50–100
Other clinical findings (optional):

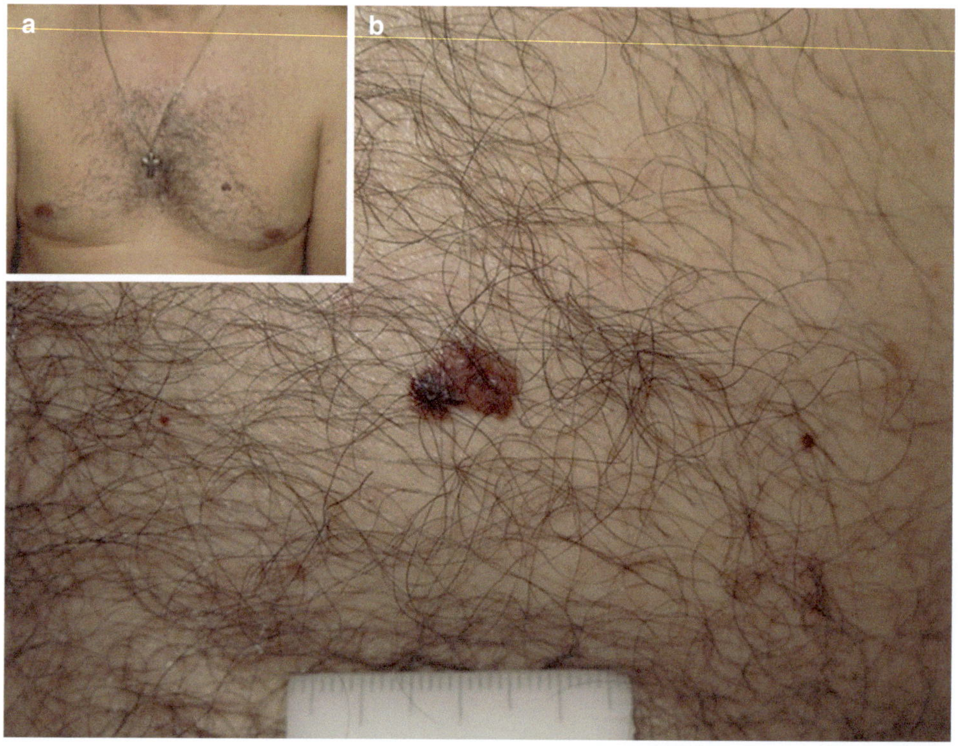

Fig. 16.10 (**a**) Clinical image; (**b**) close-up of the clinical view: pigmented palpable lesion clinically asymmetric in shape on the chest

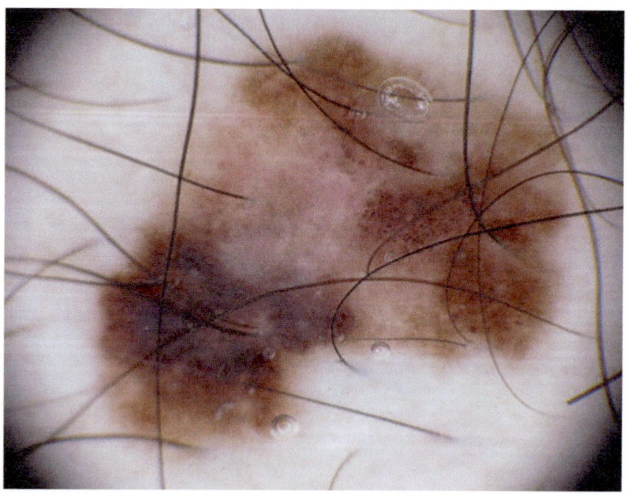

Fig. 16.11 Dermoscopy image

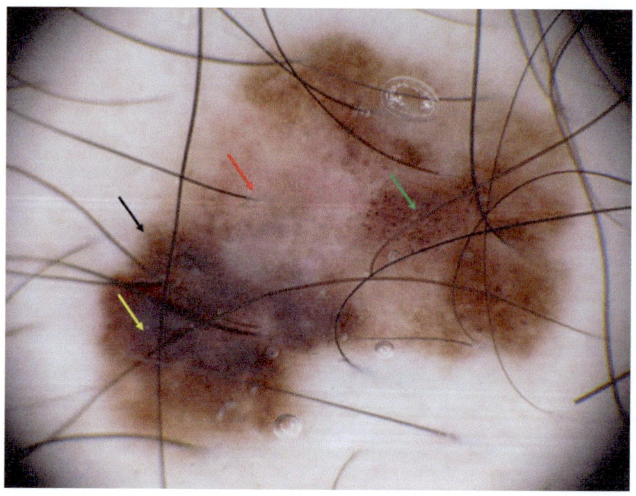

Fig. 16.12 Dermoscopically, the lesion exhibits atypical network (black arrow); regressive features in the center (red arrow); irregular dots and globules in the right side (green arrow) and a blue-white veil in the left side (yellow arrow). Asymmetry in color and shape is also visible by dermoscopy

Key Message

The asymmetry, both clinical and dermoscopical, makes the lesion suspicious. The combination of regression, blue-white veil, atypical network, and irregular dots/globules, is suggestive of superficial spreading melanoma.

Case 5: H.C.

Sex: female
Age: 47
Surface (flat/palpable/nodular): palpable
Maximum diameter: 6 mm
Duration of the lesion: >30 years
History of morphologic changes: no
Personal history of skin cancer (if yes please specify): no
Family history of skin cancer (if yes please specify): no
Skin phototype: III
Total nevus count: **(<10, 10–50, 50–100, >100)**: 50–100
Other clinical findings (optional):

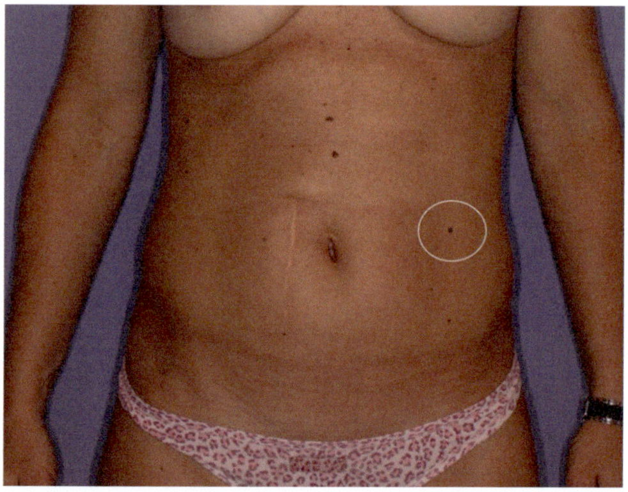

Fig. 16.13 Clinical image. Palpable brown lesion (white circle)

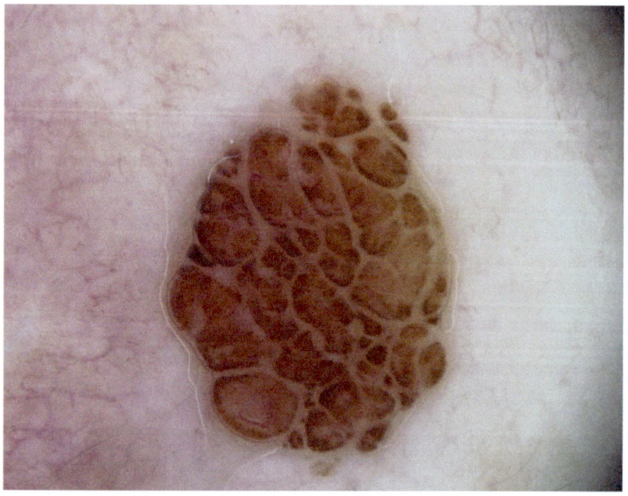

Fig. 16.14 Dermoscopy image

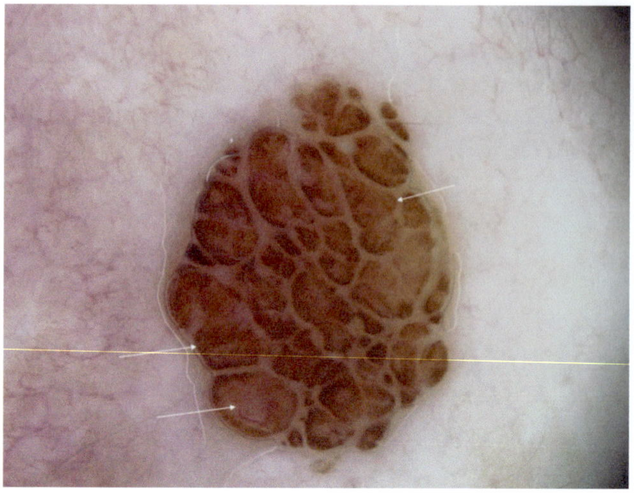

Fig. 16.15 Dermoscopy image with brown angulated globules (white arrows)

Key Message
Diagnosis: Congenital nevus with globular pattern
Globule is one of the criteria of melanocytic nevus. In this case, the pattern is globular. When these globules are angulated (cobblestone pattern), correspond to congenital melanocytic nevus.

Case 6: H.C.

Sex: female
Age: 48
Surface (flat/palpable/nodular): palpable
Maximum diameter: 10 mm
Duration of the lesion: 2 years
History of morphologic changes: yes
Personal history of skin cancer: superficial spreading melanoma B 0.5, on the right leg/2014
Family history of skin cancer (if yes please specify): no
Skin phototype: III
Total nevus count: (<10, 10–50, 50–100, >100): 10–50
Other clinical findings (optional):

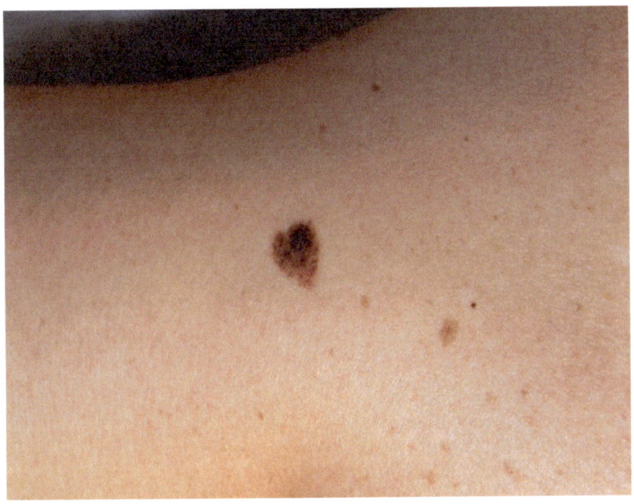

Fig. 16.16 Clinical view: asymmetric and palpable lesion in the back with three colors. The lesion changed in size and shape in the last 4 months

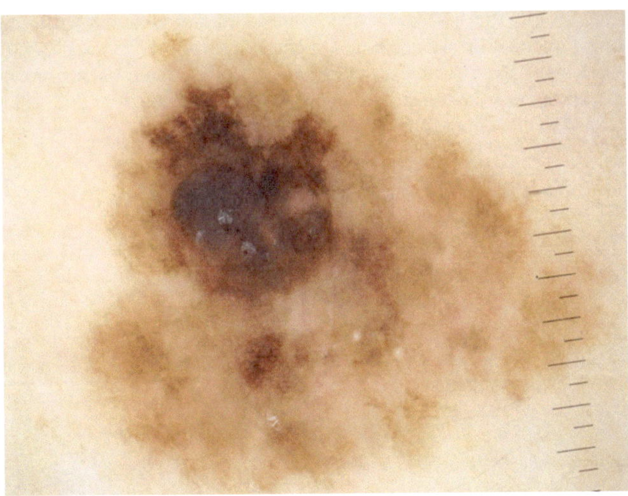

Fig. 16.17 Dermoscopy view

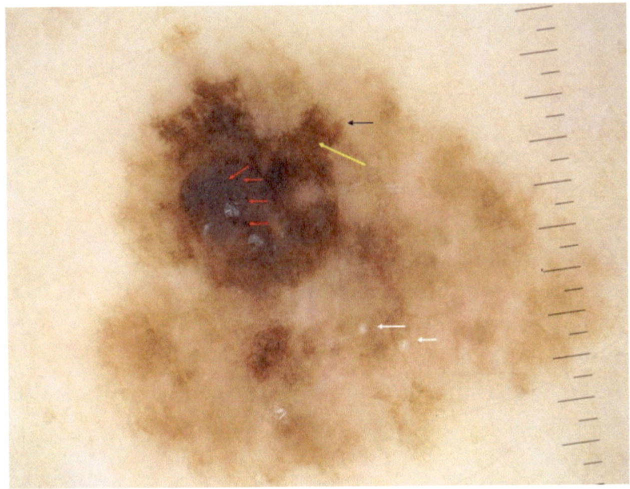

Fig. 16.18 Dermoscopy view: milia-like cysts (white arrows); pseudofollicular openings (red arrows); fat fingers (black arrow); and reticular appearance (yellow arrow)

Key Message
Diagnosis: Seborrheic keratosis
Seborrheic keratosis on occasion shows dermoscopy features that can simulate melanoma, especially flat seborrheic keratosis (solar lentigo)
Dermoscopy clues: milia-like cysts, pseudofollicular openings, fat fingers, pseudo-reticular network in the flat area (solar lentigo)

Case 7: E.N.C.S.

Sex: male
Age: 62
Surface: palpable
Maximum diameter: 1 cm
Duration of the lesion: >3 years
History of morphologic changes: unknown
Personal history of skin cancer: no
Family history of skin cancer: no
Skin phototype: III
Total nevus count: 10–50

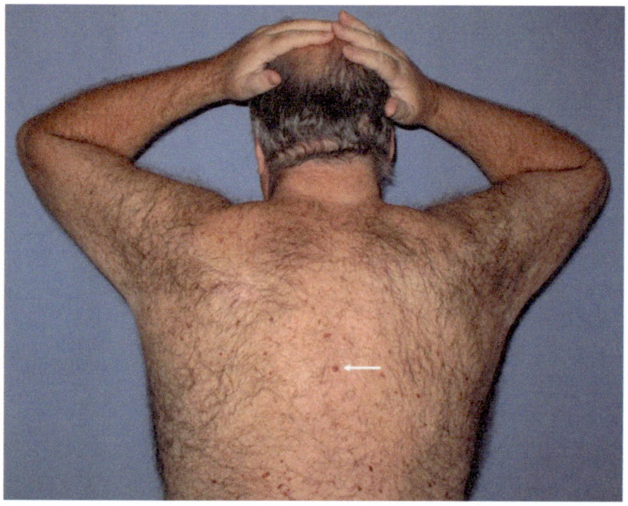

Fig. 16.19 Clinical view: asymmetric pigmented lesion on the back with different colors (white arrow)

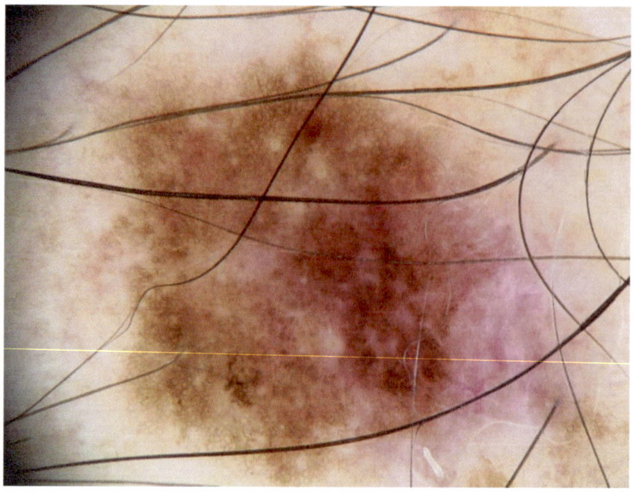

Fig. 16.20 Dermoscopy view: irregular lesion with different colors (different shades of brown, with pink and darker brown area in the right side)

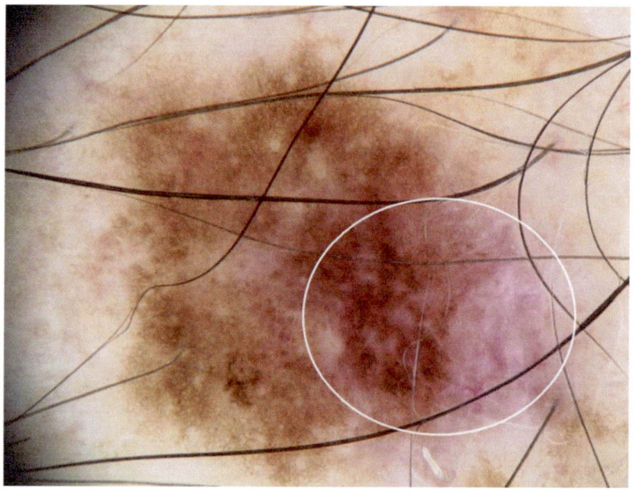

Fig. 16.21 The left side shows a mixed central pattern nevus with brown globules in the center and pigment network in the periphery of the lesion. The structures within the right circle, with darker brown globules and a pink area with linear vessels, are enough to perform a biopsy to rule out melanoma

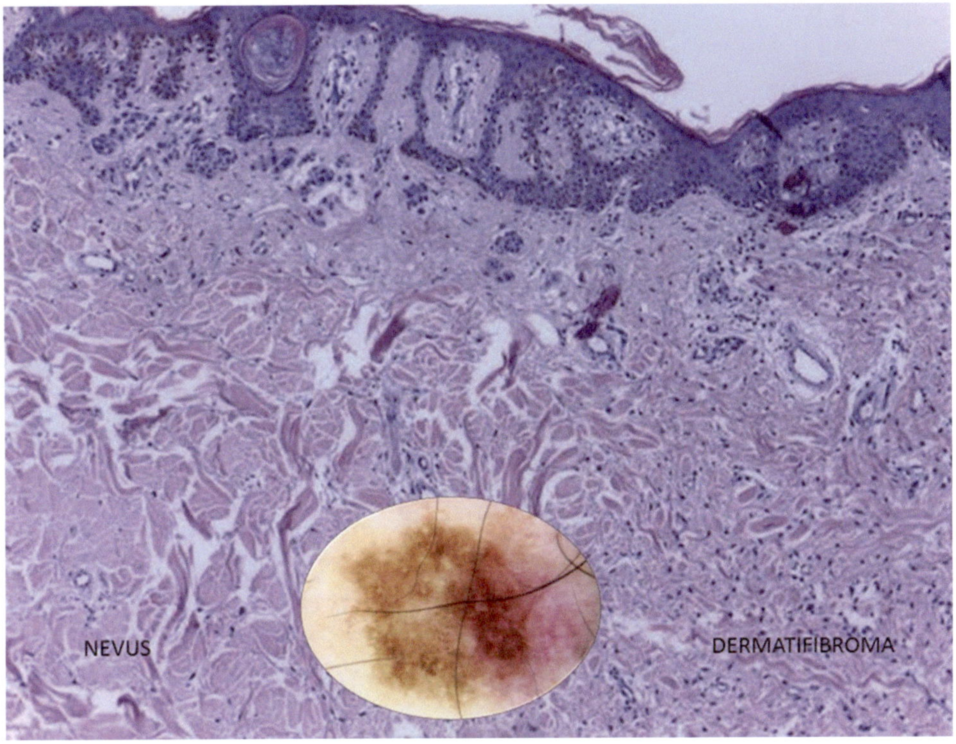

Fig. 16.22 This is a collision tumor, compound nevus, and dermatofibroma

Key Message

Collision tumors on occasion are melanoma simulators. In this case, we have recognized clearly the melanocytic lesion (left side of the lesion) but the typical dermatofibroma structures are not present (right side of the lesion), so, under dermoscopy examination, this is an atypical melanocytic lesion and we have to perform a biopsy to rule out melanoma and make the right diagnosis.

Case 8: R.P.

Sex: female
Age: 54 years
Surface (flat/palpable/nodular): palpable
Maximum diameter: 25 mm
Duration of the lesion: She hadn't noticed it previously
History of morphologic changes: –
Personal history of skin cancer (if yes please specify): no
Family history of skin cancer (if yes please specify): no
Skin phototype: III
Total nevus count: (**<10, 10–50, 50–100, >100**): 10–50
Other clinical findings (optional): –

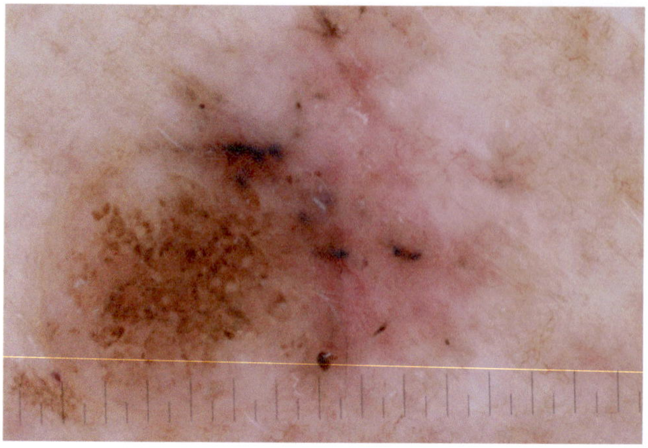

Fig. 16.24 Dermatoscopic image of the lesion

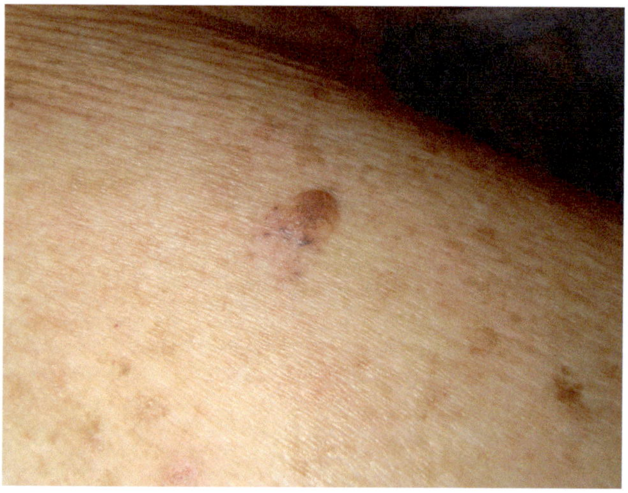

Fig. 16.23 Clinical image. Pigmented lesion on the back, measuring 20 × 25 mm, slightly elevated, smooth surface, irregular borders with pink and brown coloration

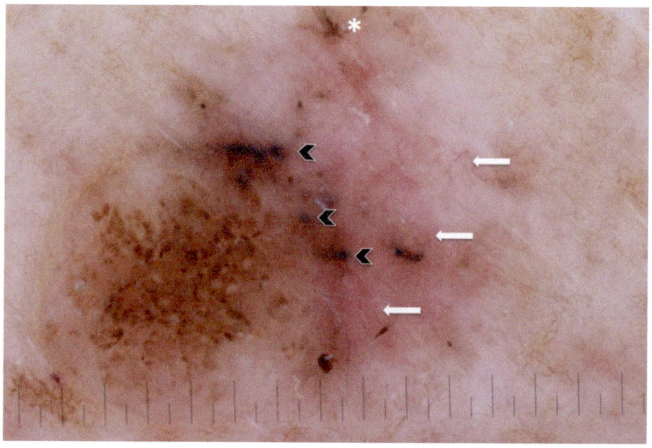

Fig. 16.25 Dermoscopy examination revealed on the left side of the lesion, brown globules in a roundish and elevated area. On the right side, a pinkish background with multiple blue-gray globules (arrowheads), maple-leaflike area (asterisk), and short fine superficial telangiectasias (arrows)

Key Message

Histology reports a collision tumor composed of a melanocytic nevus and basal cell carcinoma (BCC). Collision tumors consist of two different neoplasms occurring concurrently in the same lesion. This association has been described for both benign and malignant neoplasms. BCC and seborrheic keratosis is the most common combination; however lots of different collision tumors can be identified using dermoscopy.

Case 9: R.P.

Sex: male
Age: 60 years
Surface (flat/palpable/nodular): palpable
Maximum diameter: 30 mm
Duration of the lesion: He hadn't noticed it previously
History of morphologic changes: –
Personal history of skin cancer (if yes please specify): BCC on face.
Family history of skin cancer (if yes please specify): No
Skin phototype: III
Total nevus count: **(<10, 10–50, 50–100, >100)**: 10–50
Other clinical findings (optional): Patient with multiples angiomas and seborrheic keratosis (SK).

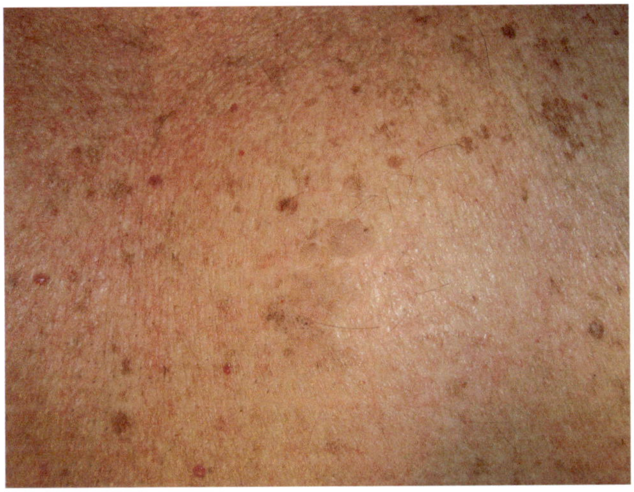

Fig. 16.26 Clinical image. Lesion located on the back with rough surface, light-brown color, and irregular borders on photodamage skin

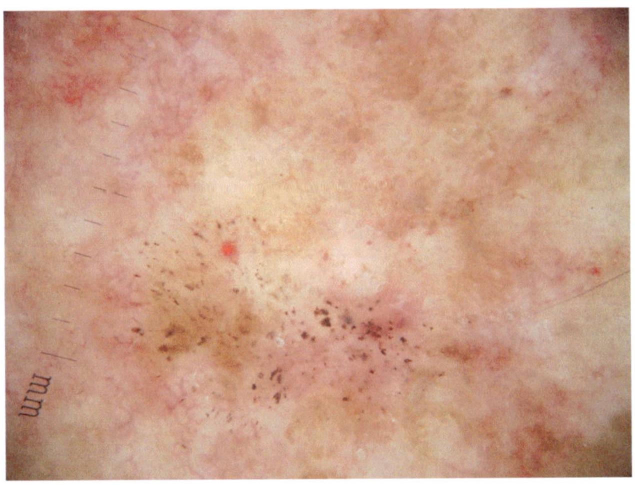

Fig. 16.27 Dermatoscopic image of the lesion

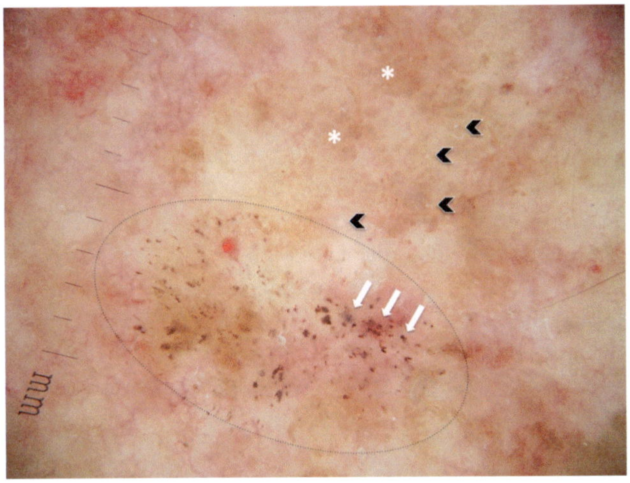

Fig. 16.28 Dermoscopy examination revealed the presence of fissures and ridges with brainlike appearance (asterisks), milia-like cysts (arrowheads), and a big area with brownish-gray dots and globules showing different kind of sizes and shapes (black circle), bluish-gray globules (arrows) on a pinkish structureless background. A small lesion with red lacunes is also observed

Key Message

Histology reports a SK with a regression area as lichenoid keratosis (LK). The LK represents a regressive response to a preexistent epidermal lesion characterized by the presence of brownish-gray, reddish-brown, bluish-gray, or whitish-gray coarse granules. The observation of these structures could simulate malignant neoplasms and histopathological examination should be performed in any doubtful cases.

Case 10: V.G.

Sex: female
Age: 44
Surface (flat/palpable/nodular): palpable
Maximum diameter: 10 mm
Duration of the lesion: Since childhood
History of morphologic changes: no
Personal history of skin cancer (if yes please specify): no
Family history of skin cancer (if yes please specify): no
Skin phototype: III
Total nevus count: **(<10, 10–50, 50–100, >100)**: 10–50
Other clinical findings (optional):

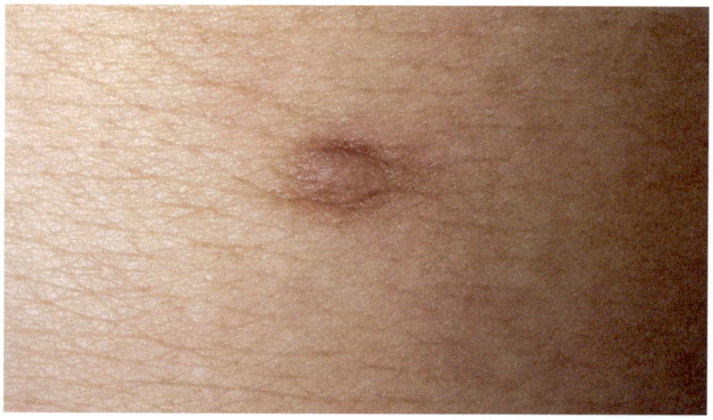

Fig. 16.29 Clinical image: unilateral, oval, slightly elevated, soft, pigmented lesion, located on the milk line of the left upper abdomen

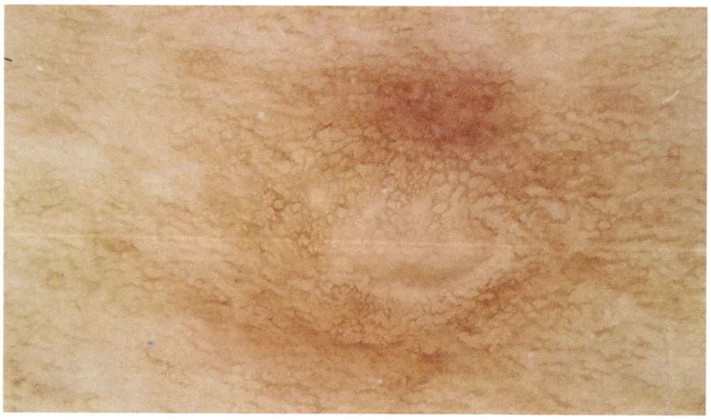

Fig. 16.30 Dermoscopy image

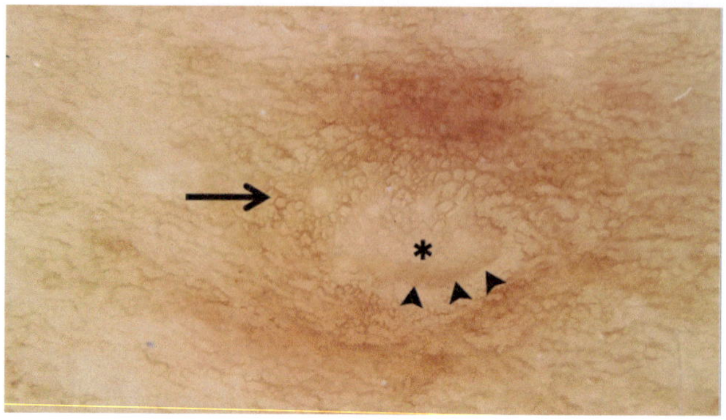

Fig. 16.31 Dermoscopy image showed a central structureless scar-like area (asterisk), a cleft-like appearance in the central area (arrowheads), and a delicate pigment network in the periphery of the lesion (arrow) on a tan to erythematous background

Key Message
Diagnosis: Supernumerary nipple
The supernumerary or accessory nipples are additional nipples with or without underlying mammary gland tissue which are located following the milk lines. Their recognition is important because they could be markers of malformations or internal malignancies. On dermoscopic observation its most frequent structures are peripheral pigment network or network-like structures and central scar-like area. Although the presence of a pigment network is a major dermoscopic criterion for melanocytic lesions, accessory nipples are an exception to the rule. Familiarity with their dermoscopic features can prevent misdiagnoses and unnecessary biopsies.

Case 11: N.E., D.M., J.M., C.C.

Sex: male
Age: 58
Surface (flat/palpable/nodular): palpable
Maximum diameter: 7 mm
Duration of the lesion: many years
History of morphologic changes: 6 months
Personal history of skin cancer (if yes please specify): no
Family history of skin cancer (if yes please specify): Yes. Sister affected with metastatic melanoma.
Skin phototype: I
Total nevus count: **(<10, 10–50, 50–100, >100)**: >100
Other clinical findings (optional): Red hair, sun-damaged skin with marked elastosis and solar lentigos.

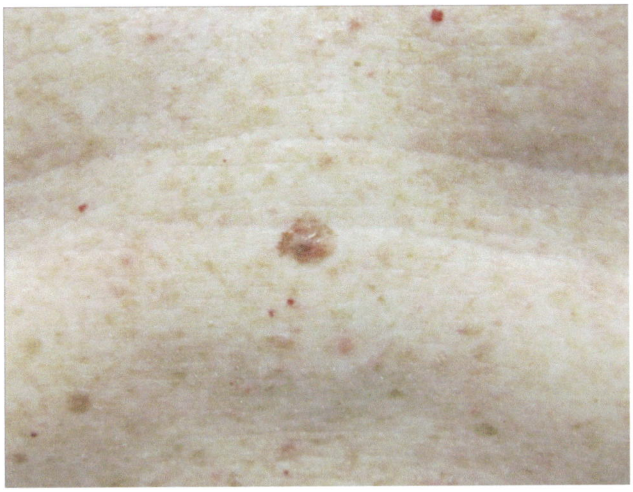

Fig. 16.32 Clinical aspect of the lesion located on sternal region. An irregular, well-demarked lesion, light brown- to pink-colored and uneven borders

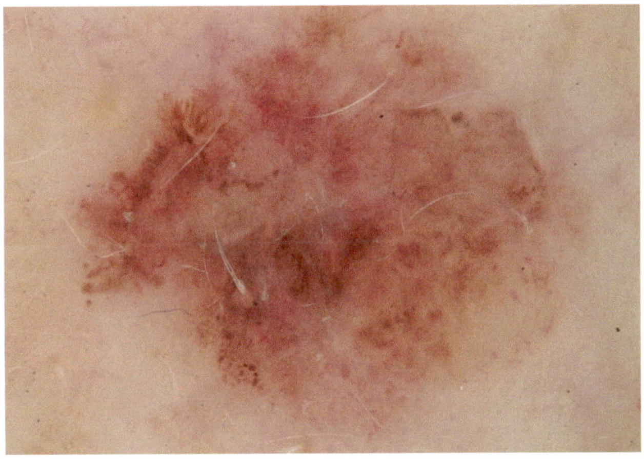

Fig. 16.33 Dermoscopy images

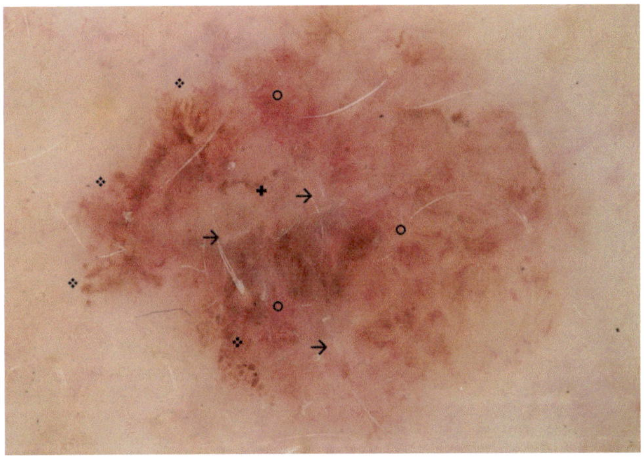

Fig. 16.34 Dermoscopic characteristics of the lesion. Asymmetric melanocytic lesion, light brown, pink, and white colored, with homogenous—globular pattern multiple focal atypical features: ❖ Streaks/Pseudopods, ✚ Blue regression/peppering, O Atypical vessels, ✜ Irregular dots and globules, → shiny white streaks (chrysalis)

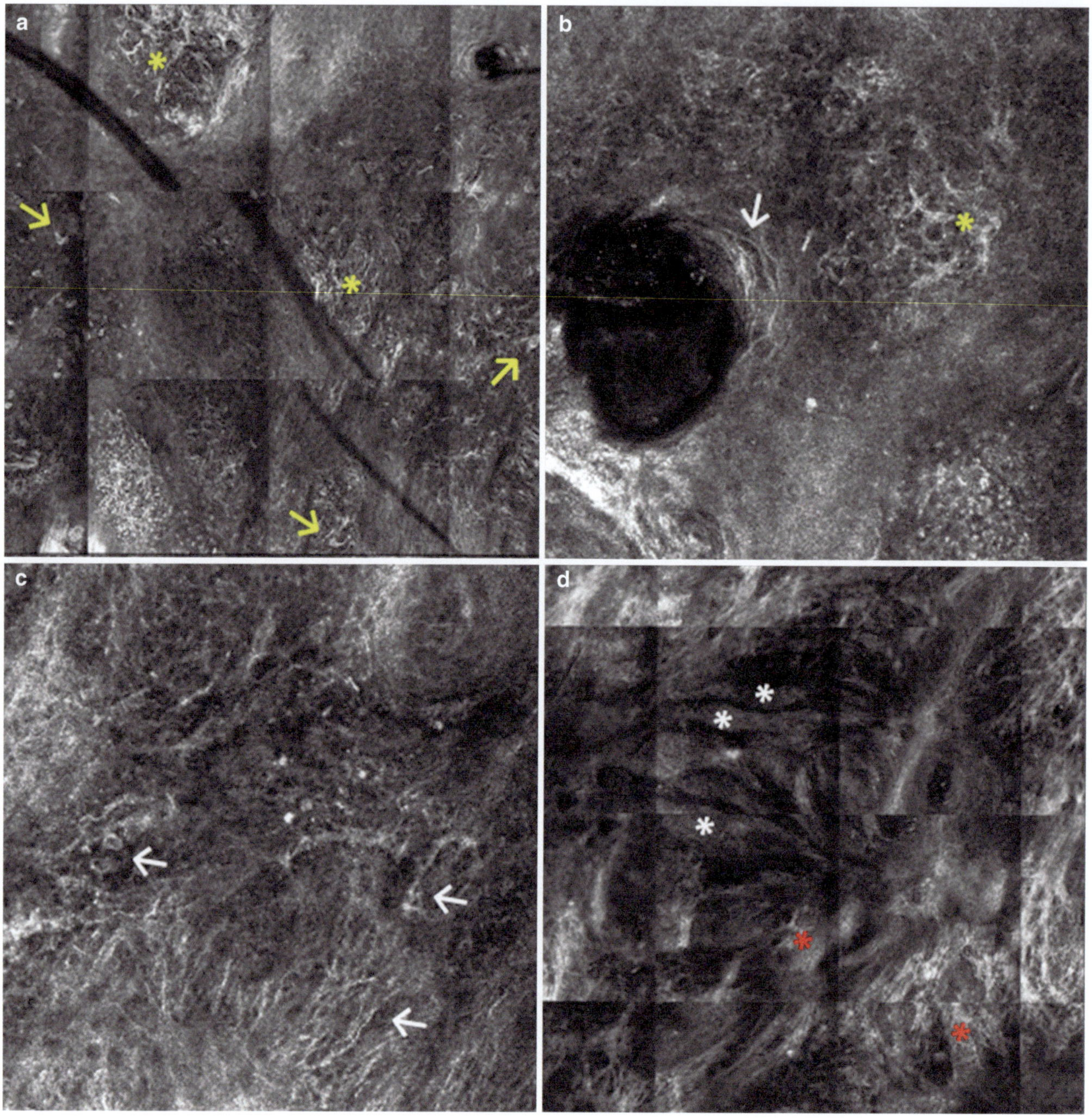

Fig. 16.35 In vivo reflectance confocal microscopy (RCM): single 500 × 500 mcs at different levels: (**a**) Epidermis: Multiple dendritic pagetoid cells within the epidermal layer forming superficial clusters (yellow*). Isolated nucleated pleomorphic cells (yellow arrow). (**b**) Epidermis: Dendritic superficial cells showing folliculotropism (white arrow). (**c**) Epidermis basal layer: Multiple dendritic atypical basal cells (white arrow). (**d**) Dermo-epidermal layer: Loss of the architecture, non-edged papillae and junctional thickenings (white*) with dendritic cells (red*)

Key Message

Definite diagnosis: Superficial spreading melanoma (Breslow 0.9 mm) arising in a dermal nevus.

The clinical and dermoscopic appearance of incipient melanoma can vary depending on the location, presence of pigmentation (phototype of patient), existence of a previous nevus, and stage of progression of the tumor. This thin melanoma arising on a dermal nevus can pose a challenge since it shows mild pigmentation and atypical vessels can lead to mistaking them as dermal nevus. However, the irregular globules and pseudopods at the periphery along with shiny white streaks and regression features in the center of the lesion are the clue to suspect melanoma. RCM allows the observation of the classical findings in superficial spreading component of melanoma: atypical pagetoid cells in the epidermis and at the basal layer.

Case 12: G.P., F.F.

Sex: male
Age: 48
Surface: palpable
Maximum diameter: 0.7
Duration of the lesion: 1 year
History of morphologic changes: In the last months the shape and the color of the lesion are changing
Personal history of skin cancer (if yes please specify): no
Family history of skin cancer (if yes please specify): no
Skin phototype: III
Total nevus count: **(<10, 10–50, 50–100, >100)**: 10–50
Other clinical findings (optional): no

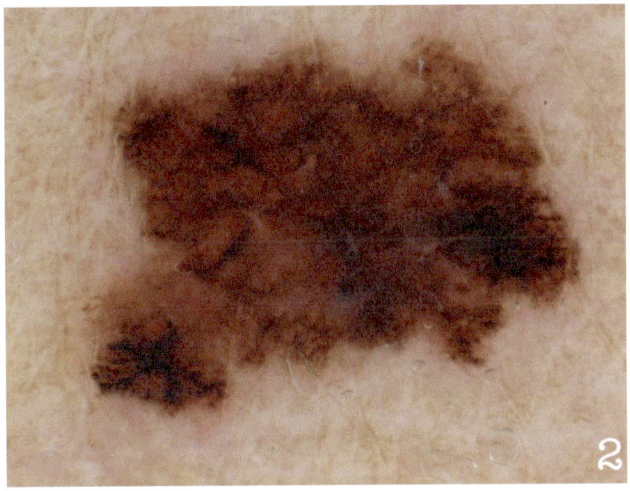

Fig. 16.37 Dermoscopy image

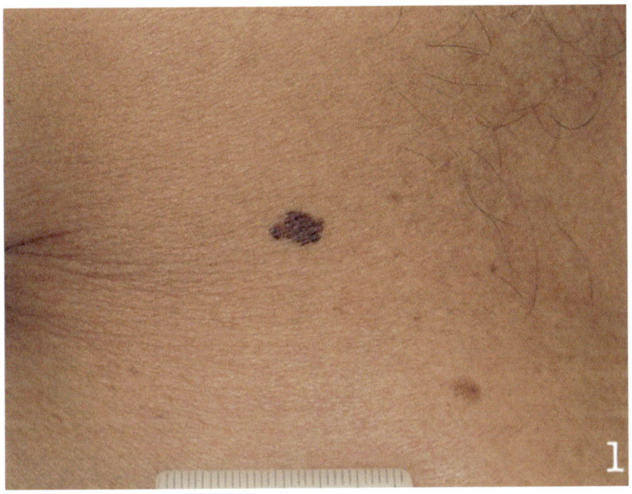

Fig. 16.36 Clinical image of pigmented melanocytic lesion on the chest. Clinically the lesion shows irregular borders, dishomogeneous color, 0.7 × 0.4 cm in diameter on sun-damaged skin

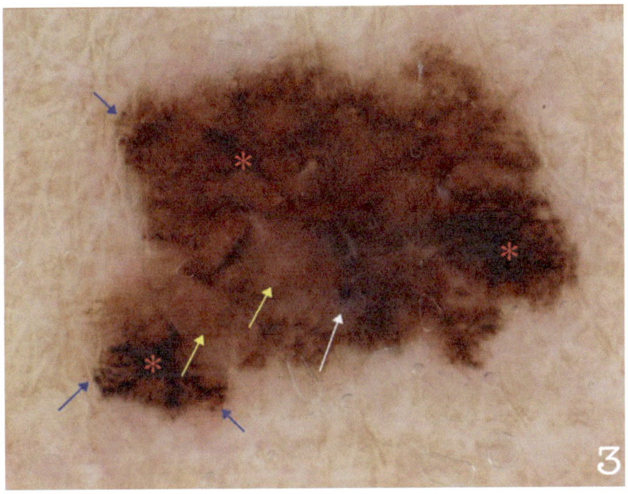

Fig. 16.38 On dermoscopy the pigmented lesion reveals irregular pigment network, gray-blue blotch (white arrow), regression area with a loss of architecture (yellow arrow), areas with an irregular hyperpigmented network (asterisk) and peripheral globules (red mark)

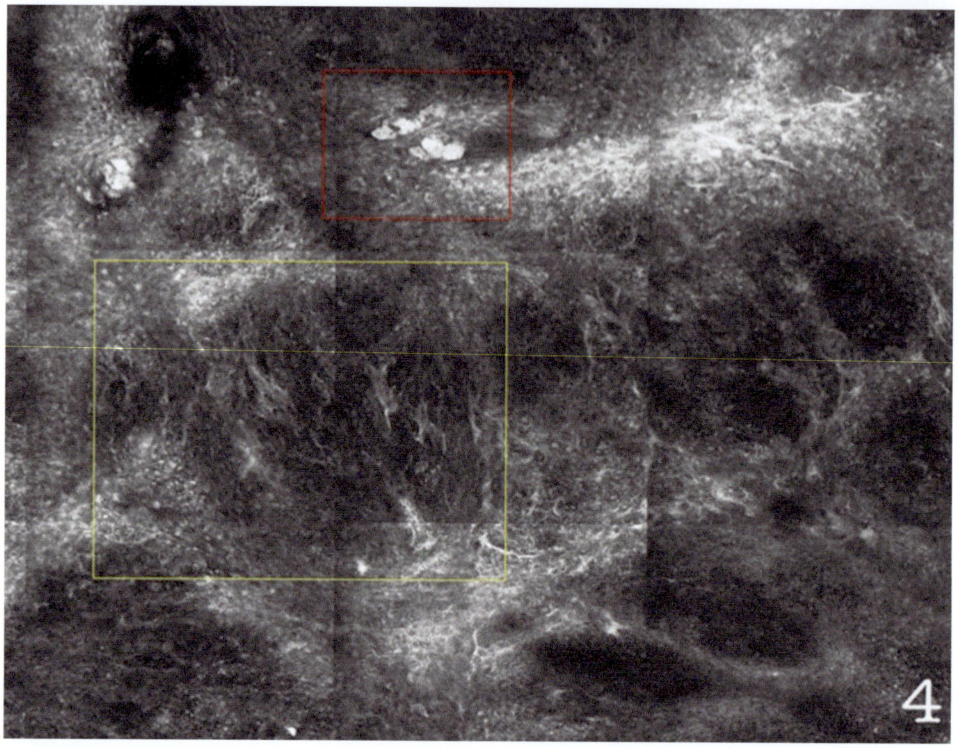

Fig. 16.39 RCM detail of dermal epidermal juction (DEJ) reveals a disarranged architecture (yellow square) with atypical cell (dendritic/round cells) infiltration (red square)

Key Message
Dermoscopic and RCM imaging reveal suggestive feature for melanoma diagnosis (0.3 mm Breslow).

Case 13: H.K.

Sex: female
Age: 43
Surface (flat/palpable/nodular): palpable
Maximum diameter: 0.6 cm
Duration of the lesion: 1 year
History of morphologic changes: Yes
Personal history of skin cancer (if yes please specify): no
Family history of skin cancer (if yes please specify): no
Skin phototype: II
Total nevus count: **(<10, 10–50, 50–100, >100)**: 10–50
Other clinical findings (optional):

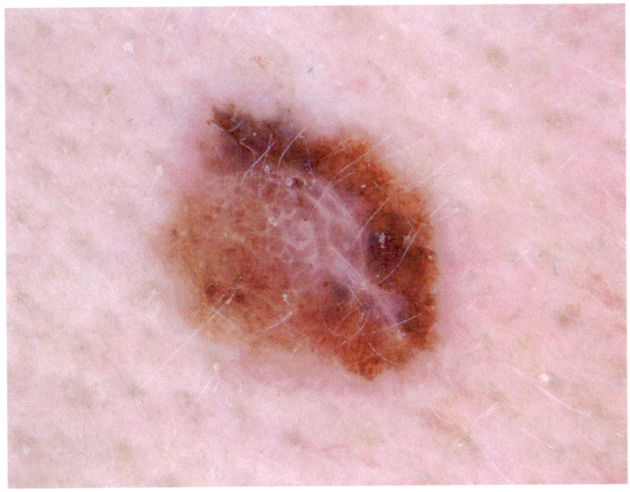

Fig. 16.41 Dermoscopy view

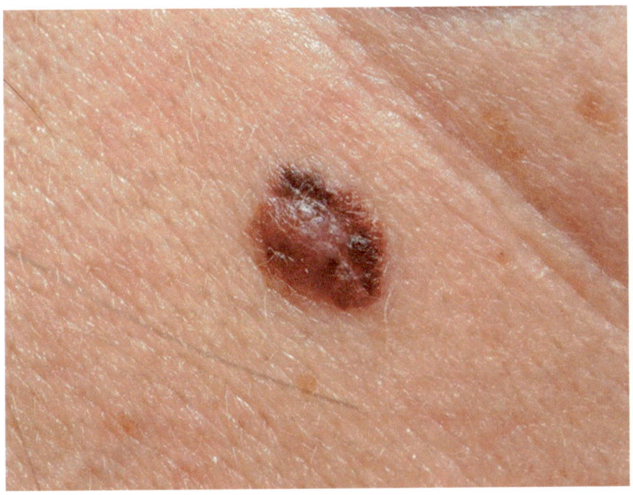

Fig. 16.40 A pigmented papule with color variegation could be a nevus or a melanoma

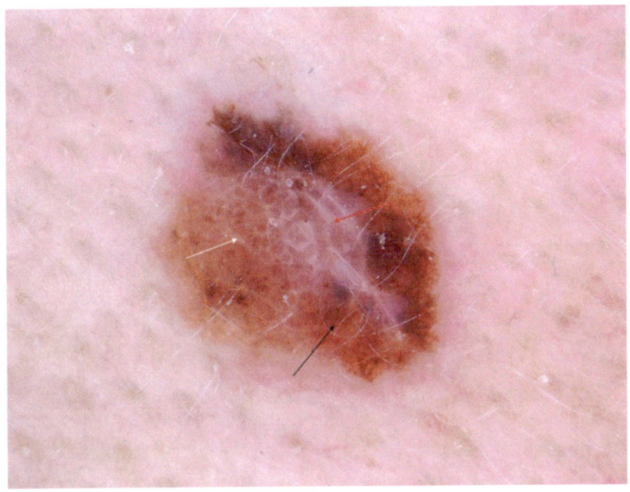

Fig. 16.42 A chaotic lesion with a pattern of clods (white arrow); structureless areas (black arrow) and white reticular lines (red arrow)

Key Message
Diagnosis: Melanoma
White reticular lines are clue to melanoma

Case 14: J.M., S.P.

Sex: female
Age: 40
Surface (flat/palpable/nodular): palpable
Maximum diameter: 5 mm
Duration of the lesion: >1 year
History of morphologic changes: The patient referred that the lesion was acquired and grew in few months with change to dark color
Personal history of skin cancer (if yes please specify):
Family history of skin cancer (if yes please specify):
Skin phototype: III
Total nevus count: **(<10, 10–50, 50–100, >100)**: 10–50
Other clinical findings (optional):

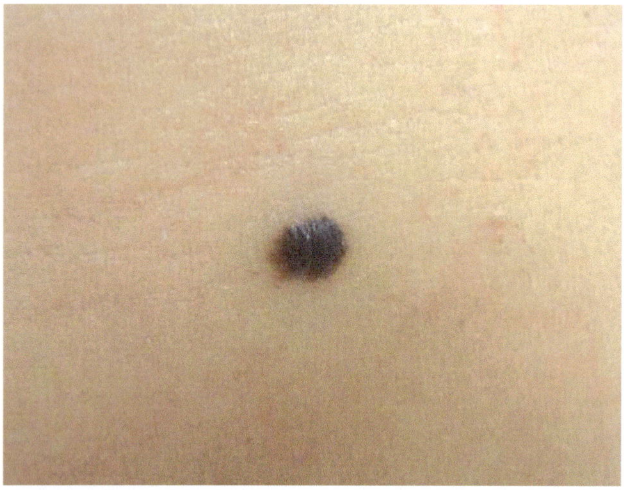

Fig. 16.43 Clinical image

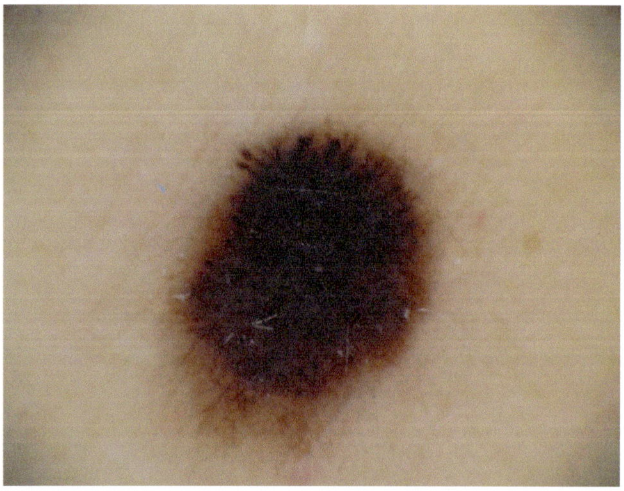

Fig. 16.44 Dermoscopy view

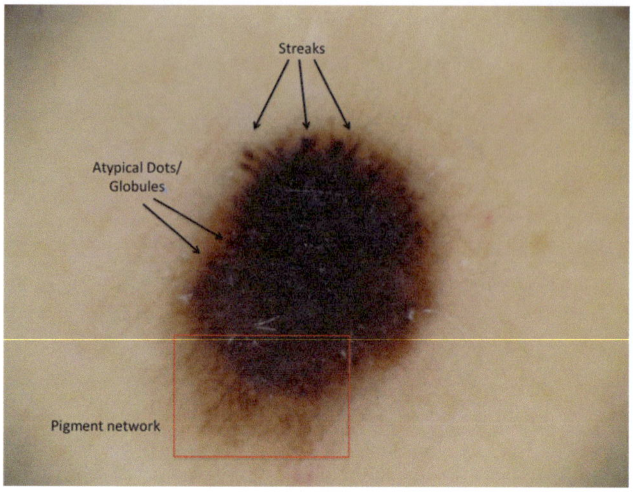

Fig. 16.45 Dermoscopy view: A melanocytic lesion with typical pigmented network (red square); atypical black dots and globules and asymmetrically distributed streaks (pseudopods) are seen (black arrows)

Key Message
Differential diagnosis: Superficial spreading melanoma (spitzoid) vs. spitzoid benign lesion (nevus or spitzoid tumor) vs. atypical nevus.
Diagnosis: Superficial spitzoid melanoma (Breslow 0.53 mm) Clark III, no mitosis.
In any melanocytic tumor with a fast growth and spitzoid features on dermoscopy in adulthood it has to be excised and confirmed by histopathology. In this case, a wide excision with 1 cm margin is recommended

Case 15: S.R.S.

Sex: male
Age: 55
Surface (flat/palpable/nodular): palpable
Maximum diameter: 8 mm
Duration of the lesion: unknown
History of morphologic changes: unknown
Personal history of skin cancer (if yes please specify): yes two melanomas, one nodular melanoma on right arm, Breslow 5.2 mm excised 1 month before
Family history of skin cancer (if yes please specify): no
Skin phototype: III
Total nevus count: (<10, 10–50, 50–100, >100): >100
Other clinical findings (optional): –

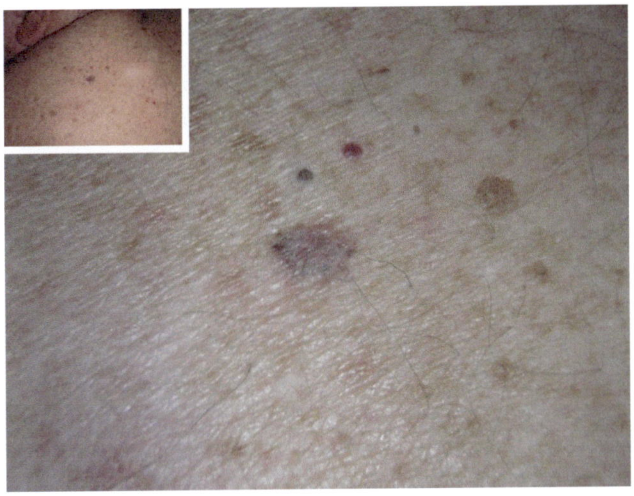

Fig. 16.46 Slightly raised, pinkish-tan lesion, on the left scapular region of a 55-year-old man

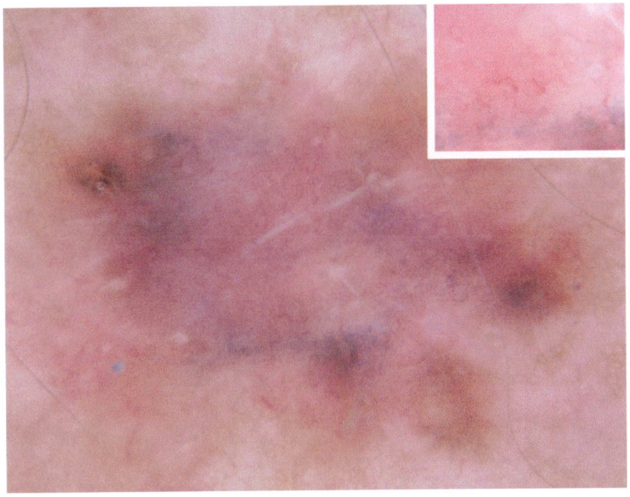

Fig. 16.47 Dermoscopy view

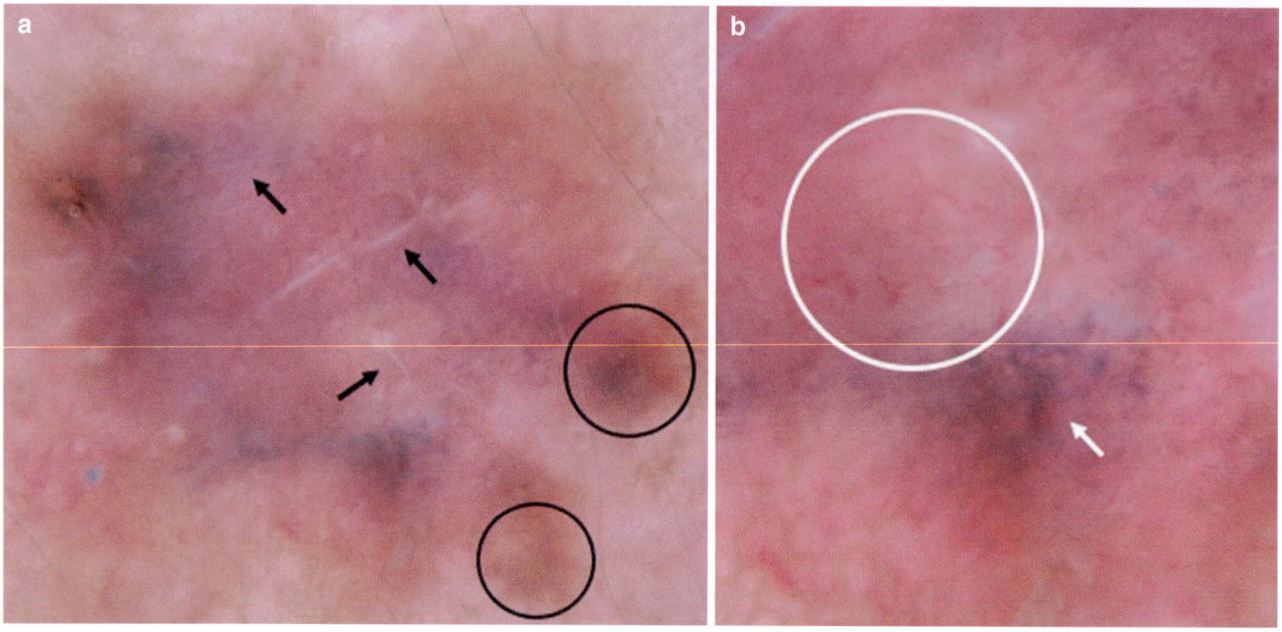

Fig. 16.48 Dermoscopy shows an atypical vascular pattern with irregular lineal vessels (white circle), on a pinkish-tan background with remnants of pigmentation that include tan-brown homogeneous areas (black circles) and multiple blue-gray dots (white arrow). Polarized dermoscopy reveals shiny white lines in an orthogonal orientation (black arrows)

Key Message

Diagnosis: Invasive hypomelanotic melanoma (Breslow thickness 1.1 mm).

Amelanotic/hypomelanotic melanomas frequently display an atypical vacular pattern (characterized by a combination of dotted and linear irregular vessels) on a pinkish or pinkish-tan background, with or without remnants of pigmentation.

Case 16: P.T.

Sex: female
Age: 70
Surface (flat/palpable/nodular): palpable
Maximum diameter: <6 mm
Duration of the lesion: unknown
History of morphologic changes: unknown
Personal history of skin cancer (if yes please specify): previous invasive melanoma
Family history of skin cancer (if yes please specify): none
Skin phototype: II/III
Total nevus count: **(<10, 10–50, 50–100, >100)**: 10–50
Other clinical findings (optional): none

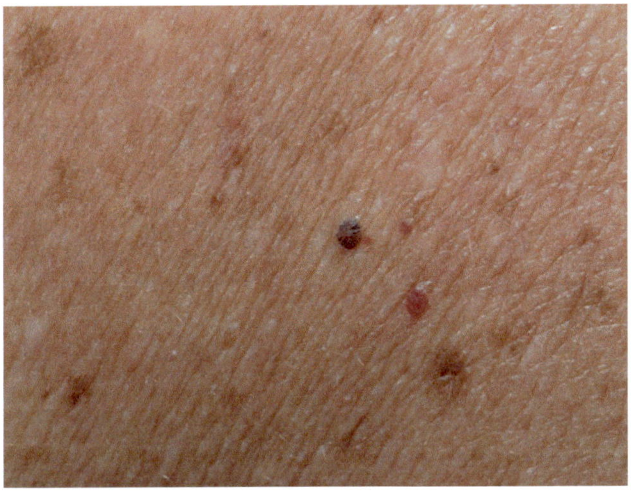

Fig. 16.49 Clinical image of a small, fairly symmetric, maculopapular pigmented lesion on the back of the patient

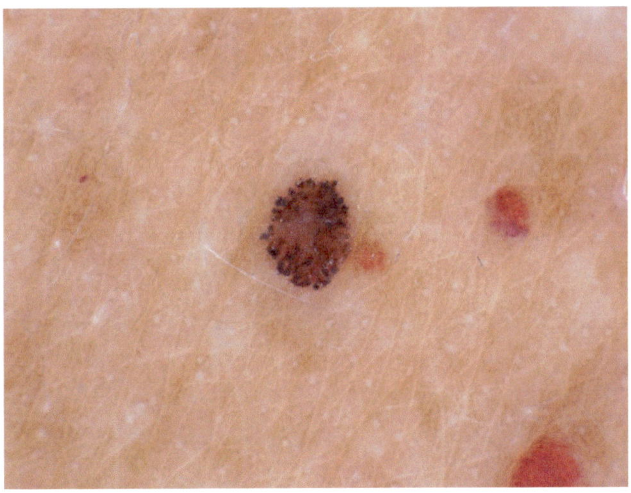

Fig. 16.50 Dermoscopy view

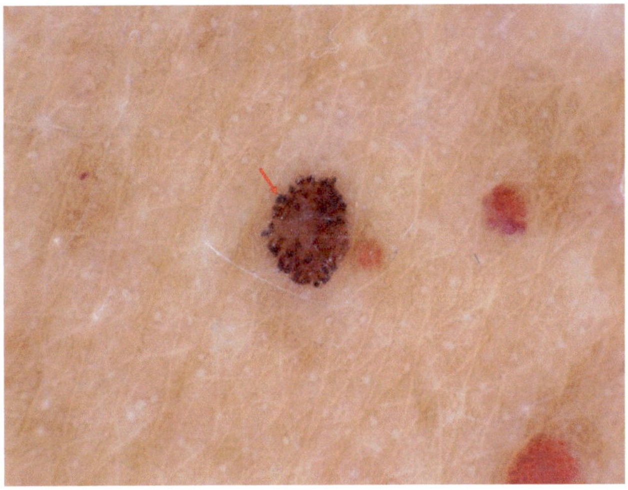

Fig. 16.51 Dermatoscopic image showing a fairly symmetric, non-chaotic, lesion composed of monomorphous brown clods. Symmetry if only disturbed by two clods (DDx: pseudopods) at the top and left side

Key Message
Diagnosis: Melanoma in situ.
Key message 1: Symmetry (or "chaos") is an important feature in detecting skin cancer by dermatoscopy. Usually symmetry has to be evaluated as a rough estimation because one deals with a biologic process where symmetry is not achievable in a perfect fashion. Though, in very small lesions as in this case, symmetry has to be evaluated more strictly, as already small breaks in the pattern can signify a malignant process.
Key message 2: A lesion with a pattern of clods should be evaluated in regard to age of the patient: Whereas in young patients clods are a common pattern for nevi, in patients >50 years of age risk of melanoma rises rapidly whenever a lesion is showing clods.

Palpable Nonpigmented Lesions on the Trunk

17

Horacio Cabo, Aimilios Lallas, Chryssoula Papageorgiou, and Pedro Zaballos

Case 1: H.C.

Sex: male
Age: 64
Surface (flat/palpable/nodular): palpable
Maximum diameter: 21 mm
Duration of the lesion: unknown
History of morphologic changes: yes
Personal history of skin cancer (if yes, please specify): melanoma
Family history of skin cancer (if yes, please specify): no
Skin phototype: III
Total nevus count (<10, 10–50, 50–100, >100): >100
Other clinical findings (optional): the lesions are bleeding spontaneously

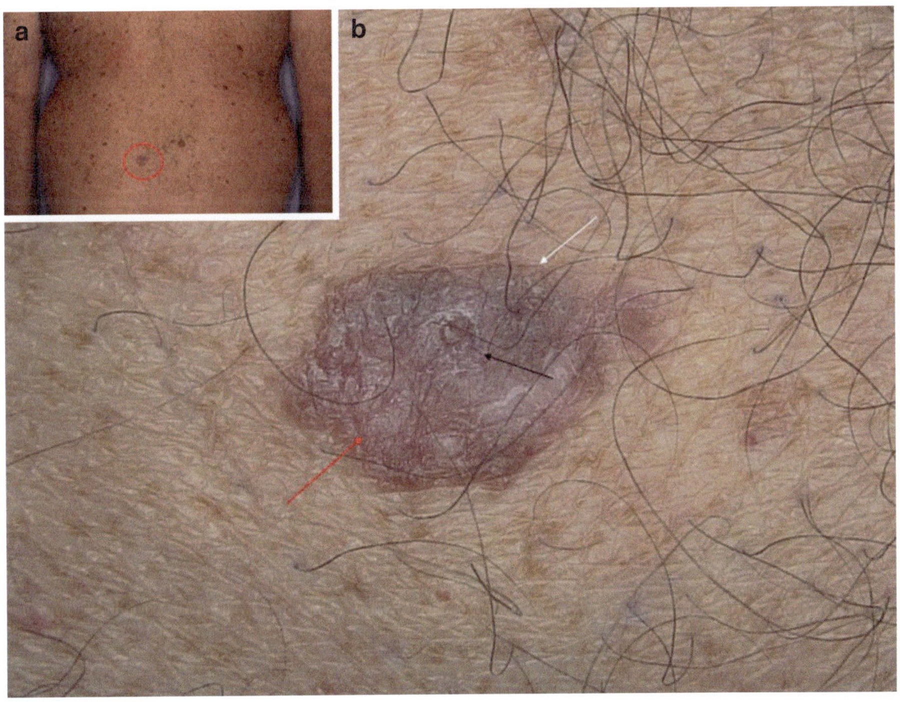

Fig. 17.1 Clinical image on the back (red circle) (**a**); close-up of the clinical image (**b**) where you can notice two different colors, pink (red arrow) and brown (white arrow) and ulceration (black arrow)

H. Cabo (✉)
Instituto de Investgaciones Médicas "A. Lanari". Dermatology Section, University of Buenos Aires, Buenos Aires, Argentina

A. Lallas · C. Papageorgiou
First Department of Dermatology, Aristotle University of Thessaloniki, Thessaloniki, Greece

P. Zaballos
University of Rovira i Virgili, Tarragona, Spain

H. Cabo, A. Lallas (eds.), *Comprehensive Atlas of Dermatoscopy Cases*, https://doi.org/10.1007/978-3-319-76932-5_17

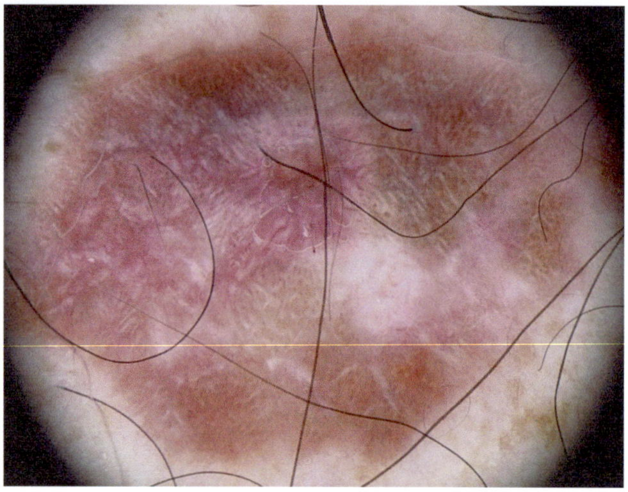

Fig. 17.2 Dermoscopy image

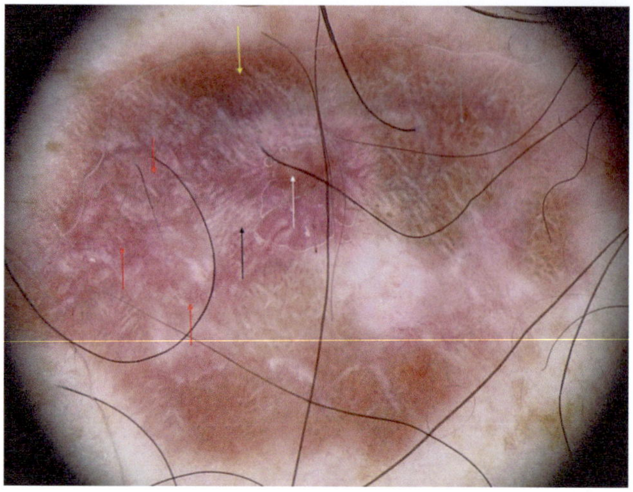

Fig. 17.3 Dermoscopy: dotted vessels and linear irregular vessels (red arrows); negative network (yellow arrow); white shining streaks (black arrow); ulceration (white arrow) and irregular brown globules (gray arrow)

Key Message

Diagnosis: Superficial spreading hypomelanotic melanoma (B 0.70 mm) with a large pink area with dotted and linear irregular vessels and negative pigment network. In addition, you can notice white shining streaks.

Case 2: A.L.

Sex: female
Age: 87
Surface (flat/palpable/nodular): palpable
Maximum diameter: 8 mm
Duration of the lesion: 8 months
History of morphologic changes: yes, slowly enlarging
Personal history of skin cancer (if yes, please specify): yes, previous BCC
Family history of skin cancer (if yes, please specify): no
Skin phototype: III
Total nevus count (<10, 10–50, 50–100, >100): <10
Other clinical findings (optional): numerous seborrheic keratosis and cherry hemangiomas

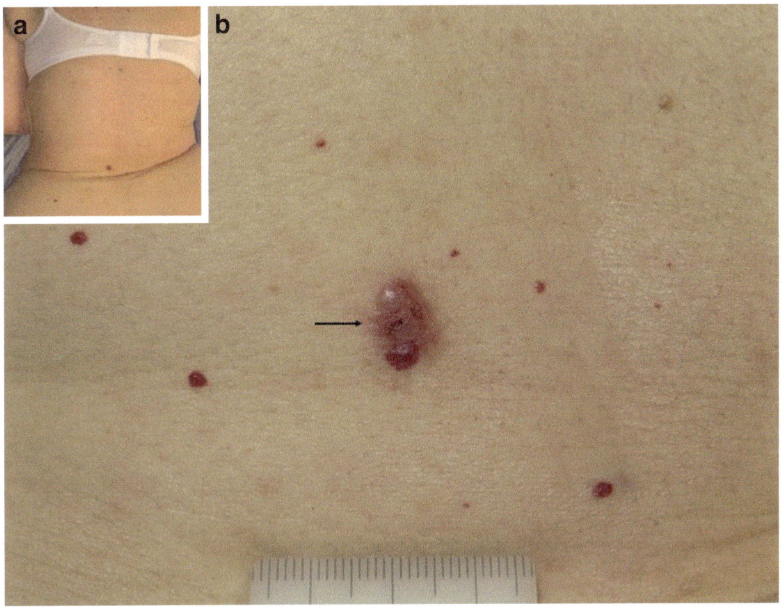

Fig. 17.4 (**a**) Clinical view; (**b**) clinically, there is a raised, reddish plaque located on the back (black arrow)

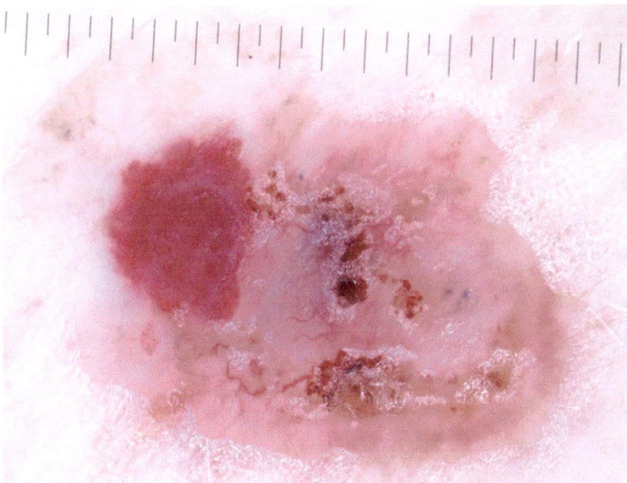

Fig. 17.5 Dermoscopy view

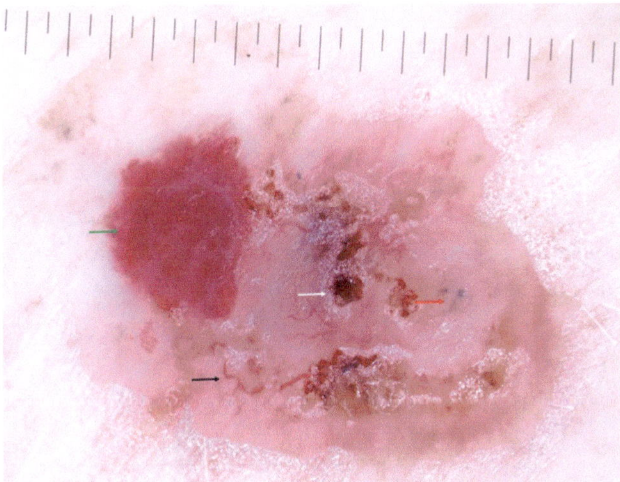

Fig. 17.6 In dermoscopy, the lesion exhibits large arborizing vessels branching irregularly into finest capillaries (black arrow); multiple erosions (white arrow) and multiple blue-gray globules/dots (red arrow). In the lower side of the lesion, there is an additional lesion characterized by red lacunas among which white lines are seen (green arrow)

Key Message

Dermoscopy allows the recognition of a collision tumor consisting of a basal cell carcinoma in the upper side and a cherry hemangioma in the lower side. Dermoscopy is very helpful for predicting the histopathologic subtype of BCC, and in this case, the large arborizing vessels and the blue-gray globules/dots are suggestive of a nodular basal cell carcinoma. The histopathologic subtype of BCC is the most crucial factor to take into account when deciding on the treatment choice for BCC with surgery to be the gold standard for the nodular BCC.

Case 3: P.Z.

Sex: female
Age: 50
Surface (flat/palpable/nodular): palpable
Maximum diameter: 1 cm
Location: Abdomen
Duration of the lesion: 8 months
History of morphologic changes: Growing
Personal history of skin cancer (if yes, please specify): None
Family history of skin cancer (if yes, please specify): None
Skin phototype: III
Total nevus count (<10, 10–50, 50–100, >100): <10
Other clinical findings (optional):

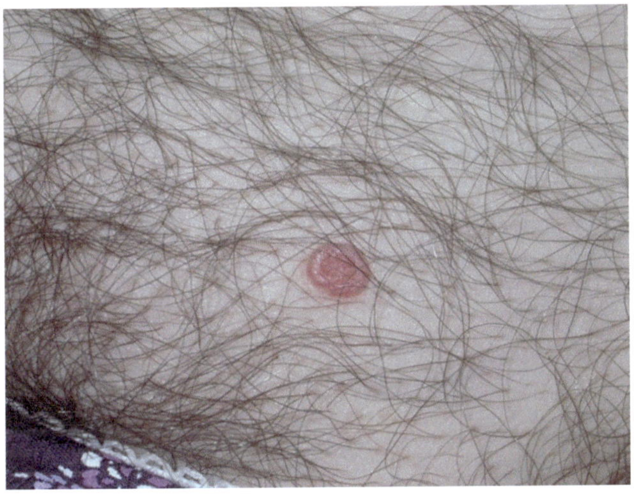

Fig. 17.7 Asymptomatic pink papule located on the abdomen of a 50-year-old woman

Key Message
Diagnosis: *Molluscum contagiosum*

Dermoscopy can improve our diagnostic accuracy of those lesions in atypical location or distribution.

The pattern composed of central polilobular yellowish amorphous structures and crown vessels is very characteristic of *Molluscum contagiosum*.

Sebaceous hyperplasias can also share this pattern.

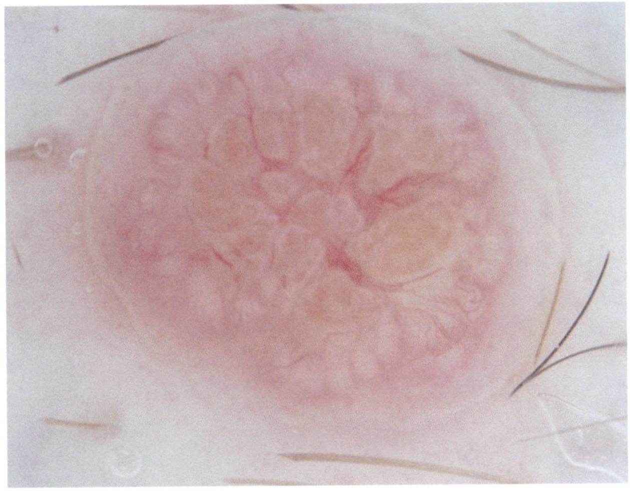

Fig. 17.8 Dermoscopy view

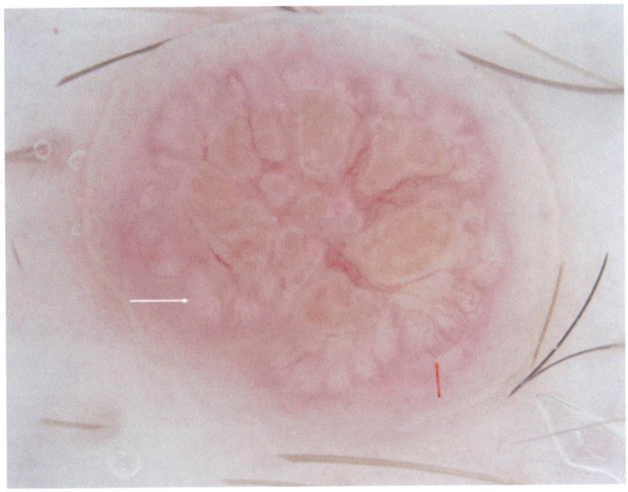

Fig. 17.9 Dermoscopically, we can observe a pattern composed of polilobular, yellowish, amorphous structures (white arrow) and crown vessels (linear or curved vessels with minimal branching situated along the periphery and extending toward the center without crossing it) (red arrow)

18 Nodular Pigmented Lesions on the Trunk

Horacio Cabo, Renato Marchiori Bakos, Dimitrios Sgouros, and Alexander Katoulis

Case 1: H.C.

Sex: female
Age: 41
Surface: nodular
Maximum diameter: 8 mm each one
Duration of the lesions: >5 years
History of morphologic changes: yes
Personal history of skin cancer: no
Family history of skin cancer: no
Skin photo type: V
Total nevus count: 10–50

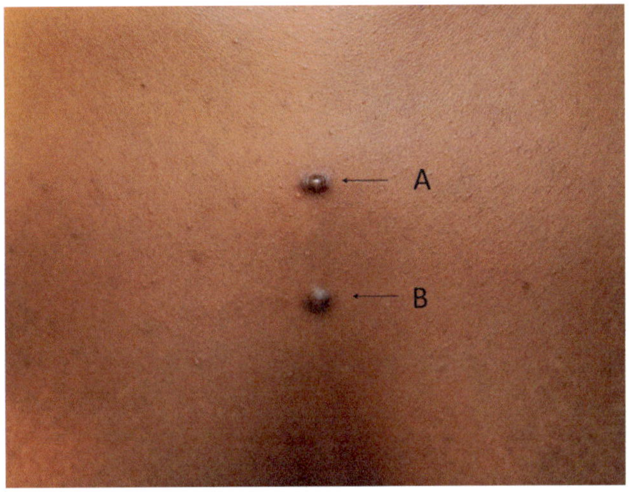

Fig. 18.1 Clinical view: two lesions on the chest. They are nodular and firms and with very dark pigmentation

H. Cabo (✉)
Instituto de Investigaciones Medicas "A. Lanari". Dermatology Section, University of Buenos Aires, Buenos Aires, Argentina

R. M. Bakos
Dermatology, Universidade Federal do Rio Grande do Sul, Porto Alegre, Brazil

D. Sgouros · A. Katoulis
2nd Department of Dermatology-Venereology, National and Kapodistrian University of Athens, "ATTIKON" University Hospital, Athens, Greece

H. Cabo, A. Lallas (eds.), *Comprehensive Atlas of Dermatoscopy Cases*, https://doi.org/10.1007/978-3-319-76932-5_18

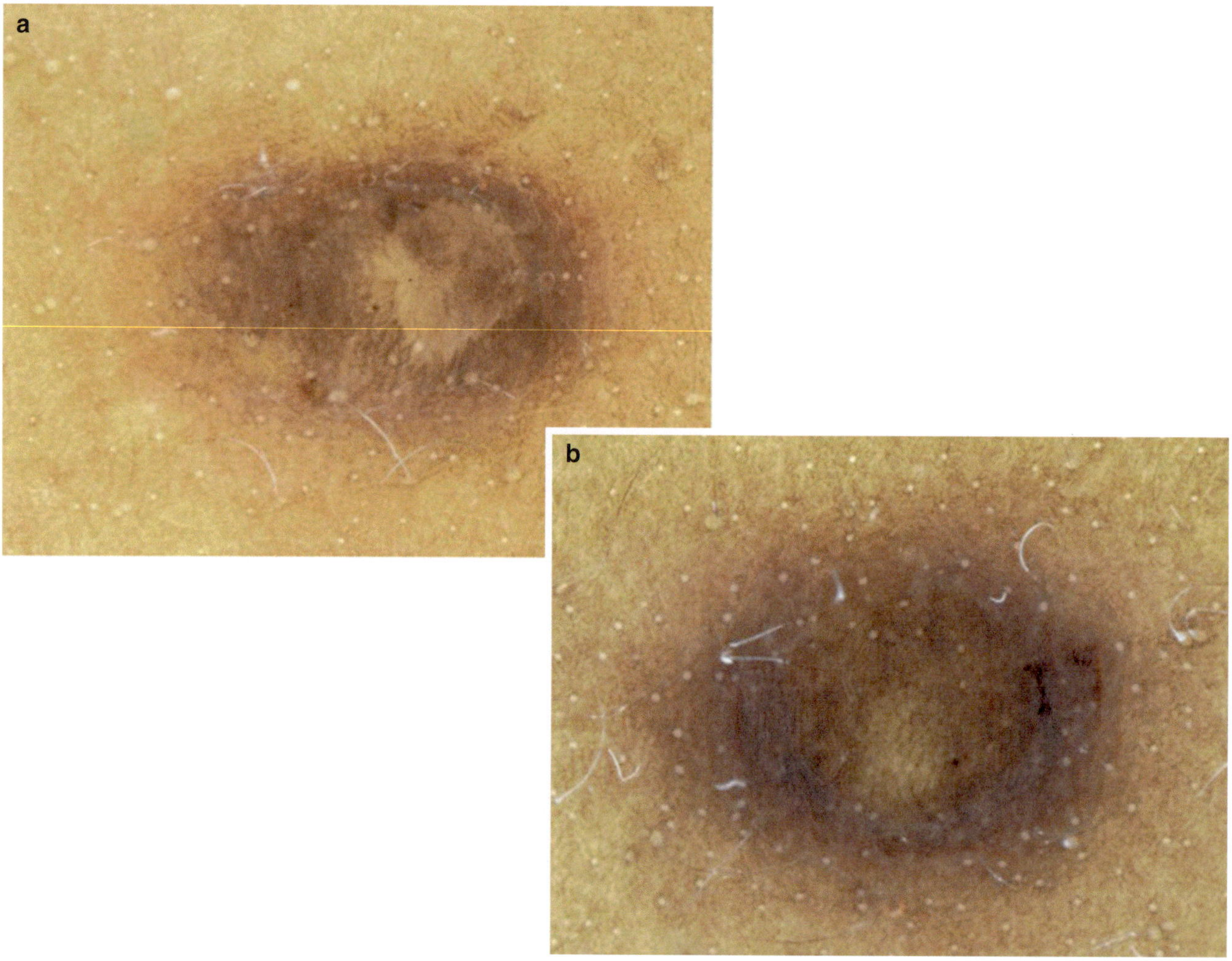

Fig. 18.2 Dermoscopy view

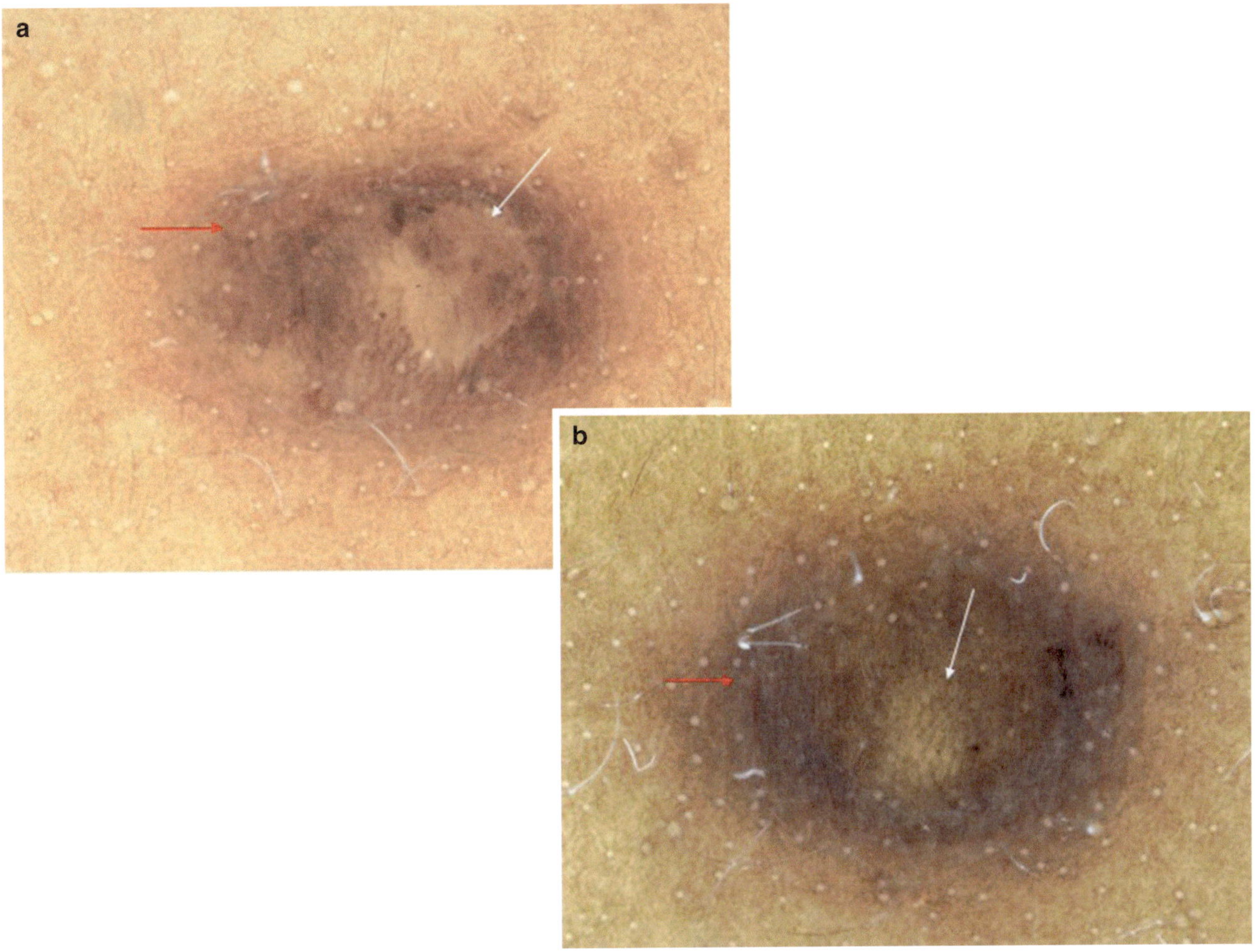

Fig. 18.3 Dermoscopy view: (**a**, **b**) show the same dermoscopy features. Pigment network (red arrows); central area with depigmentation (white arrows)

Key Message
Diagnosis: pigmented dermatofibromas
Dermoscopy clues: delicate peripheral pigment network and central white patch

In skin type V and VI, these are very pigmented lesions and on occasions can make the diagnosis difficult. The palpation of the lesion always help.

Case 2: R.M.B.

Sex: male

Age: 70 years old

Surface (flat/palpable/nodular): nodular and palpable

Maximum diameter: 1.2 cm

Duration of the lesion: 1 month

History of morphologic changes: yes

Personal history of skin cancer (if yes, please specify): no

Family history of skin cancer (if yes, please specify): no

Skin phototype: III

Total nevus count (<10, 10–50, 50–100, >100): <10

Other clinical findings (optional): lesion started to itch (patient's motivation to visit our Department)

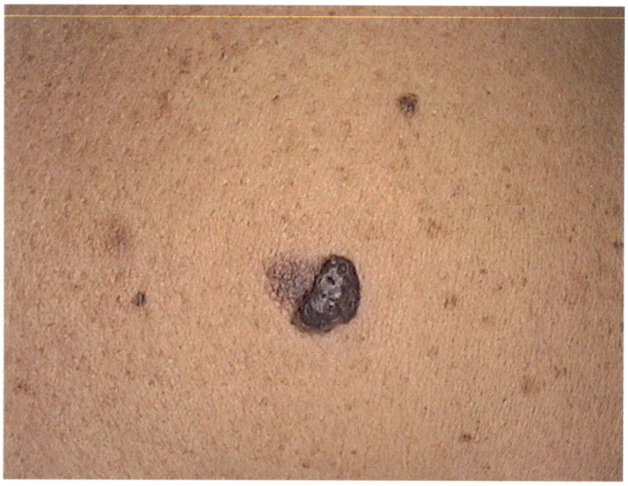

Fig. 18.4 Clinical image of the lesion on the dorsum showing an asymmetric dark brown lesion composed of a flat macule and a nodular portion with irregular surface and well-defined edges

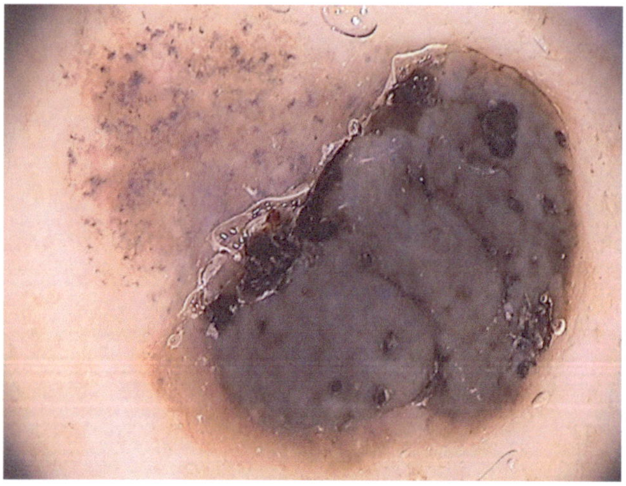

Fig. 18.5 Dermoscopy showing follicular openings and sharp edges on the nodular aspect and scattered dark globules and dots

Key Message

Lichenoid keratosis can be diagnosed based on the symptoms (changing lesion and itching sensation), the absence of melanocytic dermoscopic structures and the presence of a granular pattern and seborrheic keratosis features (follicular openings and sharp demarcation).

Case 3: D.S., A.K.

Sex: female
Age: 52 years old
Surface (flat/palpable/nodular): nodular
Maximum diameter: 7 mm
Duration of the lesion: 18 months
History of morphologic changes: enlargement of the lesion during last months
Personal history of skin cancer (if yes, please specify): No
Family history of skin cancer (if yes, please specify): No
Skin phototype: III
Total nevus count (<10, 10–50, 50–100, >100): <10
Other clinical findings (optional):

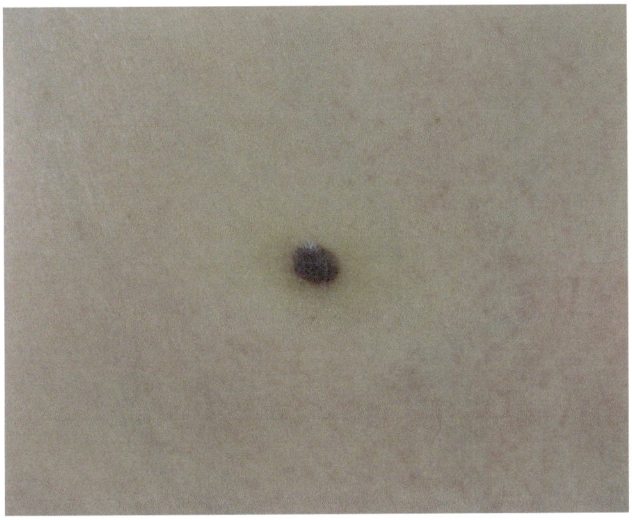

Fig. 18.6 Well-circumscribed, hard, bluish nodule on the right lateral side of the abdomen

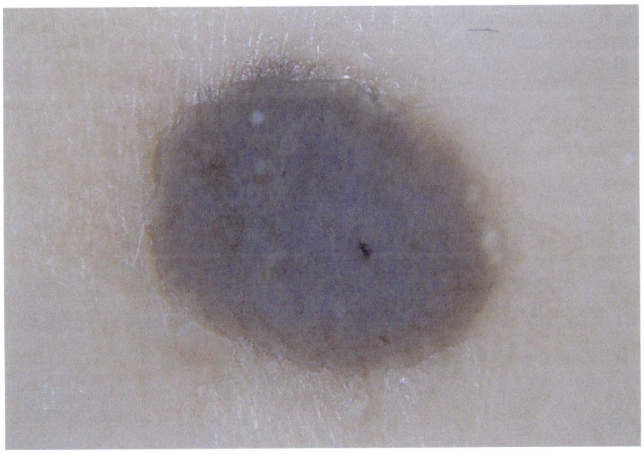

Fig. 18.7 Dermoscopy of the lesion with non-polarized light and immersion fluid. Diffuse bluish-brownish pigmentation throughout the entire surface of the lesion

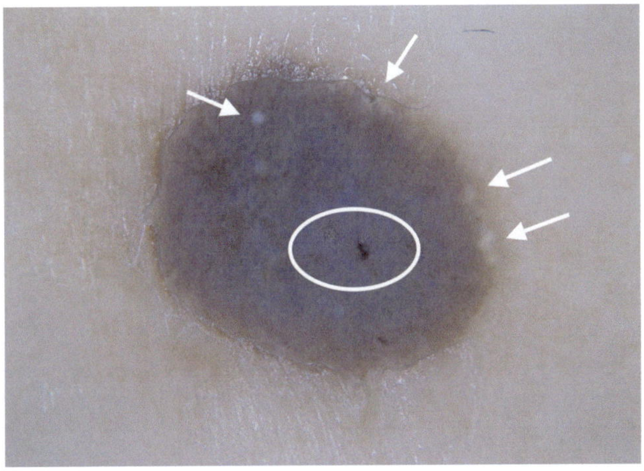

Fig. 18.8 Multiple milia-like cysts (white arrows) and comedo-like openings (white circle) along with the sharp demarcation of the lesion lead us to the diagnosis of seborrheic keratosis (SK). A few monomorphous, vascular structures on the upper part of the lesion

Key Message

Clinical history of a hard, palpable, enlarging nodule of recent onset might represent an indication for excision of the lesion in order to exclude a nodular melanoma. Bluish diffuse pigmentation can be seen in SK, blue nevus as well as nodular melanoma. Heavily pigmented SK might mimic melanoma, but the presence of typical dermoscopic features of SK usually guides to the correct diagnosis.

Case 4: D.S., A.K.

Sex: male

Age: 38 years old

Surface (flat/palpable/nodular): nodular

Maximum diameter: 6 mm

Duration of the lesion: 2 years

History of morphologic changes: history of trauma

Personal history of skin cancer (if yes, please specify): No

Family history of skin cancer (if yes, please specify): No

Skin phototype: IV

Total nevus count (<10, 10–50, 50–100, >100): 10–50

Other clinical findings (optional): no dimple sign.

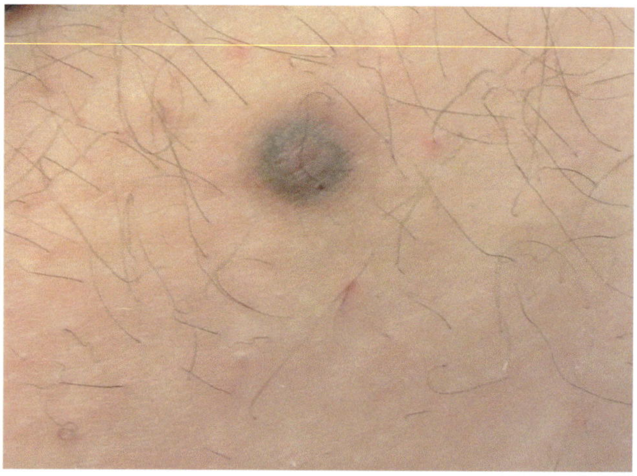

Fig. 18.9 Nodular pigmented lesion on the lateral side of the left buttock

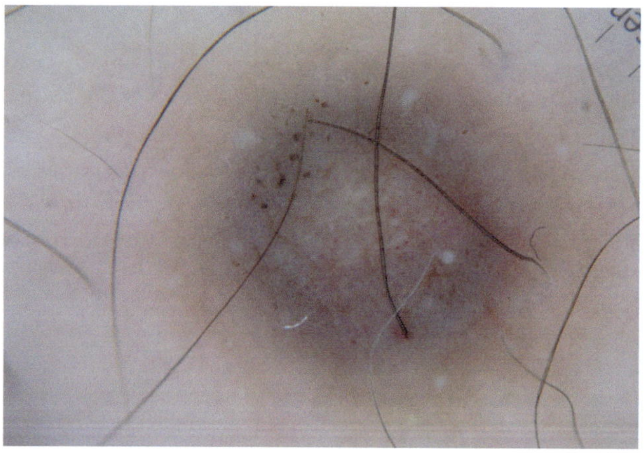

Fig. 18.10 Dermoscopically the lesion presents with a central white patch and a peripheral ring of bluish pigmentation

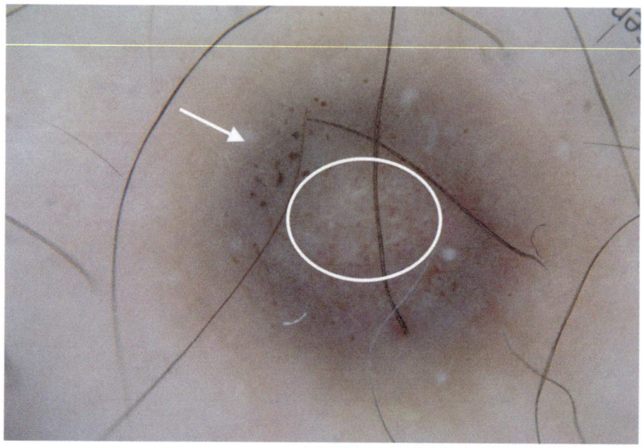

Fig. 18.11 White, shiny lines in the center of the lesion (white circle) creating a central whitish network. Periphery of the lesion showing diffuse bluish pigmentation without any features of pigment network. Monomorphous dotted vessels arranged symmetrically throughout the lesion. Globular structures in the periphery (white arrow) representing fissures. All of the above dermoscopic features are suggestive of a dermatofibroma

Key Message

Dermatofibroma might share common dermoscopic characteristics with malignant lesions such as melanoma. White, shiny lines represent a fibrotic reaction in the dermis and can be also seen in malignant lesions, such as melanoma and basal cell carcinoma. Dotted vessels in combination with polymorphous vessels are typical features of amelanotic melanoma. On the contrary, dermatofibroma follows a monomorphous vascular pattern with dotted vessels. White color and white lines in the center of a lesion as well as symmetrical distribution of the dotted vessels throughout the lesion are indicative of dermatofibroma.

Nodular Nonpigmented Lesions on the Trunk

19

Horacio Cabo, Aimilios Lallas, Chryssoula Papageorgiou, Sonia Rodriguez Saa, Josep Malvehy, Susana Puig, Giovanni Pellacani, Francesca Farnetani, and Raimonds Karls

Case 1 H.C.

Sex: male
Age: 43
Surface: nodular
Maximum diameter: 6 mm
Duration of the lesion: < 6 months
History of morphologic changes: no
Personal history of skin cancer: no
Family history of skin cancer: no
Skin photo type: III
Total nevus count: 10–50

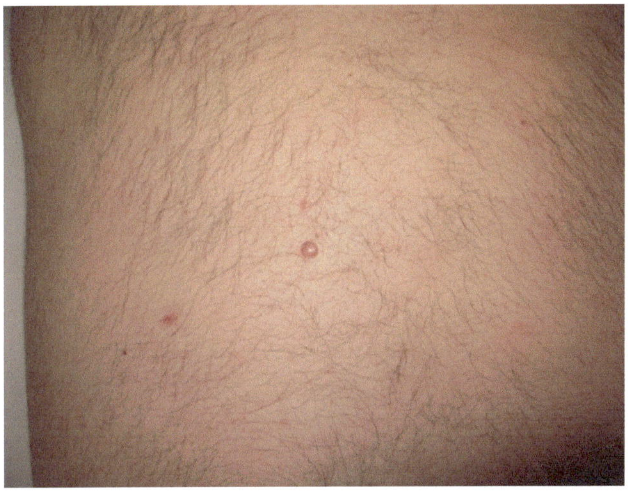

Fig. 19.1 Clinical view: elevated pink symmetric lesion on the thorax

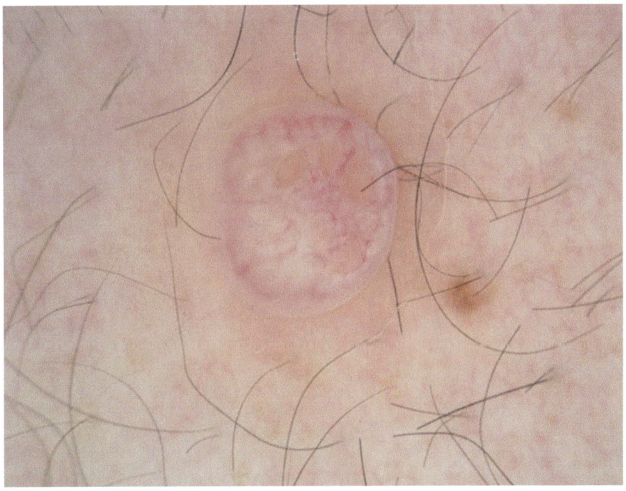

Fig. 19.2 Dermoscopy view

H. Cabo (✉)
Instituto de Investigaciones Médicas "A. Lanari". Dermatology Section, University of Buenos Aires, Buenos Aires, Argentina

A. Lallas · C. Papageorgiou
First Department of Dermatology, Aristotle University of Thessaloniki, Thessaloniki, Greece

S. R. Saa
University of Mendoza, Mendoza, Argentina

J. Malvehy · S. Puig
Dermatology Department, Barcelona, Spain

G. Pellacani · F. Farnetani
Department of Dermatology, University of Modena and Reggio Emilia, Modena, Italy

R. Karls
Department of Infectology and Dermatology, Riga Stradins University, Derma Clinic Riga, Ltd., Riga, Latvia

H. Cabo, A. Lallas (eds.), *Comprehensive Atlas of Dermatoscopy Cases*, https://doi.org/10.1007/978-3-319-76932-5_19

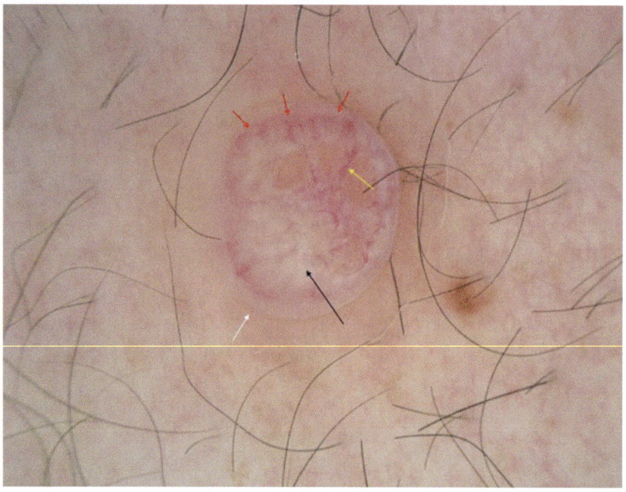

Fig. 19.3 Dermoscopy view: poly lobular amorphous white–yellow structure (black arrow); peripheral linear vessels in "red crown" arrangement (red arrows); white collared (white arrow); linear (radial) vessels arranged perpendicularly (yellow arrow)

Key Message
Diagnosis: Molluscum contagiosum
Dermoscopy Clue:

- "Fried egg" pattern, due to the presence of round structures with a central pore
- Poly lobular amorphous white–yellow structure
- Orifice: the growth of viral matter may cause a break in the skin
- Peripheral linear vessels in "red crown" arrangement
- Linear (radial) vessels arranged perpendicularly

Case 2 A.L.

Sex: male
Age: 66
Surface (flat/palpable/nodular): nodular
Maximum diameter: 9 mm
Duration of the lesion: 6 months
History of morphologic changes: no
Personal history of skin cancer (if yes, please specify): no
Family history of skin cancer (if yes, please specify): no
Skin phototype: III
Total nevus count (<10, 10–50, 50–100, >100): <10
Other clinical findings (optional):

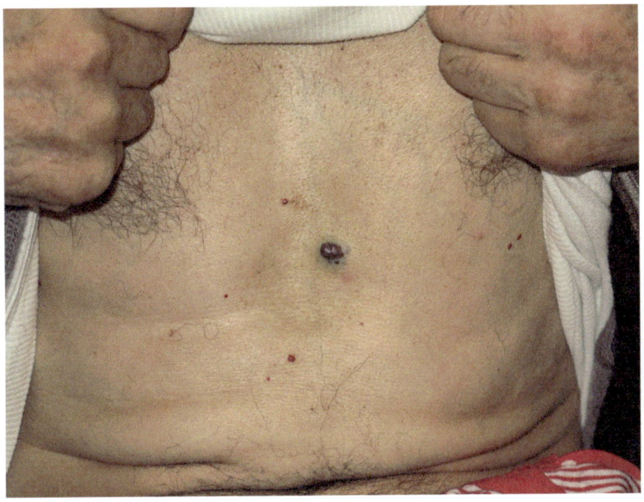

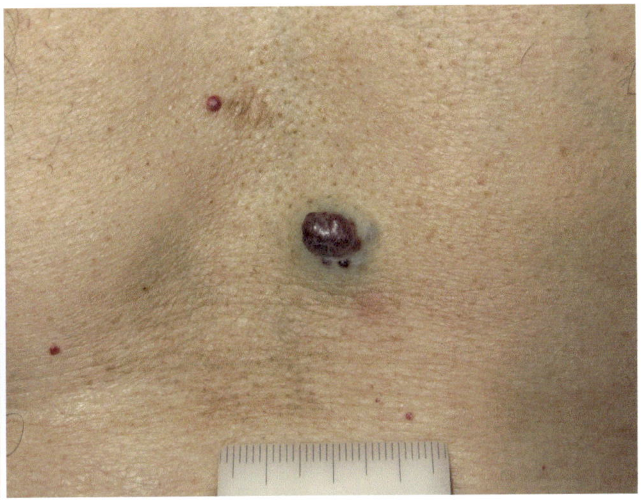

Figs. 19.4 and 19.5 Clinically, there is a red-purple, well-demarcated nodule with two smaller, similar, peripheral nodules in its lower side located on the abdomen

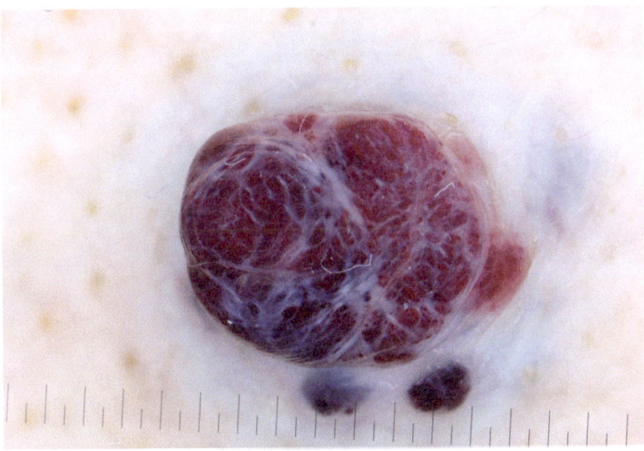

Fig. 19.6 The lesion is characterized by red to purple, well-circumscribed, round to oval structures (lacunas). White lines among the lacunas are also seen

Key Message

The clinical and dermoscopic images are suggestive of hemangioma with the red-purple globules (lacunas) corresponding to dilated, blood-filled vessels in the papillary dermis.

Case 3 S.R.S.

Sex: female
Age: 38
Surface (flat/palpable/nodular): nodular
Maximum diameter: 1.5 cm
Duration of the lesion: 6 months
History of morphologic changes: yes
Personal history of skin cancer (if yes, please specify): no
Family history of skin cancer (if yes, please specify): no
Skin phototype: III
Total nevus count (<10, 10–50, 50–100, >100): <10
Other clinical findings (optional): localized on

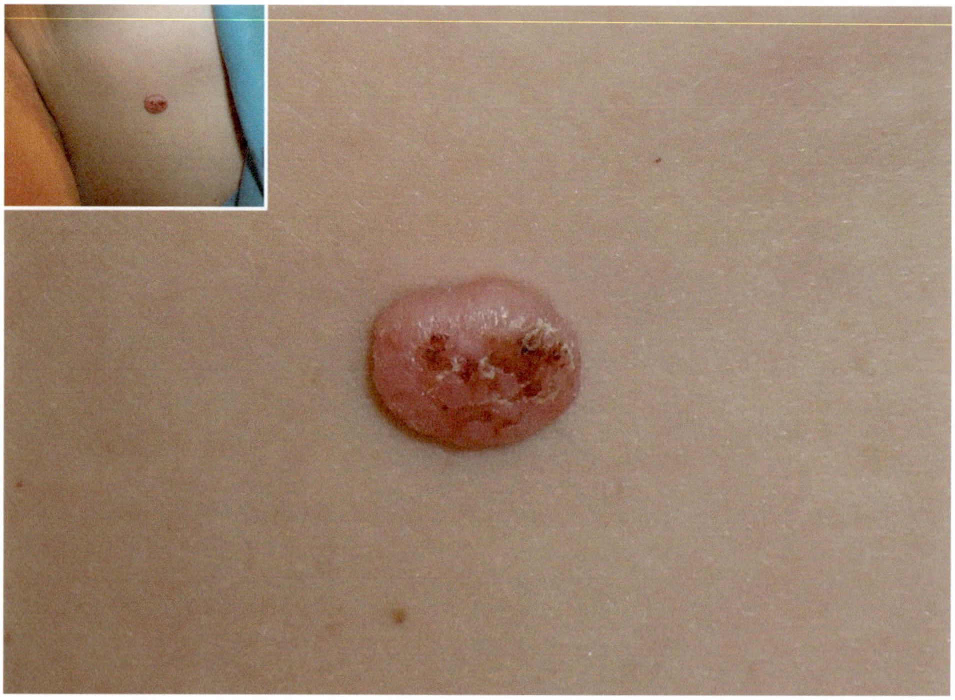

Fig. 19.7 Solitary asymptomatic erythematous tumor with central crusts, located on the right breast of a 45-year-old woman

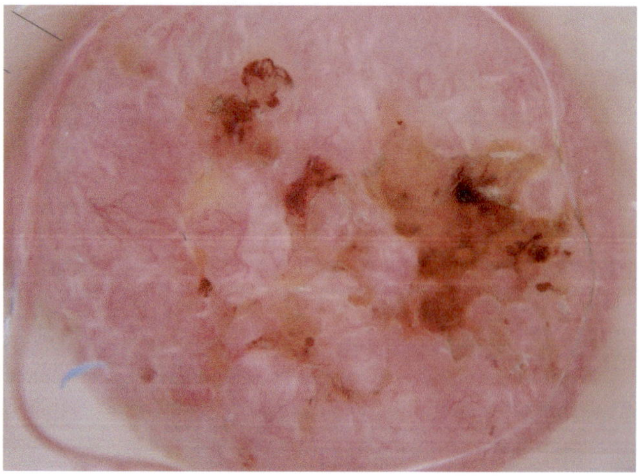

Fig. 19.8 Dermoscopic findings

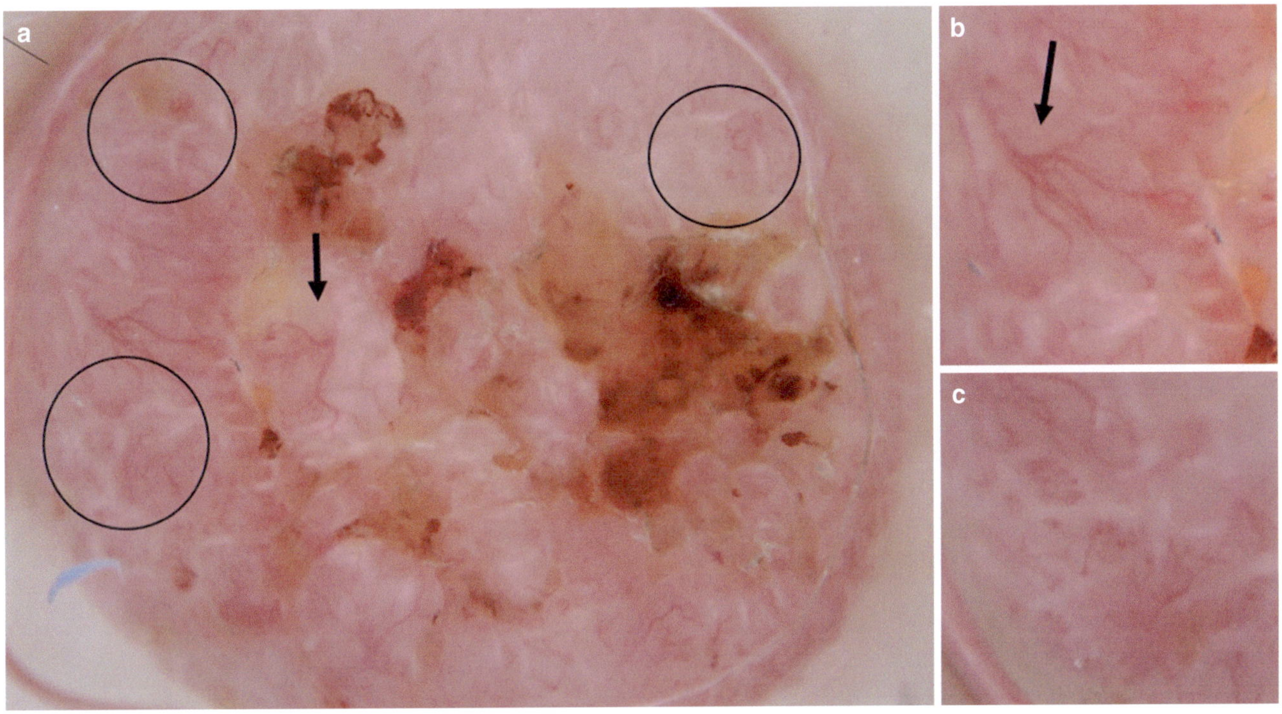

Fig. 19.9 Fibroepithelioma of Pinkus. Polarized dermoscopy demonstrates fine focused arborizing vessels (black arrows), some dotted vessels and shiny whitish streaks (black circles). Orange-red erosions and ulceration are visible in the center (red arrows)

Key Message

Fibroepithelioma of Pinkus is an uncommon subtype of basal cell carcinoma (BCC).

Dermoscopically shows shiny whitish streaks under polarized light and fine arborizing vessels that are typically smaller in caliber and have fewer ramifications than the classical treelike vessels of nodular BCC.

Erosions, ulcerations, dotted vessels, and milia cyst can also be seen.

Case 4 J.M., S.P.

Male, 52 years with personal background of diabetes mellitus. No personal or familial history of cancer

History: During a consultation in the ambulatory with his family doctor for another reason, a skin tumor on the upper right back is detected. The patient was aware of the lesion to be growing in more than 2 years without other symptoms.

The patient is referred to our center for this suspicious tumor.

Physical examination: an elevated tumor with 12 mm in diameter on the upper back with a nodular area with skin-colored nodule (soft at palpation) and a flat dark brown pigmented component at the periphery is confirmed.

No lymph nodules are present at axillary and inguinal palpation.

Dermoscopy: the tumor is composed of two different areas, a nodular amelanotic area with branched vessels and a pigmented flat area with dark brown, black, and bluish coloration and an atypical pigment network.

Differential diagnosis:

Superficial spreading melanoma versus collision tumor (basal cell carcinoma and melanoma)

Histopathology: superficial spreading melanoma, Breslow 8,01 mm, Clark III, non-ulcerated. Less than 1 mitosis/mm^2. No satellitosis.

Comment: In this tumor, the nodular component mimics in dermoscopy a collision tumor with branched vessels typically seen in a basal cell carcinoma. This dermoscopic finding is exceptional in a melanoma. However, in case on nodular lesions with this feature in dermoscopy, conformation with histopathology is recommended to rule out an amelanotic melanoma.

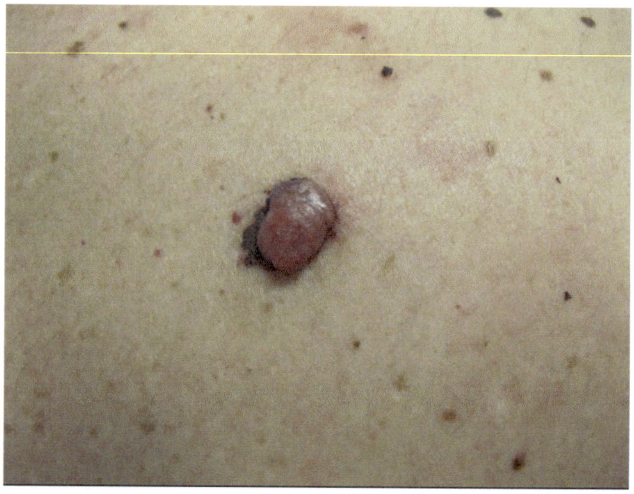

Fig. 19.10 Clinical view

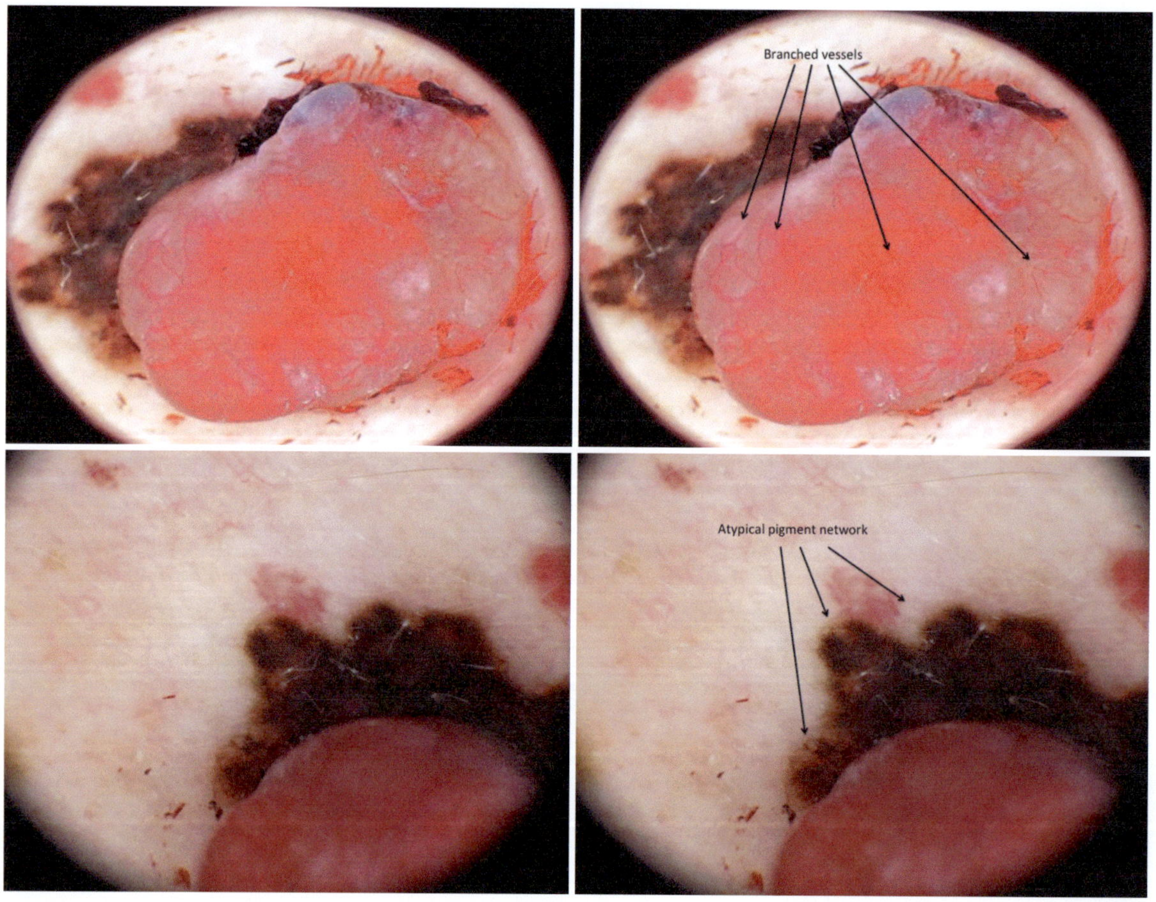

Figs. 19.11–19.14 Dermoscopy view

Case 5 G.P., F.F.

Sex: F
Age: 67
Surface: nodular
Maximum diameter: 1.2 × 0.5
Duration of the lesion: 8 months
History of morphologic changes: it's increasing in size.
Personal history of skin cancer (if yes, please specify): no
Family history of skin cancer (if yes, please specify): no
Skin phototype: 2
Total nevus count (<10, 10–50, 50–100, >100): 10–50
Other clinical findings (optional): no

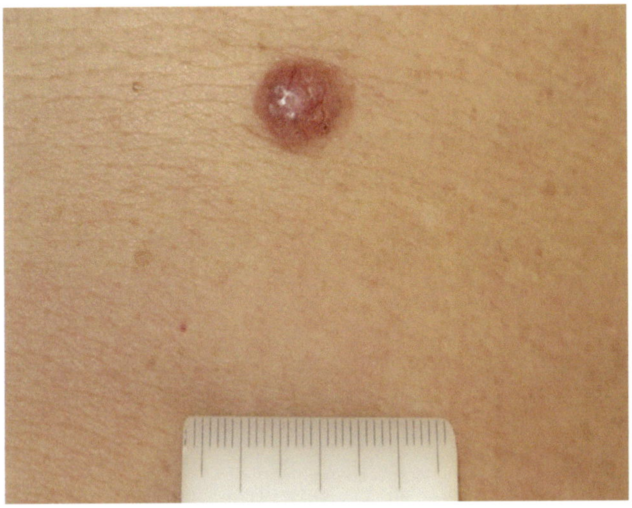

Fig. 19.15 A clinically nonpigmented nodular lesion on the back shows regular borders, pink color, 0.7 × 0,4 cm in diameter on sun-damaged skin.

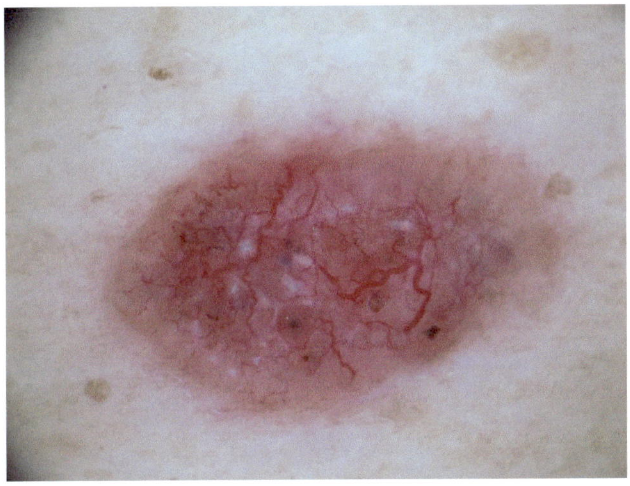

Fig. 19.16 Dermoscopy image

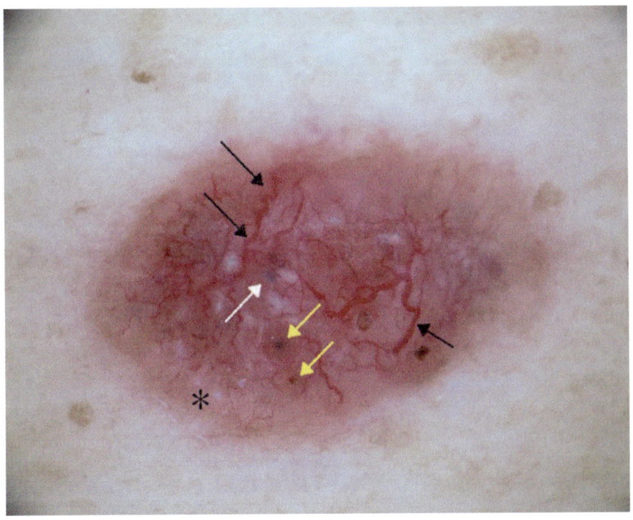

Fig. 19.17 Dermoscopy revels the presence of blue-gray ovoid nest (white arrows) corresponding to pigmented dermal basaloid nests, focused arborizing vessels (black arrows), short white streaks (asterisk), and concentric structures (yellow arrows)

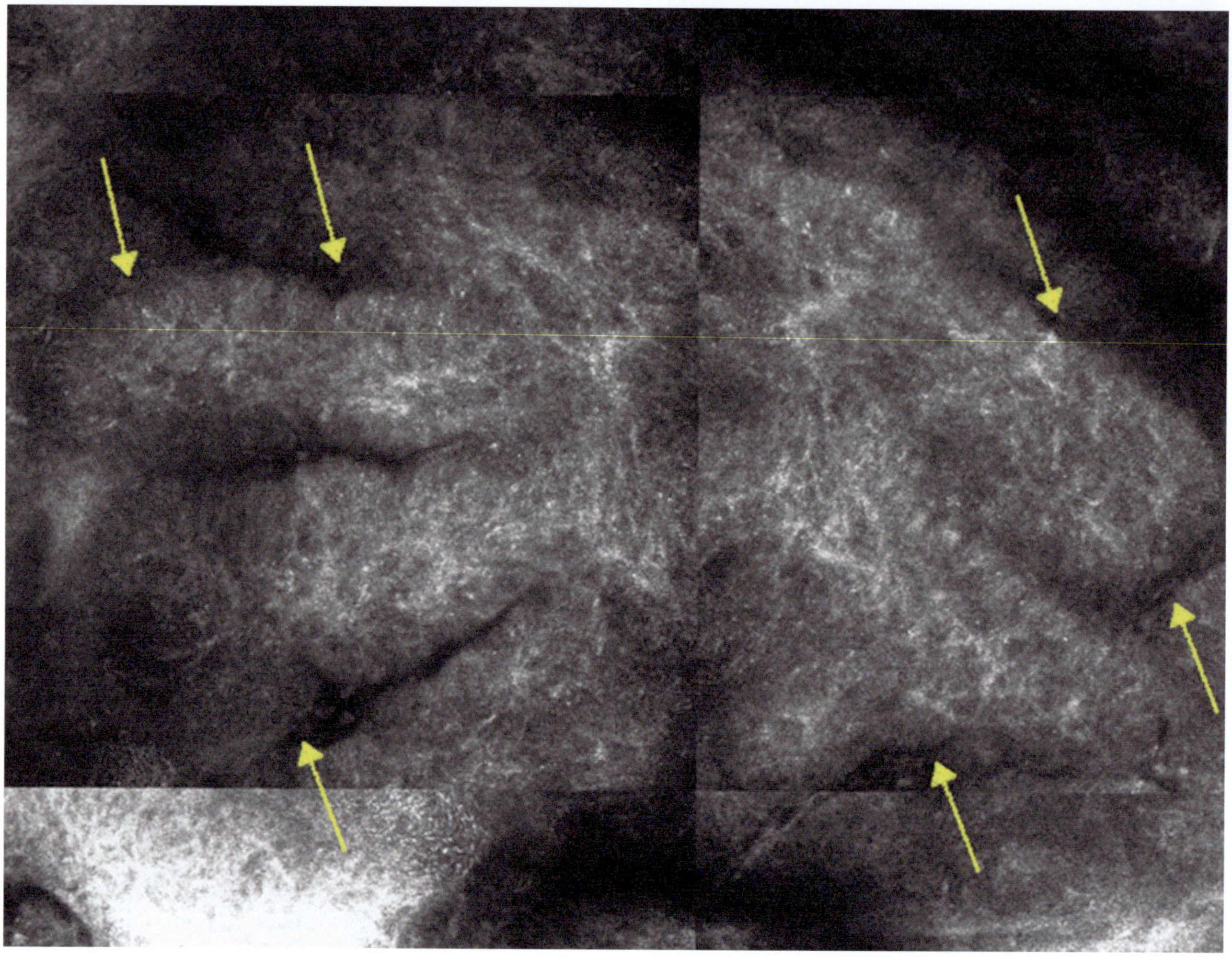

Fig. 19.18 Reflectance confocal microscopy shows a basaloid tumor islands (yellow arrows), with palisading cells at the periphery of the island

Key Message

Arborizing focused vessels represent the dermoscopic hallmark of nonpigmented nodular basal cell carcinoma.

Case 6 R.K.

Sex: female
Age: 39
Surface (flat/palpable/nodular): palpable
Maximum diameter: 7 mm
Duration of the lesion: less than 2 years
History of morphologic changes: slow, regular growing
Personal history of skin cancer (if yes, please specify): no data about the skin malignancies in personal history
Family history of skin cancer (if yes, please specify): no data about skin cancer in family history
Skin phototype: II
Total nevus count (<10, 10–50, 50–100, >100): total nevus count 10–50
Other clinical findings (optional): no specific data about other clinical findings; the lady visited clinic due to other dermatological problem.

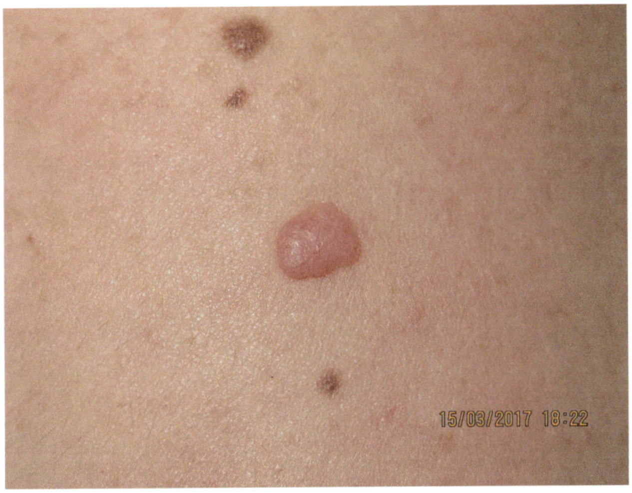

Fig. 19.19 Clinical picture of the lesion. Palpable lesion with sharply demarcated borders, well defined with smooth surface

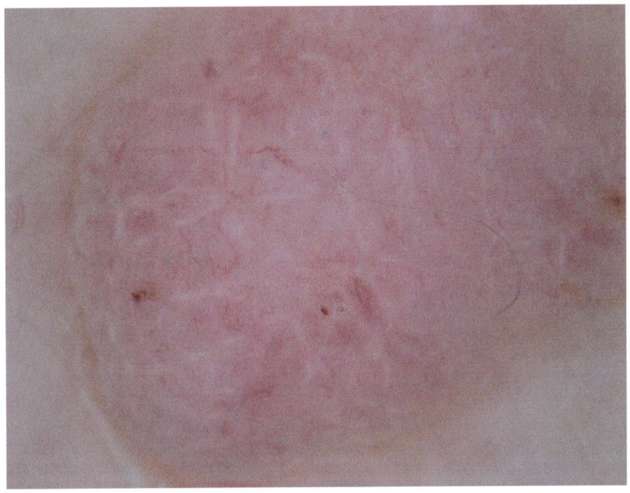

Fig. 19.20 Polarized dermoscopy—polymorphous vessels, chrysalis structures. There is no other significant dermatoscopic structures

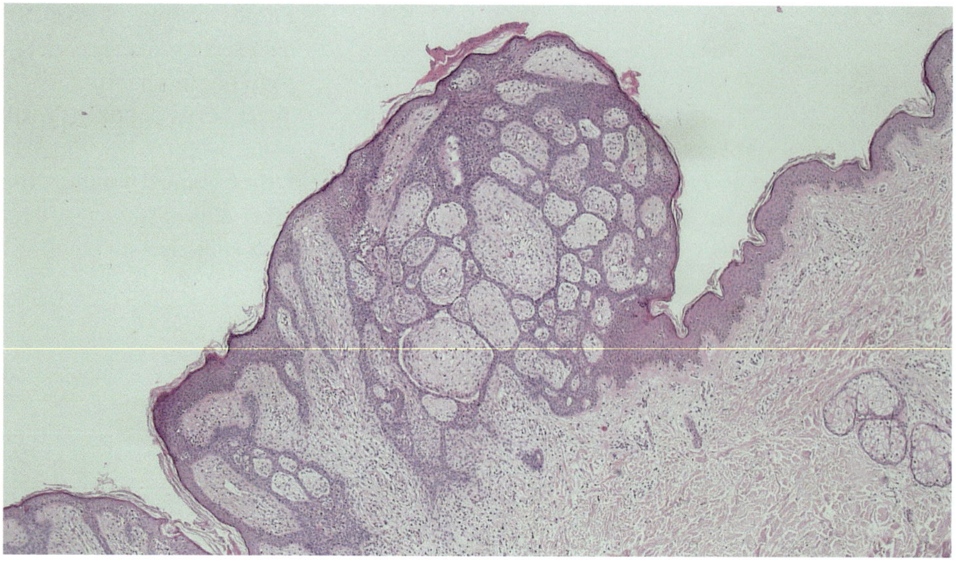

Fig. 19.21 The epidermis without ulceration symptoms. Arrangement consists of basaloid cell proliferates mesh with peripheral palisades and moderate cell atypia

Key Message

Slowly growing, skin-colored lesion must be examined with care.

Chrysalis structures under polarized dermatoscopy in combination with polymorph vessels are suspicious features.

Skin-colored papula in middle-age person with chrysalis structures and polymorph vessels could not be left without attention.

Case 7 R.K.

Sex: male
Age: 70
Surface (flat/palpable/nodular): nodular surface; without ulceration, scales, and crusts
Maximum diameter: 7 mm
Duration of the lesion: duration of the lesion could not be defined. Patient visited clinic with another dermatological problem.
History of morphologic changes: slow-growing lesion
Personal history of skin cancer (if yes, please specify): nodular basal cell carcinoma on the face (2004, 2006, 2012); superficial basal carcinoma on the back (2012). Multiple actinic keratosis on the scalp and face.
Family history of skin cancer (if yes, please specify): no data about family malignancies
Skin phototype: skin type II
Total nevus count (<10, 10–50, 50–100, >100): 10–15
Other clinical findings (optional): several senile angiomas surrounding the skin

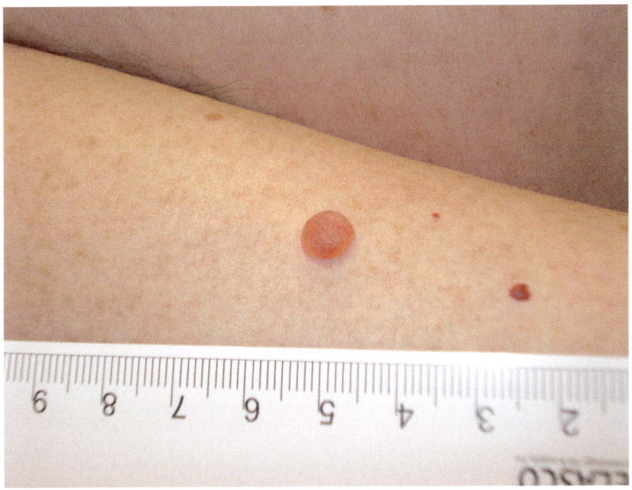

Fig. 19.22 Asymptomatic, pink, nodular lesion on the ventral aspect of the right shoulder. No more similar lesions on the skin

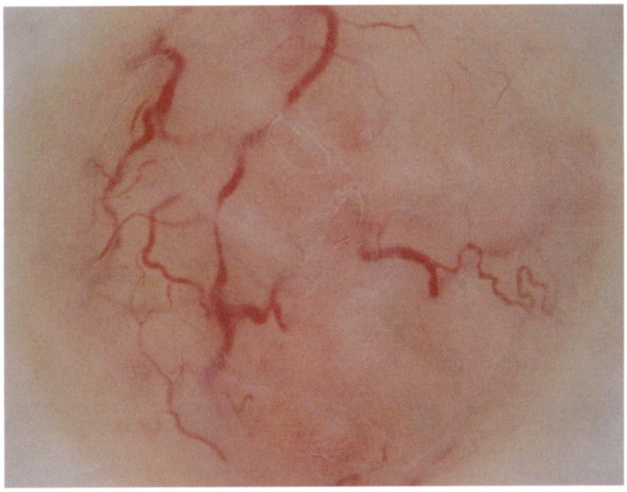

Fig. 19.23 True arborizing, sharply focused vessels, pinkish background, and the absence of any other significant features under dermatoscopy

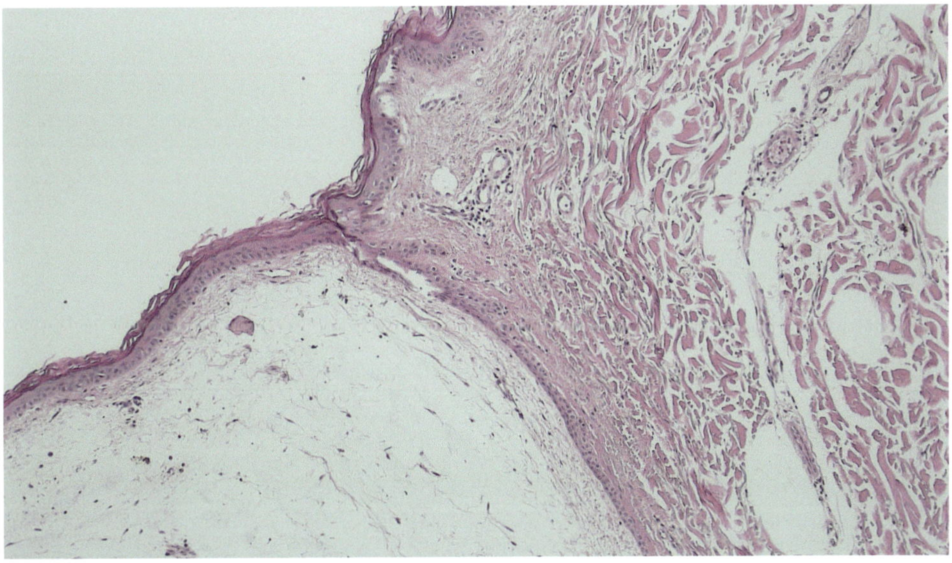

Fig. 19.24 Beneath the epidermis colorless structure, mutually well marked by atrophic epidermis, but distally blend into the dermis. Rare fibroblasts and capillaries with thicken walls. Inflammatory elements are not seen, in some areas rare lymphocytes

Key Message

Nodular pink lesion in elderly patients must be evaluated in details.

True arborizing vessels are most common finding in nodular basal cell carcinoma.

Dermatoscopy of clinically typical lesions is helpful.

20 Flat Pigmented Lesions on the Upper Limbs

Chryssoula Papageorgiou and Aimilios Lallas

Case 1

Sex: male
Age: 8
Surface (flat/palpable/nodular): flat
Maximum diameter: 4 mm
Duration of the lesion: 3 months
History of morphologic changes: yes, slowly enlarging
Personal history of skin cancer (if yes please specify): no
Family history of skin cancer (if yes please specify): no
Skin phototype: III
Total nevus count: (<10, 10–50, 50–100, >100): 10–50
Other clinical findings (optional):

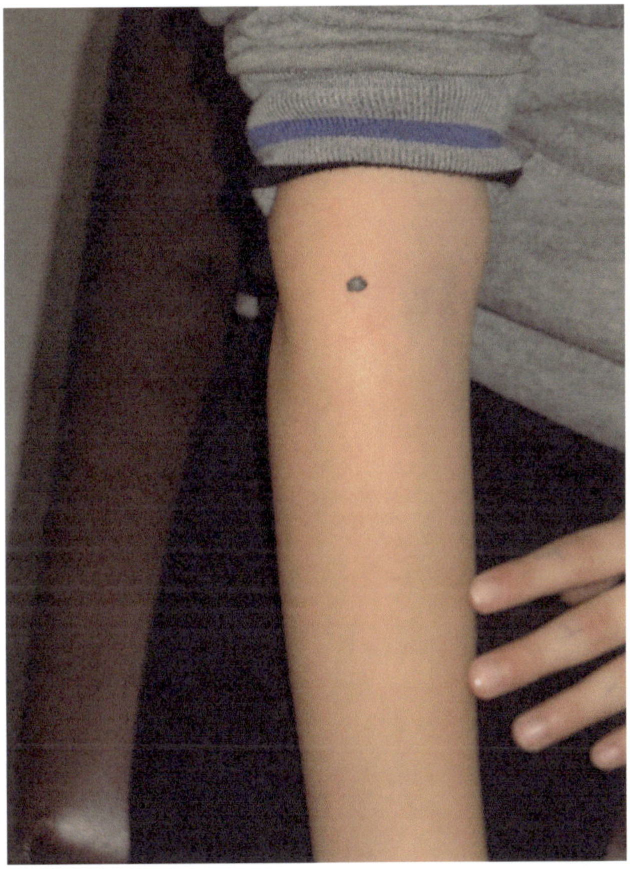

Fig. 20.1 On clinical examination, there is a symmetric heavily pigmented lesion located on the flexural surface of the right elbow

C. Papageorgiou · A. Lallas (✉)
First Department of Dermatology, Aristotle University of Thessaloniki, Thessaloniki, Greece

H. Cabo, A. Lallas (eds.), *Comprehensive Atlas of Dermatoscopy Cases*, https://doi.org/10.1007/978-3-319-76932-5_20

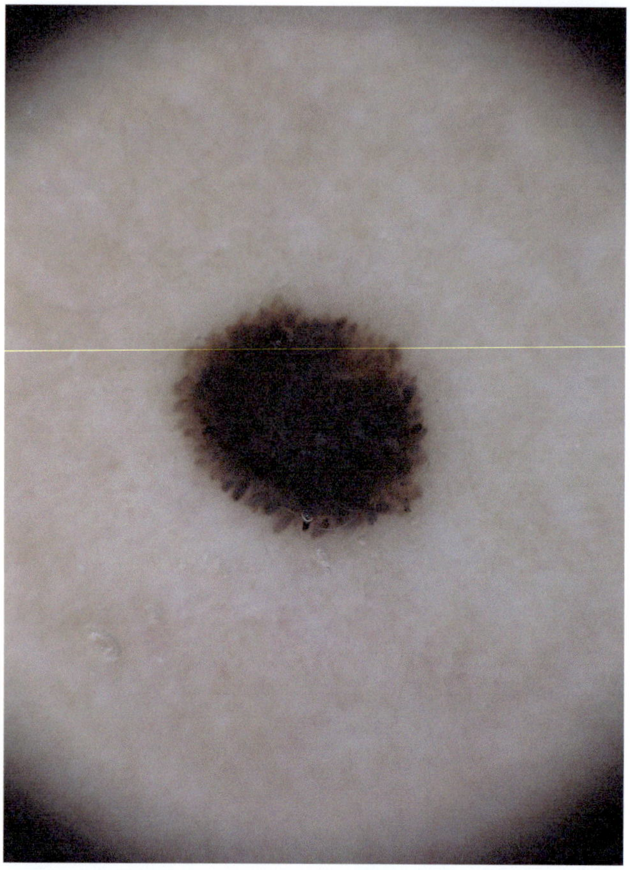

Fig. 20.2 Dermoscopically, there is a symmetric spitzoid-looking lesion that exhibits a starburst pattern composed of a central homogeneous black-blue pigmented area and peripheral regularly and radially arranged pigmented streaks (giving the impression of an exploding star)

Key Message

Spitzoid lesions represent a challenging group of tumors as they can biologically be either nevi or melanomas. It seems that the age plays an important role on the nature of the lesion and is the key when managing these lesions. In symmetric flat spitzoid lesions, excision is highly recommended when developing after the age of 12 years, while when developing before this age, the recommended management is follow-up until stabilization. In this case, dermoscopy revealed a symmetric spitzoid lesion. Taking also into account the age of the patient suggests a pigmented Spitz nevus. After the 18 months of follow-up, the lesion is still growing but in a symmetric way to all directions.

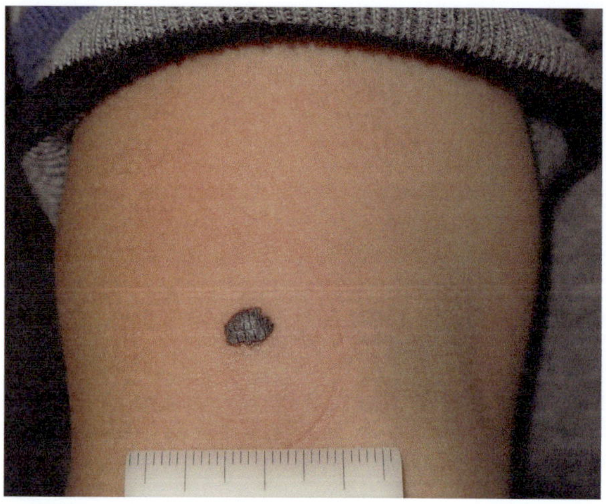

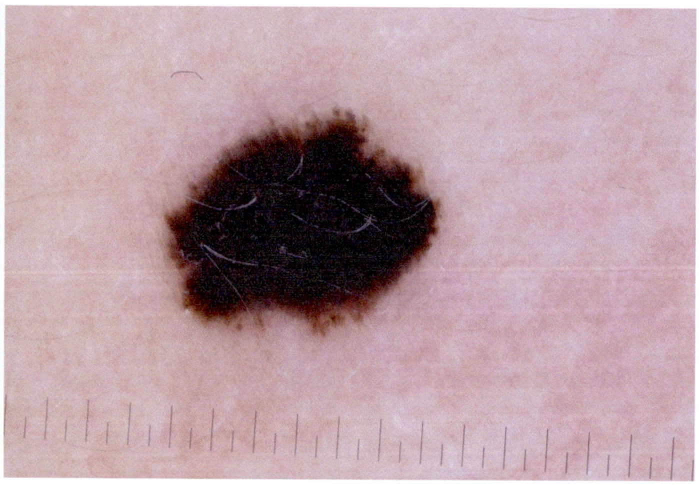

Figs. 20.3 and 20.4 Same lesion after 18 months follow-up. Both clinically and dermoscopically, the lesion has symmetrically grown to all directions maintaining the starburst pattern

Flat Nonpigmented Lesions on the Upper Limbs

21

Horacio Cabo

Case 1

Sex: female
Age: 73
Surface: flat
Maximum diameter: 9 mm
Duration of the lesion: > 1 year
History of morphologic changes: yes
Personal history of skin cancer: no
Family history of skin cancer: no
Skin phototype: II
Total nevus count: <10
Other clinical findings: the patient had a burning sensation

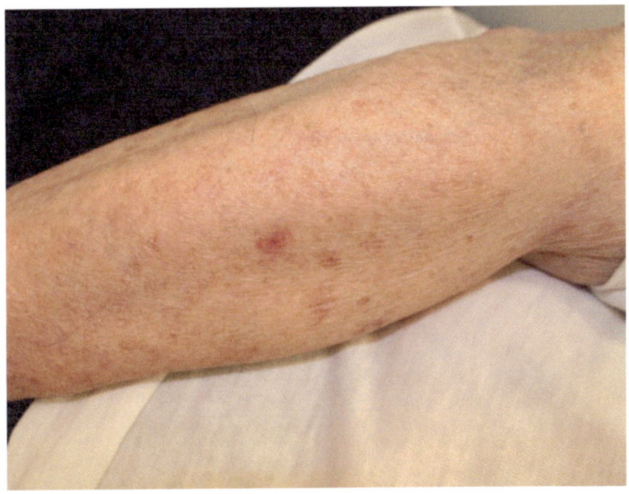

Fig. 21.1 Clinical view: flat red lesion; the patient had a burning sensation, and she noticed that the lesion was growing in the last months

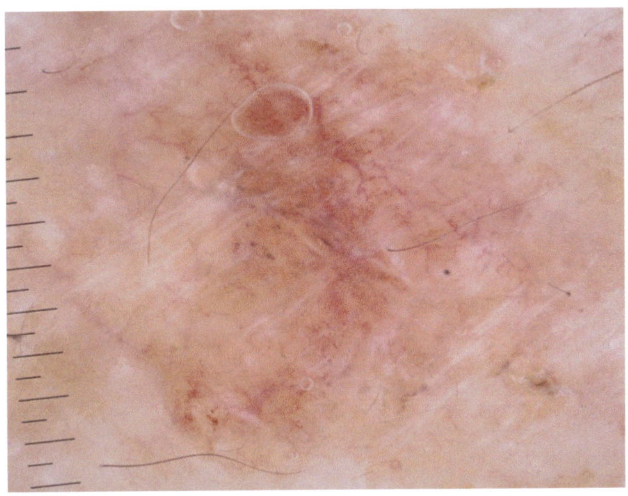

Fig. 21.2 Dermoscopy image

H. Cabo
Instituto de Investigaciones Medicas "A. Lanari". Dermatology Section, University of Buenos Aires, Buenos Aires, Argentina

H. Cabo, A. Lallas (eds.), *Comprehensive Atlas of Dermatoscopy Cases*, https://doi.org/10.1007/978-3-319-76932-5_21

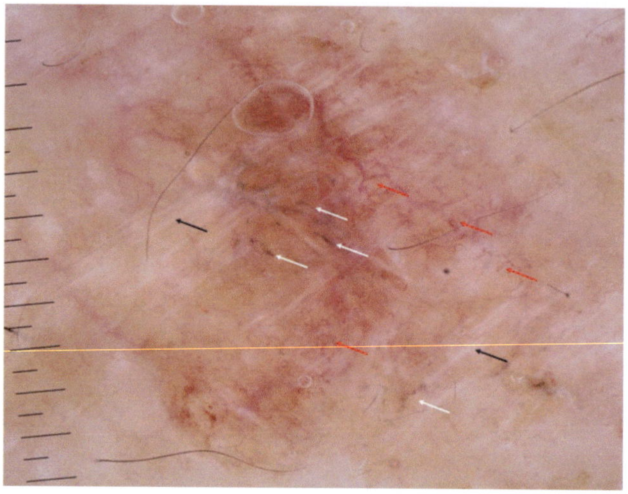

Fig. 21.3 Dermoscopy view: asymmetric lesion, with different colors, red, light brown, white, and blue-gray. Notice the blue-gray with peppering appearance (white arrows), irregular linear-branching vessels (red arrows), and the white shiny streaks

Key Message

Diagnosis: Lichen planus-like keratosis

In the presence of a pink lesion, we must consider these following differential diagnoses: superficial basal cell carcinoma, actinic keratosis, Bowen's disease, hypomelanotic melanoma, and lichen planus-like keratosis.

The vascular pattern is different in these lesions. The presence of blue-gray color with peppering appearance with the other dermoscopy features such as white shiny streaks and the vascular pattern is frequent in lichen planus-like keratosis.

In addition, the absence of dermoscopy features for basal cell carcinoma (blue-gray color, arborizing vessels, and ulceration), Bowen's disease (glomerular vessels with focal distribution), hypomelanotic melanoma (pigment traces and dotted vessels, linear irregular vessels with polymorphic pattern and random distribution), and actinic keratosis (undulated vessels around the hair follicle, strawberry pattern, and rough surface) helps us to make the diagnosis of lichen planus-like keratosis

Palpable Pigmented Lesions on the Upper Limbs

22

Horacio Cabo and Virginia Mariana Gonzalez

Case 1: H.C.

Sex: male
Age: 47
Surface: palpable
Maximum diameter: 12 mm
Duration of the lesion: >1 year
History of morphologic changes: yes
Personal history of skin cancer: no
Family history of skin cancer: no
Skin phototype: III
Total nevus count: 10–50

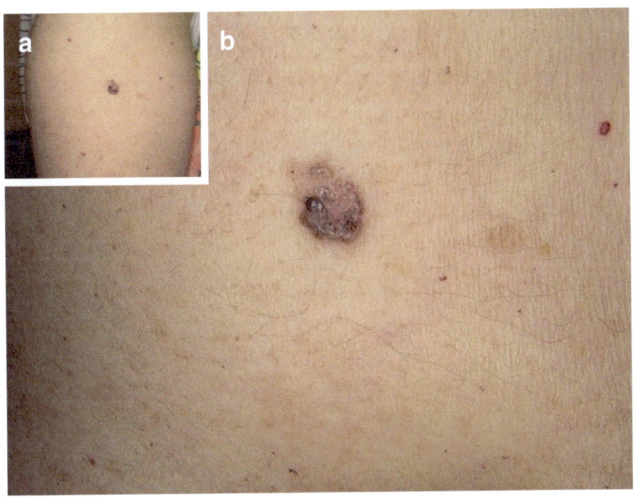

Fig. 22.1 Clinical view: (**a**) asymmetric lesion with different colors and an elevated edge in the lower part of the lesion, (**b**) close-up of clinical view

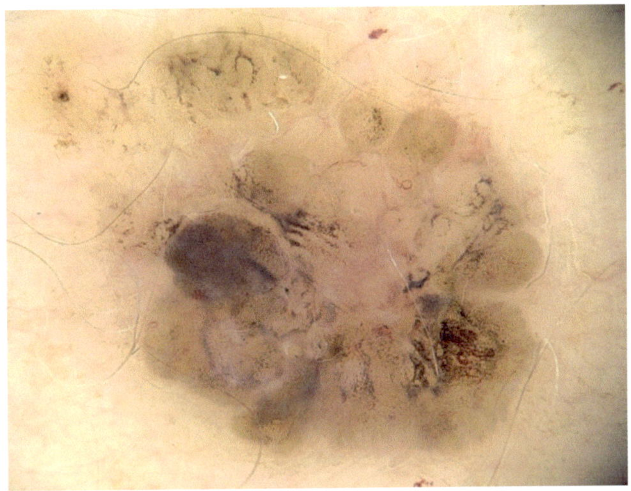

Fig. 22.2 Dermoscopy view (polarized light)

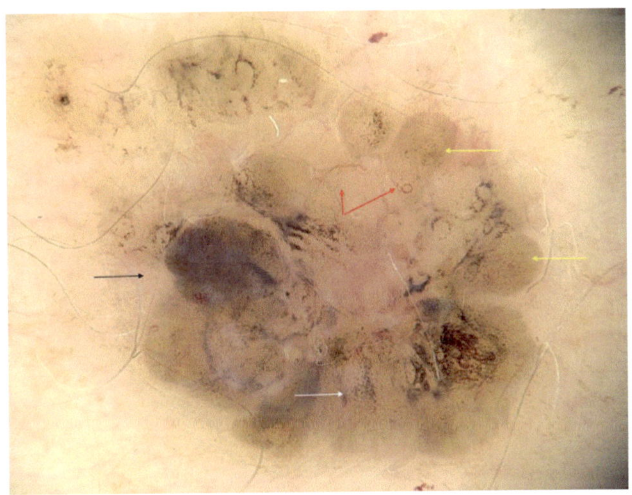

Fig. 22.3 Dermoscopy view: blue-gray areas (black arrow); thick and irregular vessels (red arrows); multiple blue-dots (white arrow); leaf-like structures (yellow arrows)

Key Message

Diagnosis: basal cell carcinoma

Notice the presence of two of the major criteria, blue-gray pigmentation (Globules, dots and leaf-like structures) and vascular pattern with thick irregular and arborizing vessels.

H. Cabo (✉)
Instituto de Investigaciones Medicas "A. Lanari". Dermatology Section, University of Buenos Aires, Buenos Aires, Argentina

V. M. Gonzalez
Hospital Alemán, Buenos Aires, Argentina

H. Cabo, A. Lallas (eds.), *Comprehensive Atlas of Dermatoscopy Cases*, https://doi.org/10.1007/978-3-319-76932-5_22

Case 2: H.C.

Sex: male
Age: 36
Surface: palpable
Maximum diameter: 8 mm

Duration of the lesion: >10 years
History of morphologic changes: no
Personal history of skin cancer: no
Family history of skin cancer: no
Skin phototype: III
Total nevus count: 10–50

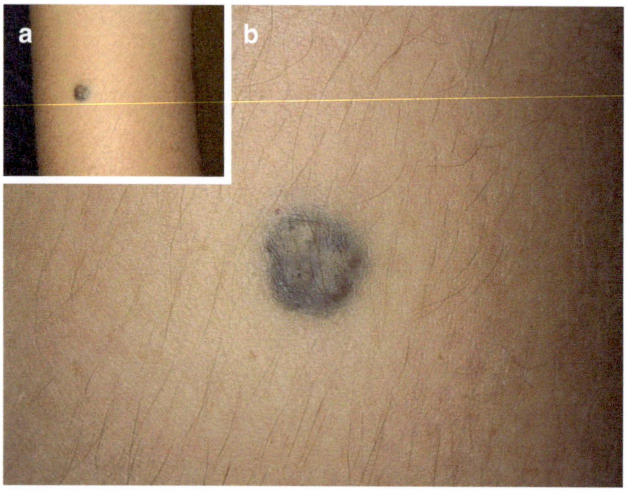

Fig. 22.4 Clinical image (**a**); close-up of the clinical image (**b**). The lesion has two different colors; at the periphery it is blue and in the central part is brown

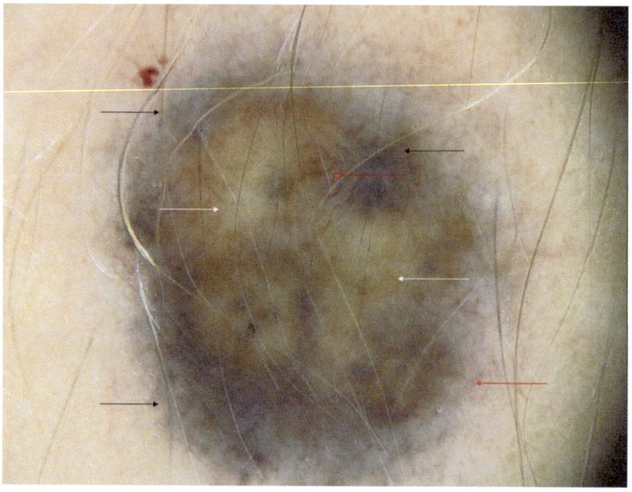

Fig. 22.6 Dermoscopy image: notice the blue areas at the periphery of the lesion (black arrows), the brown and yellow areas in the central part of the lesion (white arrows), and the vascular pattern with linear branching and reticular vessels (red arrows)

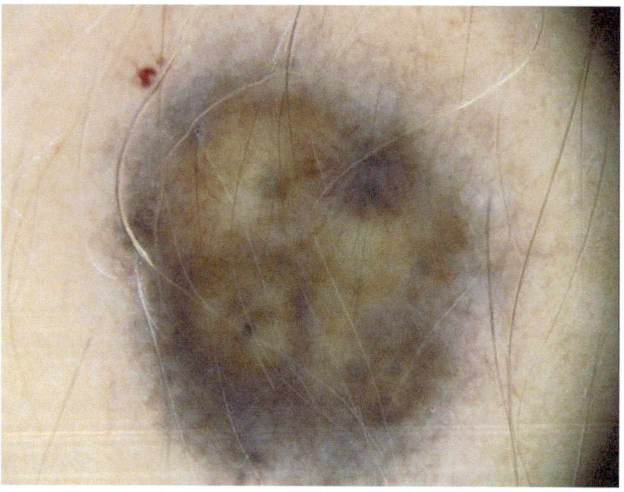

Fig. 22.5 Dermoscopy image (polarized light)

Key Message

Diagnosis: sclerotic blue nevus

With polarized light dermatoscope shows brown yellow areas.

The vascular pattern of the lesion made us think in a collision tumor (BCC & Blue nevus), but it was discard for the pathologist study.

Case 3: V.G.

Sex: female
Age: 62
Surface (flat/palpable/nodular): palpable
Maximum diameter: 4 mm
Duration of the lesion: unknown
History of morphologic changes:
Personal history of skin cancer (if yes, please specify):
Family history of skin cancer (if yes, please specify):
Skin phototype: III
Total nevus count (<10, 10–50, 50–100, >100): 10–50
Other clinical findings (optional): she had personal history of multiple basal cell carcinomas.

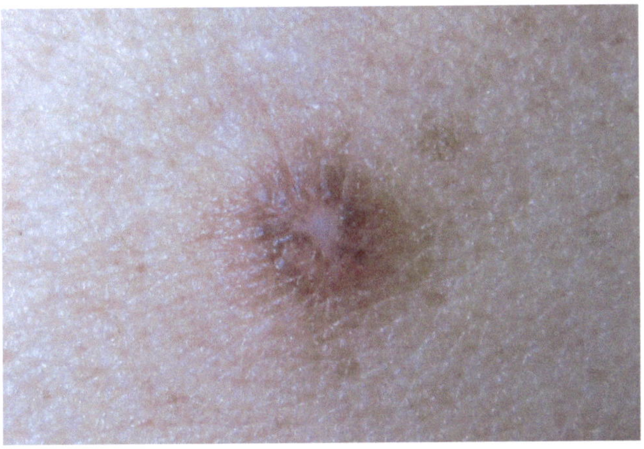

Fig. 22.7 Clinical image. Slightly elevated pigmented lesion, located on the left arm

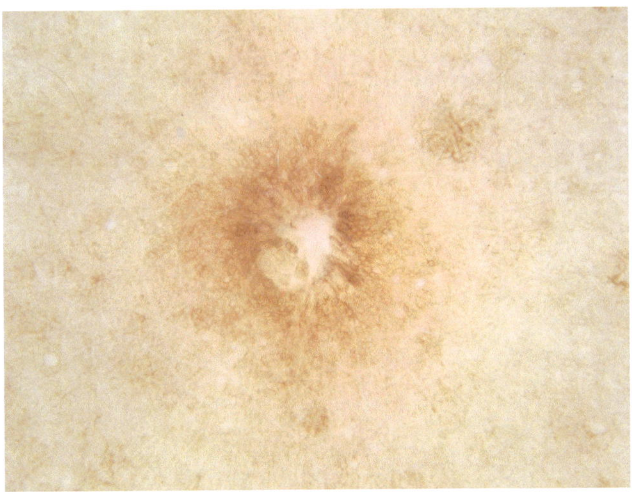

Fig. 22.8 Dermoscopic image

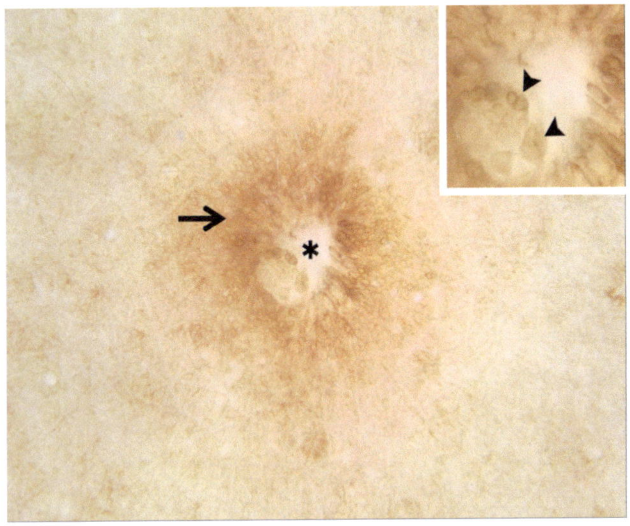

Fig. 22.9 Dermoscopic examination with polarized light dermoscope showed a central scar-like white patch (asterisk), pseudo globular structures in the central area (arrowheads), and delicate peripheral pigment network (arrow)

Key Message
Diagnosis: dermatofibroma

Dermatofibromas are frequent benign cutaneous fibrohistiocytic tumors which clinically exhibit a "dimple sign." More common in females than males, these lesions may be single or multiple and are preferentially located on the legs. Although its clinical manifestations are usually typical, dermoscopy improves diagnosis. There are several dermoscopic types of dermatofibromas. The most common is characterized by a central white scar-like patch and a peripheral thin pigment network (or network-like structure).Even though the presence of a pigment network is a major dermoscopic criterion for melanocytic lesions, dermatofibromas and accessory nipples are exceptions to the rule.

Palpable Nonpigmented Lesions on the Upper Limbs

23

Gabriel Salerni

Case 1: G.S.

Sex: male
Age: 33 years
Surface (flat/palpable/nodular): palpable
Maximum diameter: 5 mm
Duration of the lesion: 6 months
History of morphologic changes: increase in size since occurrence
Personal history of skin cancer (if yes, please specify): no
Family history of skin cancer (if yes, please specify): no
Skin phototype: 3
Total nevus count (<10, 10–50, 50–100, >100): 50–100
Other clinical findings (optional):

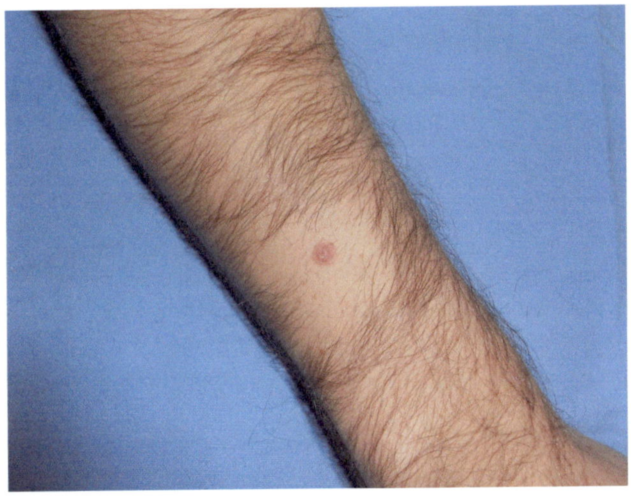

Fig. 23.1 Lesion in the forearm, slightly elevated, symmetric with pink coloration

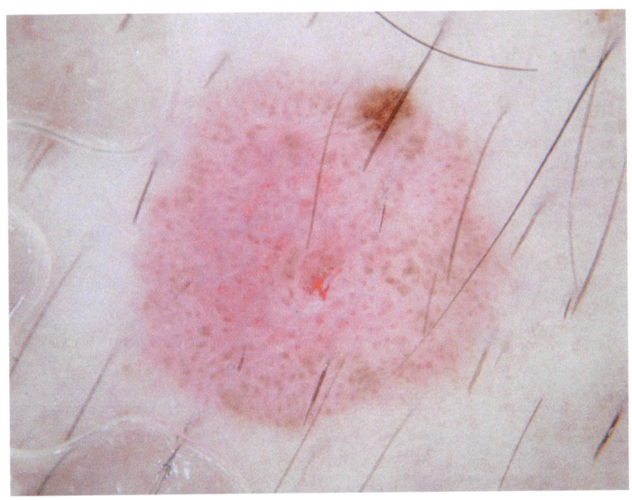

Fig. 23.2 Dermoscopy view

G. Salerni
Dermatologist Doctor in Medicine Universidad Nacional de Rosario and Hospital Provincial del Centenario de Rosario
Santa Fe, Santa Fe, Argentina
e-mail: gabrielsalerni@gmail.com

H. Cabo, A. Lallas (eds.), *Comprehensive Atlas of Dermatoscopy Cases*, https://doi.org/10.1007/978-3-319-76932-5_23

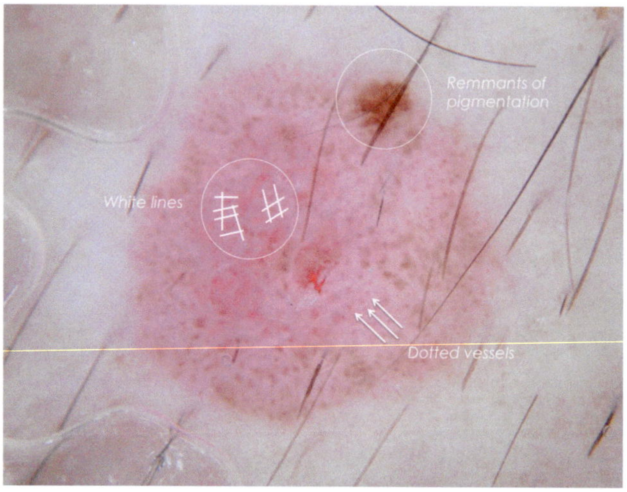

Fig. 23.3 Dermoscopy examination revealed a homogeneous vascular pattern with dotted vessels, pink (milky red) background with white lines. An eccentric focus of brown pigmentation is also observed

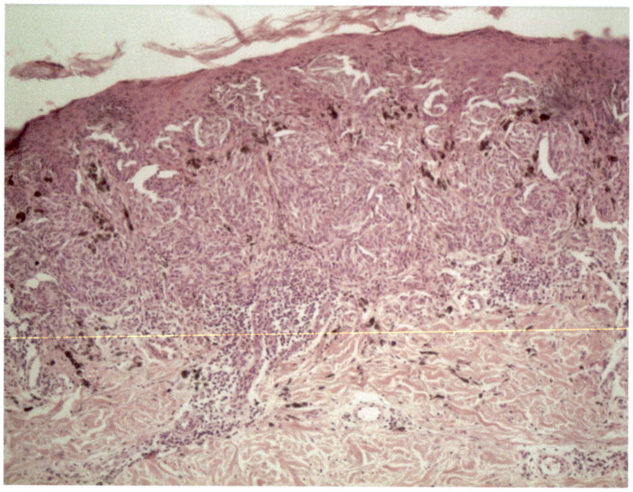

Fig. 23.4 Histology revealed a melanocytic proliferation with junctional component forming vertical oval nests. There is slight epidermal hyperplasia, as well as shrinkage artifacts surrounding junctional nests. Overall, the architecture is regular (cellular features, arrangement of cells, type and degree of reactive changes). The diagnosis is Spitz nevus, spindle cell type

Key Message

A lesion with dotted vessels in a regular arrangement when additional criteria, such as reticular depigmentation, crystalline structures, and remnants of pigmentation, are present is suggestive of Spitz nevus or thin amelanotic melanoma, and excision is recommended.

Nodular Pigmented Lesions on the Upper Limbs

24

Horacio Cabo

Case 1: H.C.

Sex:
Age:
Surface: nodular
Maximum diameter: 8 mm
Duration of the lesion: 6 month
History of morphologic changes: yes
Personal history of skin cancer: no
Family history of skin cancer:
Skin phototype: III
Total nevus count: 10–50

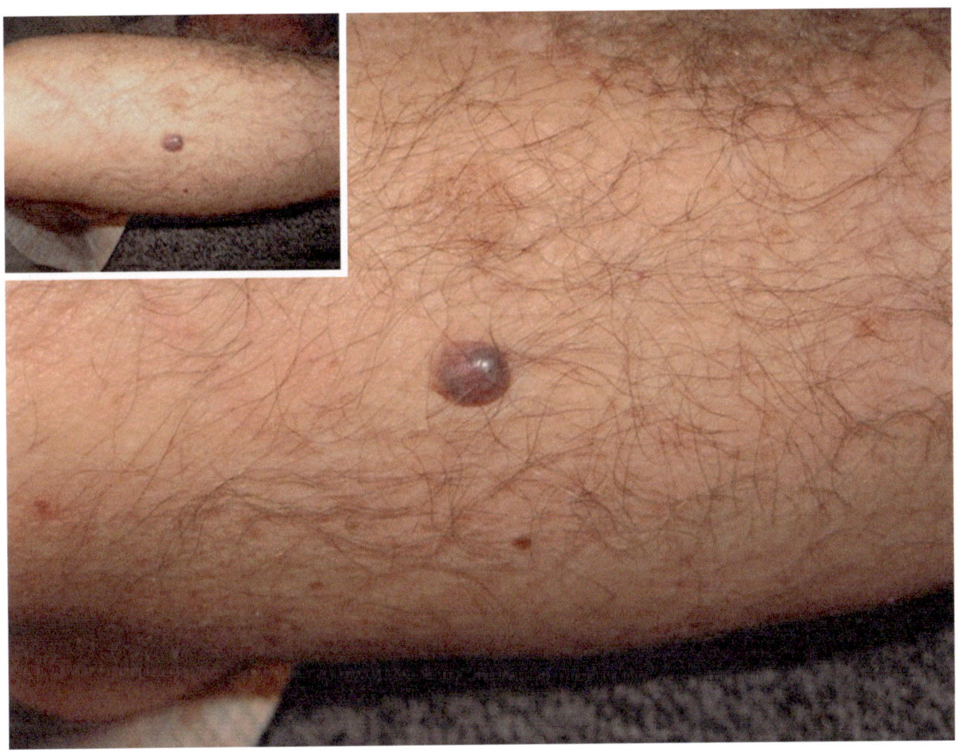

Fig. 24.1 Clinical image: firm, dark bluish nodular lesion

H. Cabo
Instituto de Investigaciones Medicas "A. Lanari". Dermatology Section, University of Buenos Aires, Buenos Aires, Argentina

H. Cabo, A. Lallas (eds.), *Comprehensive Atlas of Dermatoscopy Cases*, https://doi.org/10.1007/978-3-319-76932-5_24

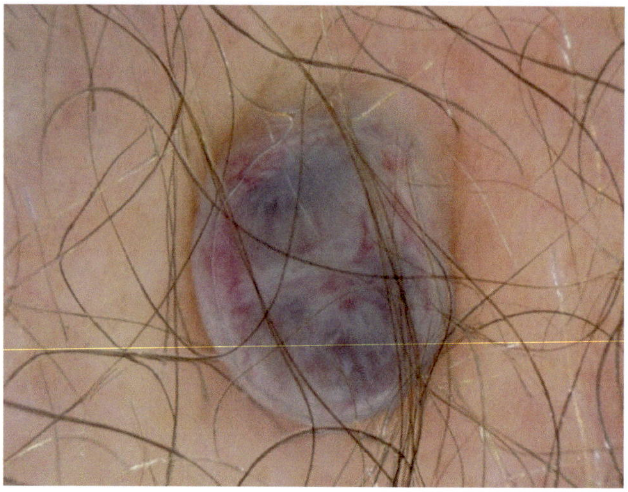

Fig. 24.2 Dermoscopy image

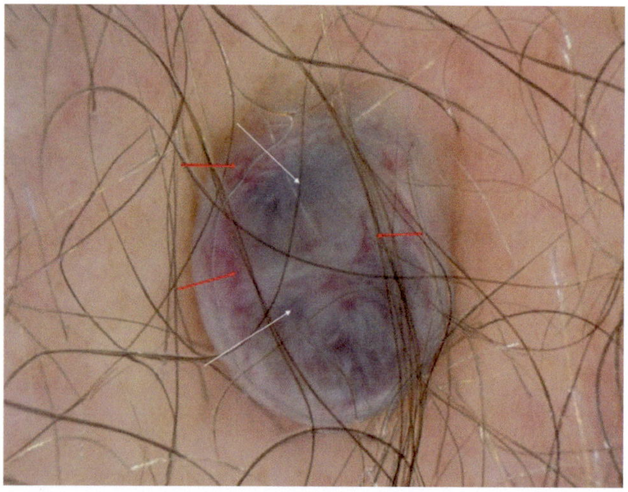

Fig. 24.3 Dermoscopy image: blue areas (white arrows); branching vessels (red arrows)

Key Message

Diagnosis: Dermal eccrine acrospiroma

A benign adnexal neoplasm that grows fast

The blue hue is a clue to malignancy especially in clinically equivocal melanocytic skin lesions.

The main differential diagnoses are basal cell carcinoma and nodular melanoma because both can show blue-red color and irregular lineal and branching vessels.

Nodular Nonpigmented Lesions on the Upper Limbs

25

Horacio Cabo

Case 1

Sex: male
Age: 69
Surface: nodular
Maximum diameter: 9 mm
Duration of the lesion: >1 year
History of morphologic changes: yes
Personal history of skin cancer: no
Family history of skin cancer: no
Skin phototype: III
Total nevus count: 10–50
Other clinical findings: no

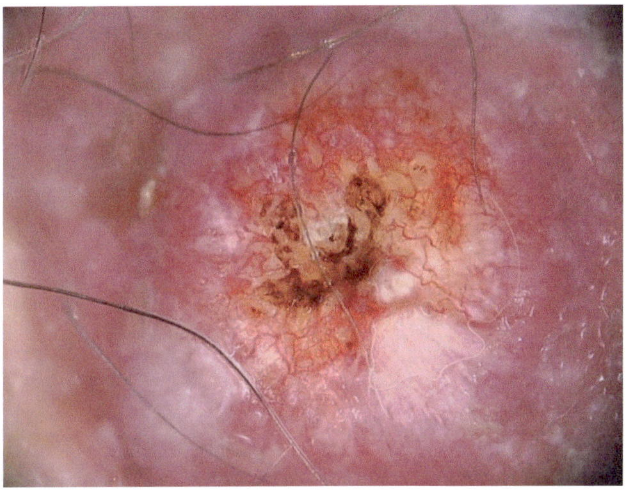

Fig. 25.1 Clinical view. Elevated lesion on dorsum of the right hand, with central hyperkeratosis

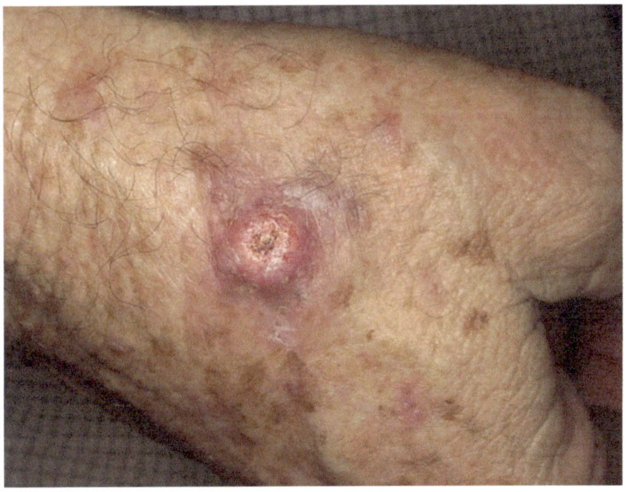

Fig. 25.2 Dermoscopy view

H. Cabo
Instituto de Investigaciones Medicas "A. Lanari". Dermatology Section, University of Buenos Aires, Buenos Aires, Argentina

H. Cabo, A. Lallas (eds.), *Comprehensive Atlas of Dermatoscopy Cases*, https://doi.org/10.1007/978-3-319-76932-5_25

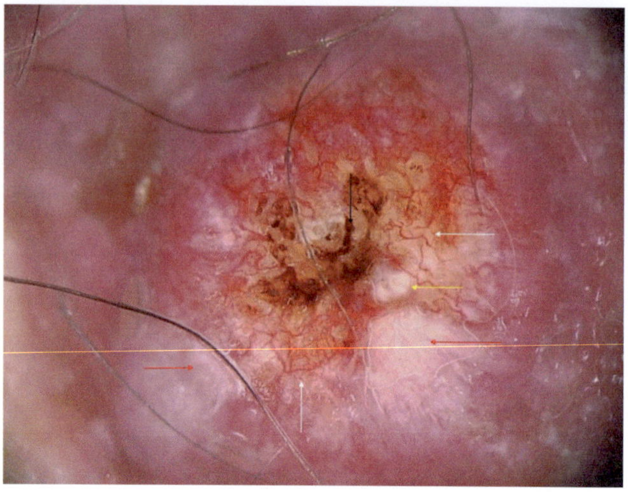

Fig. 25.3 Dermoscopy view. Central hyperkeratosis (black arrow); white areas (red arrows); white circle (yellow arrow); peripheral linear irregular vessels (white arrows)

Key Message

Diagnosis: Squamous cell carcinoma.

The major criteria are white areas and circles, peripheral irregular vessels, and central hyperkeratosis

Flat Pigmented Lesions on the Lower Limbs

26

Horacio Cabo, Oriol Yélamos, Manu Jain,
Ashfaq A. Marghoob, Romana Kupsa, Roberta Giuffrida,
Georg Richtig, Teresa Deinlein, Cesare Massone,
Erika Richtig, and Iris Zalaudek

Case 1 H.C.

Sex: female
Age: 54
Surface: flat
Maximum diameter: 9 mm
Duration of the lesion: > 5 years
History of morphologic changes: no
Personal history of skin cancer: no
Family history of skin cancer: no
Skin photo type: II
Total nevus count: 10–50
Other clinical findings: the patient has multiple lesions on the legs that are worsening with the UV exposition

Key Message
Diagnosis: Porokeratosis (disseminated actinic porokeratosis)

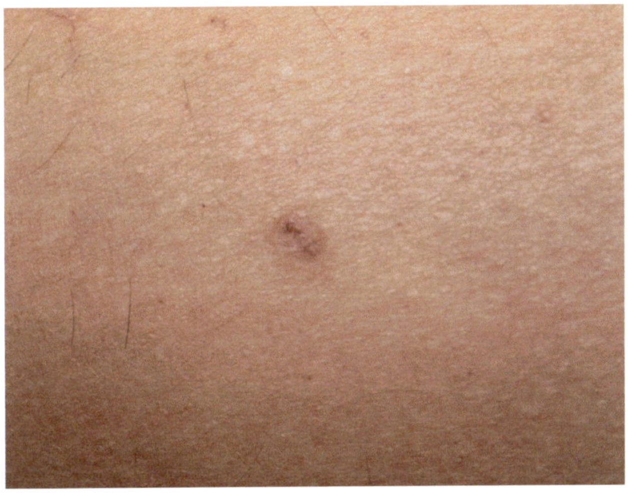

Fig. 26.1 Clinical view: light brown-colored lesion with peripheral elevated border and rough surface

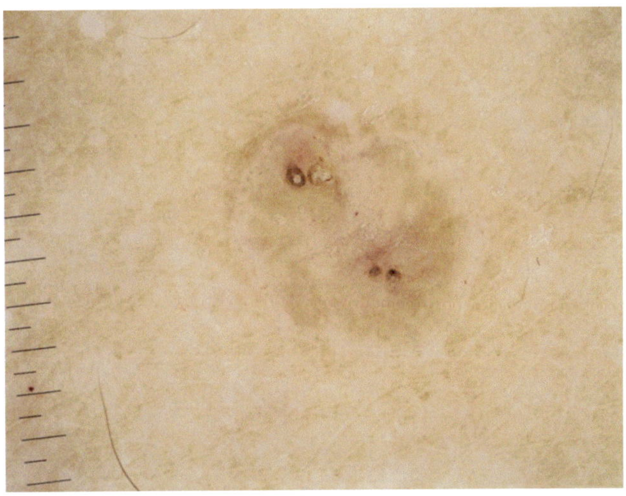

Fig. 26.2 Dermoscopy view

H. Cabo (✉)
Instituto de Investigaciones Medicas "A. Lanari". Dermatology Section, University of Buenos Aires, Buenos Aires, Argentina

O. Yélamos · M. Jain · A. A. Marghoob
Memorial Sloan Kettering Cancer Center, New York, NY, USA
e-mail: yelamoso@mskcc.org; jainm@mskcc.org

R. Kupsa · T. Deinlein · E. Richtig · I. Zalaudek
Department of Dermatology, Medical University of Graz, Graz, Austria

R. Giuffrida
Department of Clinical and Experimental Medicine, Section of Dermatology, University of Messina, Messina, Italy

G. Richtig
Department of Dermatology, Medical University of Graz, Graz, Austria

Institute of Experimental and Clinical Pharmacology, Medical University of Graz, Graz, Austria

C. Massone
Department of Dermatology, Medical University of Graz, Graz, Austria

Department of Dermatology, Galliera Hospital, Genoa, Italy

H. Cabo, A. Lallas (eds.), *Comprehensive Atlas of Dermatoscopy Cases*, https://doi.org/10.1007/978-3-319-76932-5_26

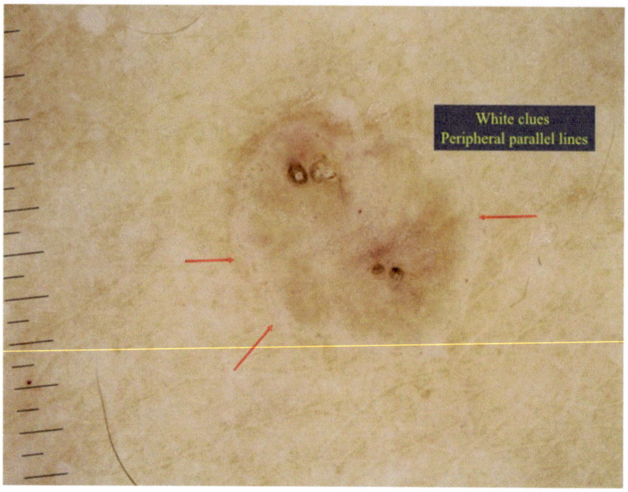

Fig. 26.3 Dermoscopy view: notice the peripheral white parallel lines (red arrows)

The dermoscopy clue are the peripheral white parallel lines (white tract) that correspond to the cornoid lamella.

In addition, we can observe brown color in the central area, some dotted vessels, and rough surface.

Case 2 O.Y., M.J., A.M.

Sex: male
Age: 67
Surface (flat/palpable/nodular): flat
Maximum diameter: 4 mm
Duration of the lesion: unknown
History of morphologic changes: During routine skin cancer surveillance examination, an isolated pigmented lesion was noted on this 67-year-old male's leg. He was unaware of the presence of this lesion. He denied sustaining any trauma to the area. Close inspection of his baseline clinical images obtained 2 years prior disclosed a slightly raised skin-colored lesion at the same location.
Personal history of skin cancer (if yes, please specify): Yes. One melanoma in situ on the abdomen excised 4 years ago and one infiltrative basal cell carcinoma on his right chest excised 5 years ago.
Family history of skin cancer (if yes, please specify): No.
Skin phototype: III
Total nevus count: (<10, 10–50, 50–100, >100): 50–100
Other clinical findings (optional): The lesion revealed an atypical starburst pattern with streaks when viewed with dermoscopy (Fig. 26.4). A dermoscopy pattern consisting of streaks distributed in a centrifugal fashion leads to a differential diagnosis consisting mainly of melanoma, Spitz/Reed nevi, and recurrent/traumatized nevus. On rare occasions, the peripherally located leaf-like or spoke-wheel-like structures in a pigmented BCC can mimic the streaks seen in melanocytic lesions. Based on the dermoscopy pattern and the overview clinical images (Fig. 26.5), the diagnosis of a recurrent nevus was favored. Histologic examination confirmed that the lesion was indeed a recurrent/traumatized nevus (Fig. 26.6).

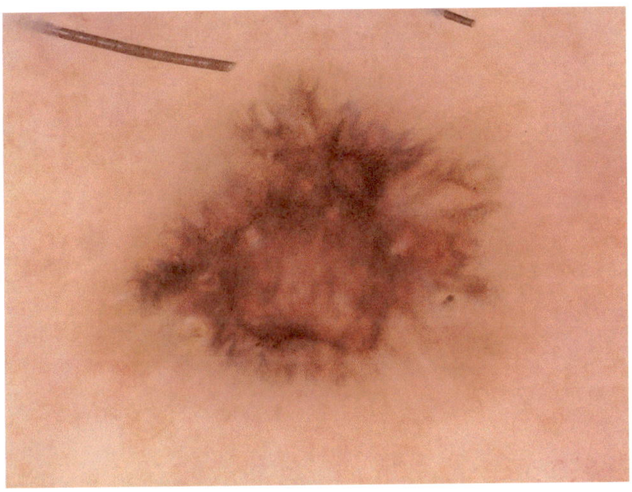

Fig. 26.4 Dermoscopically, the lesion revealed an atypical starburst pattern with radial lines and irregular dots arranged in a centrifugal fashion. The overall pattern was not that of a pigmented BCC. The differential diagnosis was narrowed down to melanoma versus Spitz/Reed nevus versus recurrent/traumatized nevus

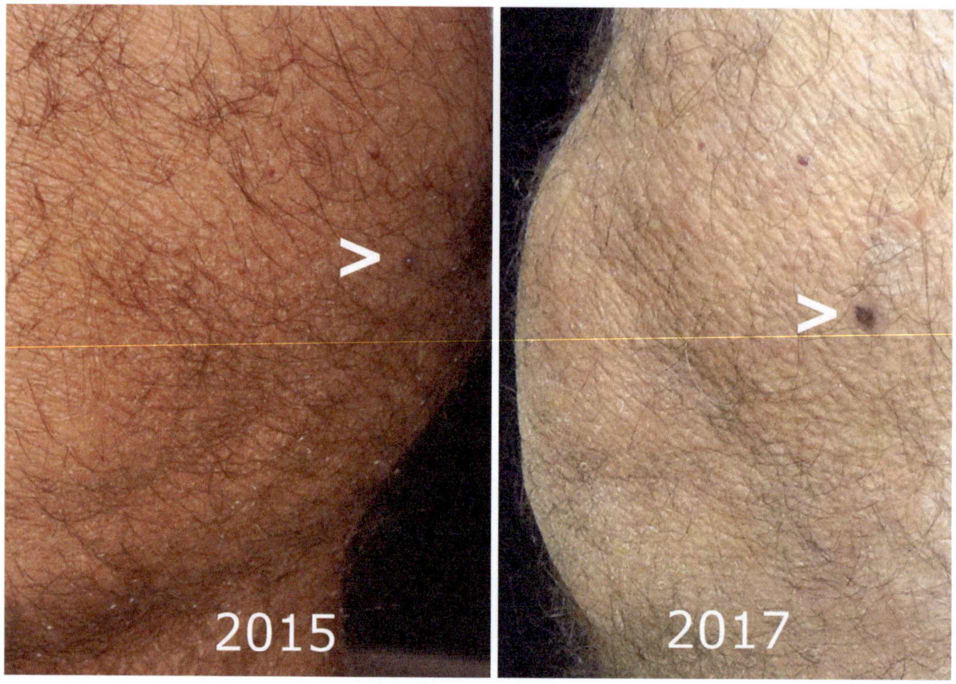

Fig. 26.5 After careful review of the baseline clinical images obtained 2 years previously, a presumed intradermal nevus was noted to have been present in the same area

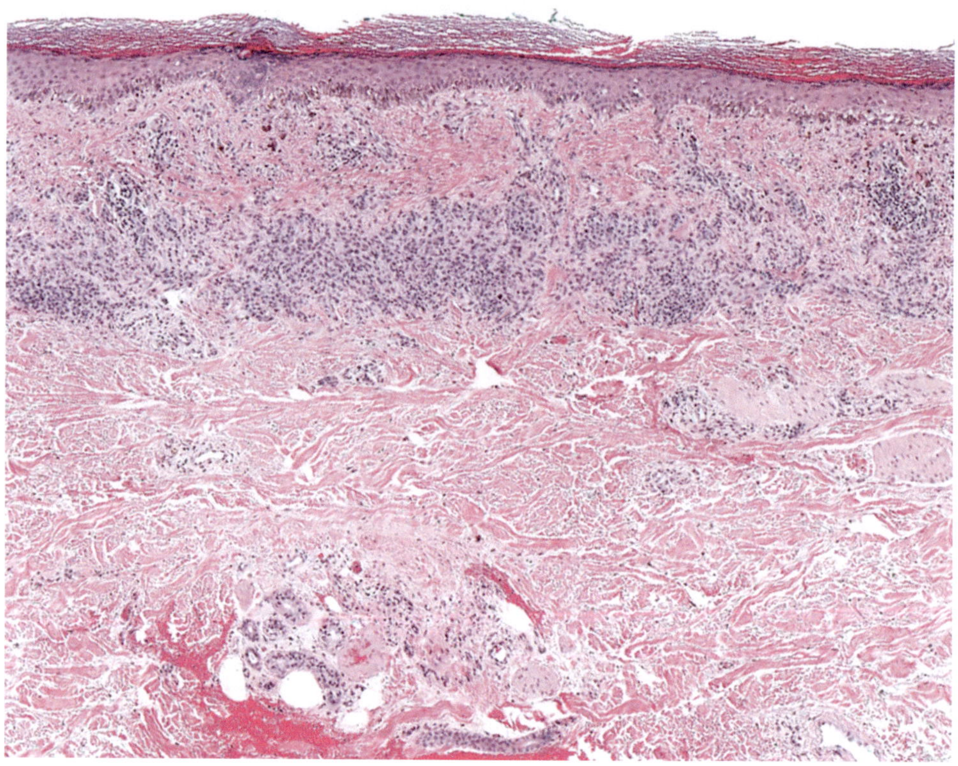

Fig. 26.6 Histologic examination of the case revealed a compound melanocytic nevus with fibrosis suggestive of a recurrent/traumatized nevus (hematoxylin and eosin)

Key Message

Radial lines arranged in a centrifugal pattern at the periphery are associated most commonly with Spitz/Reed nevi and recurrent nevi but can also be seen on rare occasions in superficial spreading melanoma and on extremely rare occasions in superficial pigmented BCC. Clues to the diagnosis of recurrent/traumatized nevi include a previous history of trauma/biopsy and the confinement of pigment to within the scar when evaluated with dermoscopy [1]. Without such a history, one needs to more seriously consider the possibility that the lesion may represent a melanoma (or perhaps a superficial pigmented BCC). Since Spitz/Reed nevi occur infrequently in adults and since superficial spreading melanomas can manifest a morphology mimicking Spitz/Reed nevi, lesions with streaks in adults should generally be biopsied [2].

Case 3 R.K., R.G., G.R., T.D., C.M., I.Z.

Sex: male
Age: 80
Surface (flat/palpable/nodular): flat
Maximum diameter: 1 cm in diameter
Duration of the lesion: approximately 3 years
History of morphologic changes: The lesion was first noticed by the patient 3 years before and has slowly enlarged over the time. One month prior to the current visit, he noticed a progressive hypopigmentation around the pigmented macule. Clinically, the lesion on his arm presented as central ill-defined, gray-bluish-black macule with shades of red that was surrounded by a white halo. Dermoscopically, a structureless gray, white, and red-to-brown pattern was seen. In some areas, gray dots forming lines were additionally noted. Furthermore, a circular, white, symmetrical halo was seen. Taking into account the history and the clinical-dermoscopic features, a diagnosis of halo melanoma was made, and the lesion was biopsied.
Personal history of skin cancer (if yes, please specify): none
Family history of skin cancer (if yes, please specify): none
Skin phototype: 2
Total nevus count: (<10, 10–50, 50–100, >100): 50–100
Other clinical findings (optional):
The punch biopsy of the pigmented area revealed a nonconclusive, fully regressed lesion. Based on the history, the clinical and dermoscopic features, and the histopathology showing a completely regressed tumor, we suspected the diagnosis of fully regressed halo melanoma and excised the lesion completely, but also histopathology of the completely excised tumor was not conclusive as only regression was seen.
Histopathology revealed a normal epidermis without a melanocytic proliferation. A band-like lymphohistiocytic inflammatory infiltrate with numerous melanophages was observed in both the papillary dermis and upper dermis. Results of HMB-45, S100, and Melan-A stainings were negative.

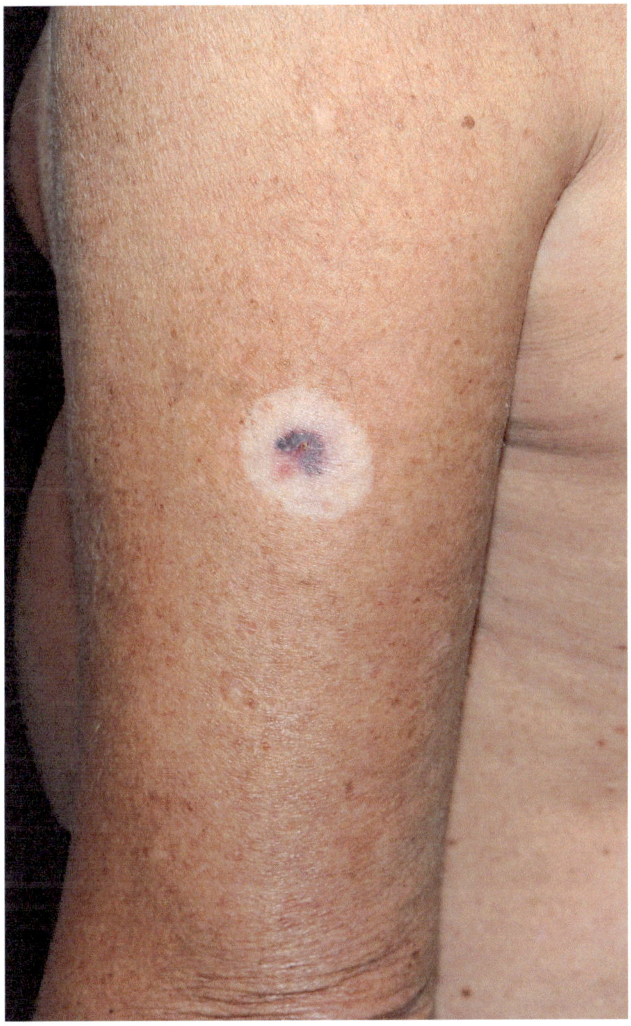

Fig. 26.7 Clinical image of a halo melanoma located on the left lateral upper arm. An asymmetric bluish-black-reddish macule measuring 1 cm in diameter and an evident white halo is seen

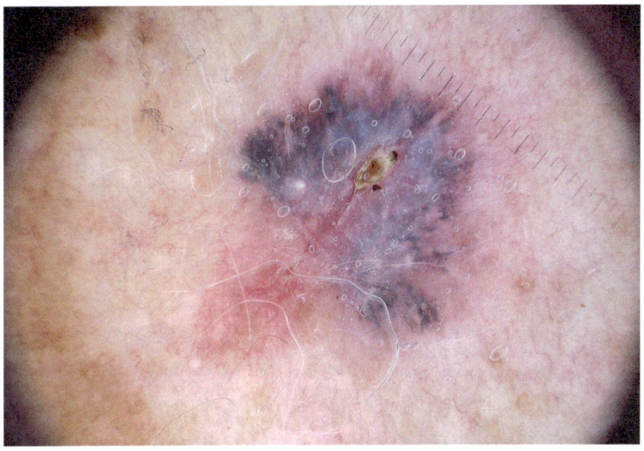

Fig. 26.8 Dermatoscopic image of the same suspicious melanoma. Evidence of the previously taken punch biopsy is observable as a yellowish crust in the center of the lesion. Gray dots that formed unstructured areas as well as lines, a whitish veil, and nonpigmented areas with atypical vascular pattern are visible

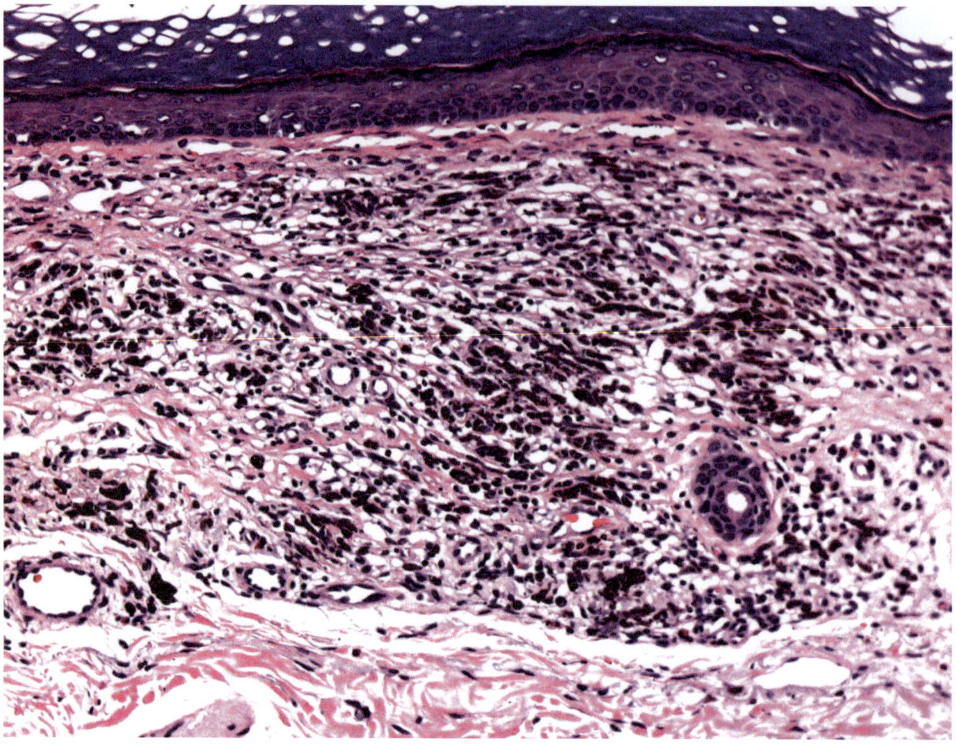

Fig. 26.9 Histopathologic picture

Key Message

The immunogenic response resulting in the so-called halo phenomenon occurs frequently in benign nevi of youth while being uncommon in melanoma. Nevertheless, it is important to differentiate a halo nevus from halo melanoma. The clinical history, the patients' age, and the number of affected lesions are important criteria for the differential diagnosis. Dermoscopy often allows recognizing benign nevus pattern within the halo, while melanoma often shows a chaotic arrangement of colors. Despite the clinical difficulties, also histopathology may face troubles in an accurate differentiation between both entities. As in our case, a conclusive diagnosis was impossible due to complete regression of specific features allowing to assign the lesion to any specific diagnosis.

Special caution is always warranted for solitary lesions in adults with a history of enlargement and with a sudden onset of a halo phenomenon.

Flat Non-pigmented Lesion on the Lower Limbs

27

Danica Tiodorovic

Case 1

Sex: female
Age: 28
Surface (flat/palpable/nodular): flat
Maximum diameter: 13 mm
Duration of the lesion: 6 weeks
History of morphologic changes: slightly increasing in diameter over the time
Personal history of skin cancer (if yes, please specify): no
Family history of skin cancer (if yes, please specify): no
Skin phototype: III
Total nevus count: (<10, 10–50, 50–100, >100): 10–50
Other clinical findings (optional): none

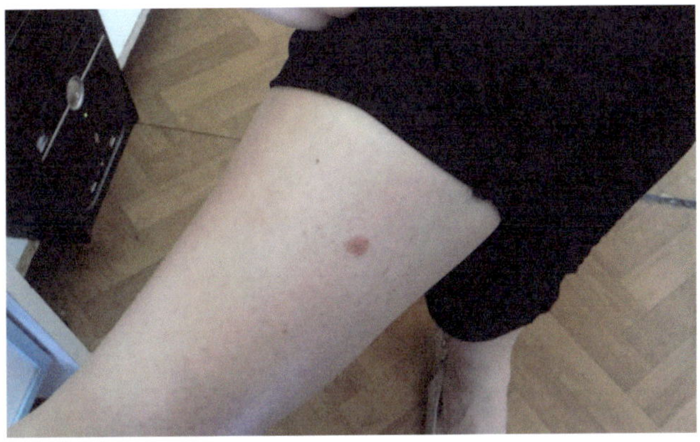

Fig. 27.1 Clinical image of lesion located on the left lower leg revealed a pigmented reddish macule resembling an inflammatory lesion

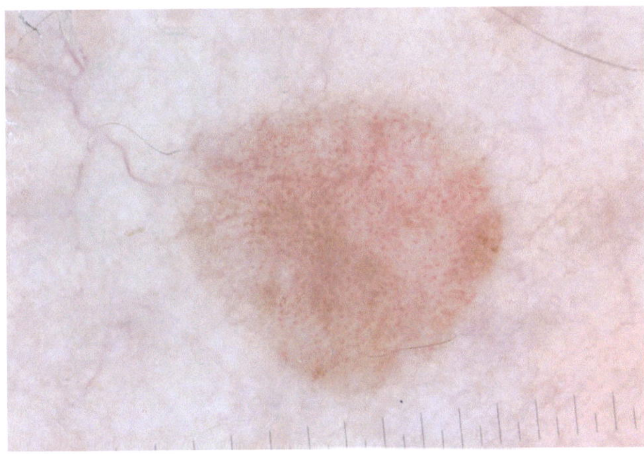

Fig. 27.2 Dermoscopic image of the lesion revealed absence of typical pigmented network and presence of dotted vessels together with remnants of the pigmentation on the milky red background, indicating the diagnosis of hypomelanotic melanoma

D. Tiodorovic
Medical Faculty of Nis, Serbia, Clinic of Dermatology,
Clinical Center Nis, Nis, Serbia
e-mail: danica.dr@gmail.com

H. Cabo, A. Lallas (eds.), *Comprehensive Atlas of Dermatoscopy Cases*, https://doi.org/10.1007/978-3-319-76932-5_27

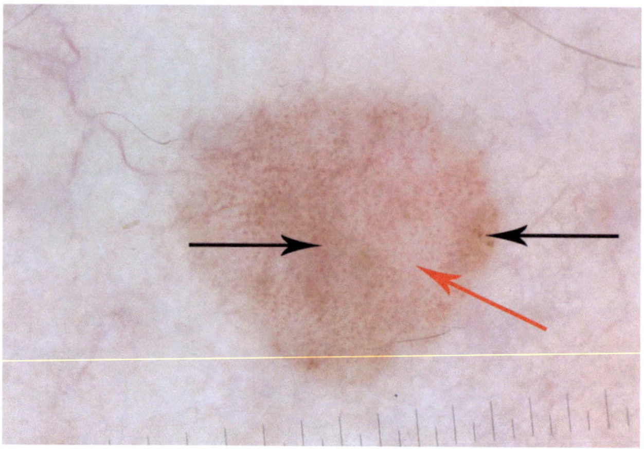

Fig. 27.3 Black arrow indicates dotted vessels, while red arrow shows remnants of pigmentation

Key Message

Milky red coloration together with vessels and remnants of pigmentation represent a clue to diagnosis of hypomelanotic melanoma

Palpable Pigmented Lesion of the Lower Limbs

28

Giuseppe Argenziano, Gabriella Brancaccio, Antonia Laino, and H. Peter Soyer

Case 1: G.A., G.B.

Sex: male
Age: 82
Surface (flat/palpable/nodular): palpable
Maximum diameter: 9 mm
Duration of the lesion: 1 year
History of morphologic changes: no
Personal history of skin cancer (if yes, please specify): yes, a previous basal cell carcinoma
Family history of skin cancer (if yes, please specify): no
Skin phototype: III
Total nevus count (<10, 10–50, 50–100, >100): 10–50
Other clinical findings (optional): presence of numerous seborrheic keratosis, freckles, and actinic keratosis on the scalp

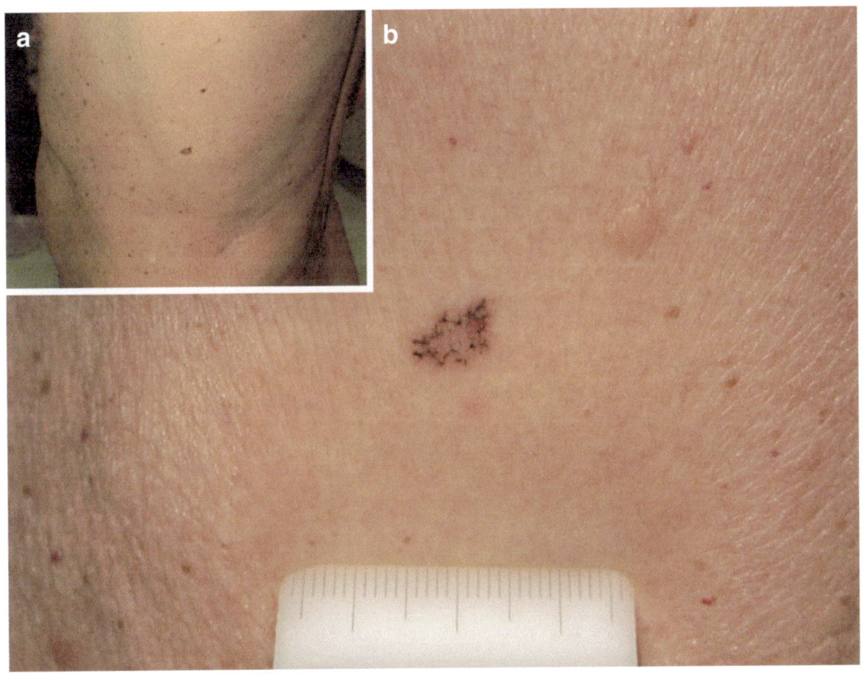

Fig. 28.1 (**a**) Clinical image: on clinical examination, there is a symmetric lesion located on the upper leg, unevenly pigmented. (**b**) Close-up of the clinical view

G. Argenziano (✉) · G. Brancaccio
Dermatology Unit, University of Campania, Naples, Italy
e-mail: g.argenziano@gmail.com

A. Laino
University of Queensland (UQ), St Lucia, QLD, Australia

H. Peter Soyer
Department of Dermatology, The University of Queensland (UQ), St Lucia, QLD, Australia

H. Cabo, A. Lallas (eds.), *Comprehensive Atlas of Dermatoscopy Cases*, https://doi.org/10.1007/978-3-319-76932-5_28

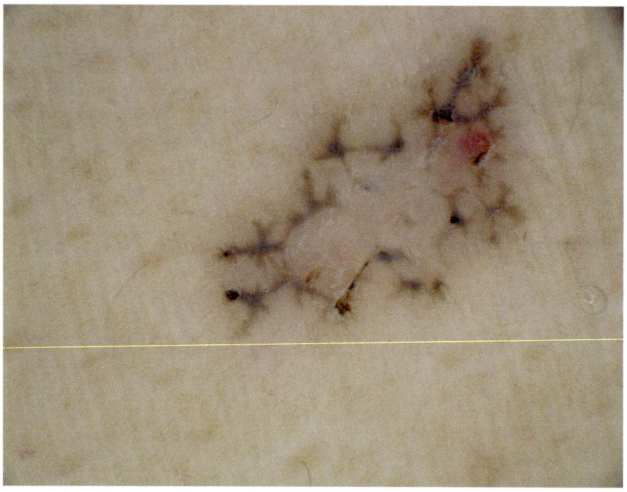

Fig. 28.2 Dermoscopy view

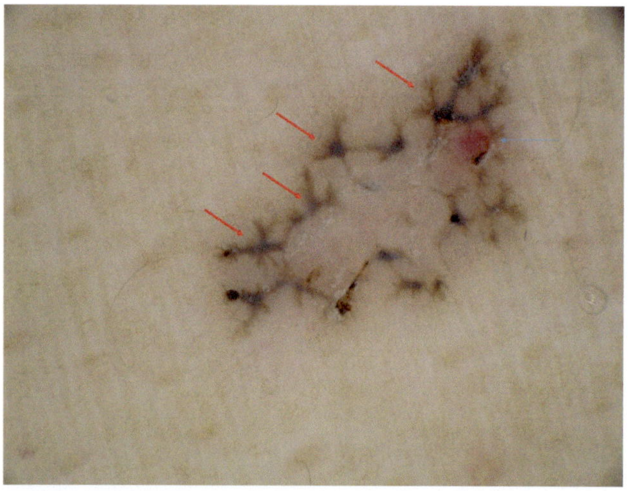

Fig. 28.3 Dermoscopy view: spoke wheel projections meeting a darker central axis (red arrows) and ulceration (white arrow)

Key Message

Spoke wheel areas are a pathognomonic feature of basal cell carcinoma.

Case 2: A.L., H.P.S.

Sex: female
Age: 49 years old
Surface (flat/palpable/nodular): palpable
Maximum diameter: 7.5 mm
Duration of the lesion: long-standing, patient reported lesion present for more than 20 years.
History of morphologic changes: yes, lesion had developed a central dark-brown clod over the course of 4 months.
Personal history of skin cancer (if yes, please specify): two prior melanoma diagnoses: left upper arm Clark level 2 superficial spreading melanoma 2008; right elbow Clark level 1 melanoma 2011
Family history of skin cancer (if yes, please specify): yes, father was diagnosed with melanoma at age 40 years.
Skin phototype: Fitzpatrick skin type I
Total nevus count (<10, 10–50, 50–100, >100): 50–100

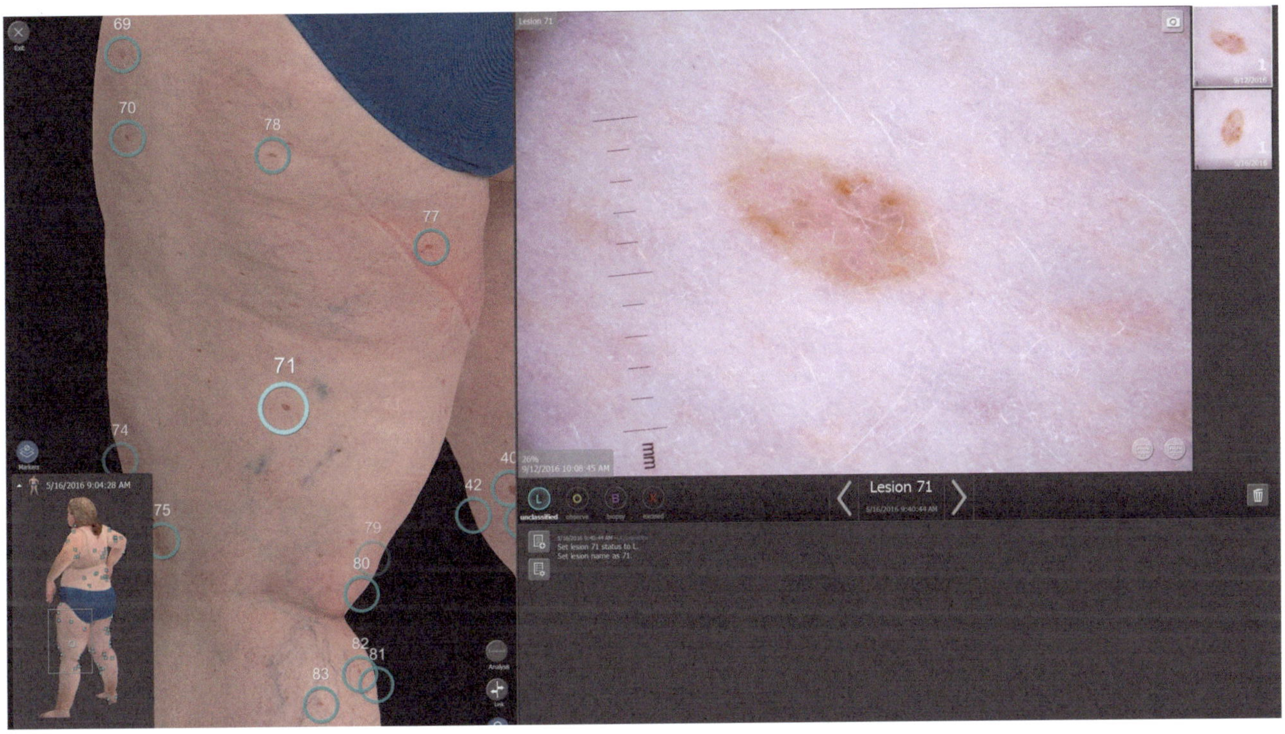

Fig. 28.4 3D body image taken with VECTRA whole body 360 system and associated dermoscopic image of lesion

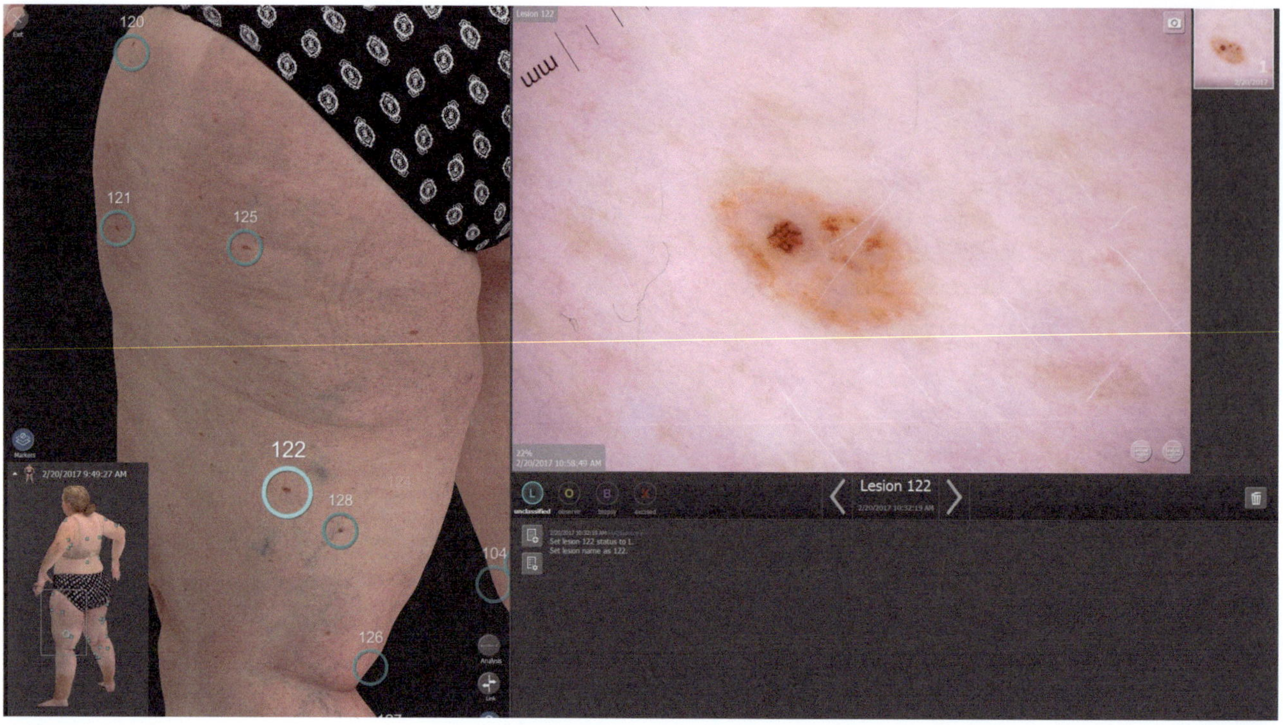

Fig. 28.5 3D body image taken with VECTRA whole body 360 system and associated dermoscopic image of lesion, 4 months after initial imaging. New area of pigmentation noted in the upper left quadrant of lesion

Key Message

The lesion was excised and histopathology showed a severely dysplastic compound nevus, with changes in one area falling just short of level 1 melanoma. This case demonstrates the rapid rate at which nevi change, and the importance of early identification of these changes. The patient had not noted any morphologic changes in the nevus between imaging sessions, and as such this lesion may have been followed up as an "atypical nevus" without immediate excision. Sequential dermoscopic imaging systems aid dermatologists in determining which lesions have undergone substantial changes over time and assist in the early diagnosis of melanoma.

Palpable Nonpigmented Lesion of the Lower Limbs

29

Horacio Cabo, Chryssoula Papageorgiou, and Aimilios Lallas

Case 1: H.C.

Sex: female
Age: 63
Surface: palpable
Maximum diameter: 11 mm
Duration of the lesion: >1 year
History of morphologic changes: yes
Personal history of skin cancer: no
Family history of skin cancer: no
Skin photo type: II
Total nevus count: 10–50
Other clinical findings: very sun-damaged skin

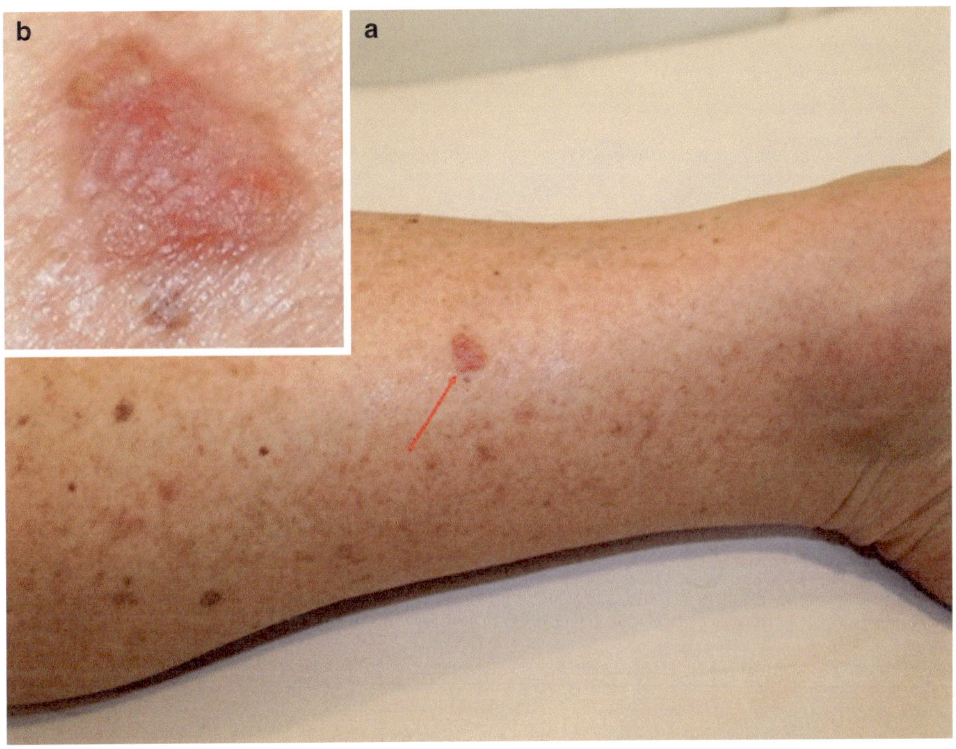

Fig. 29.1 Clinical view: (**a**) asymmetric pink lesion with rough surface on the left leg (red arrow); (**b**) close-up of the clinical view

H. Cabo (✉)
Instituto de Investigaciones Medicas "A. Lanari". Dermatology Section, University of Buenos Aires, Buenos Aires, Argentina

C. Papageorgiou · A. Lallas
First Department of Dermatology, Aristotle University of Thessaloniki, Thessaloniki, Greece

H. Cabo, A. Lallas (eds.), *Comprehensive Atlas of Dermatoscopy Cases*, https://doi.org/10.1007/978-3-319-76932-5_29

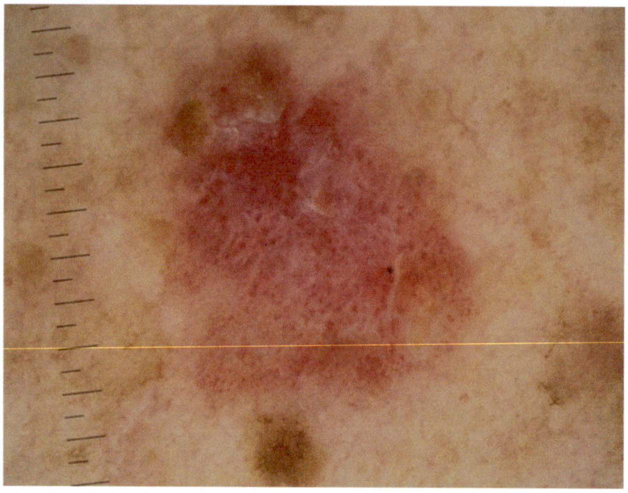

Fig. 29.2 Dermoscopy view

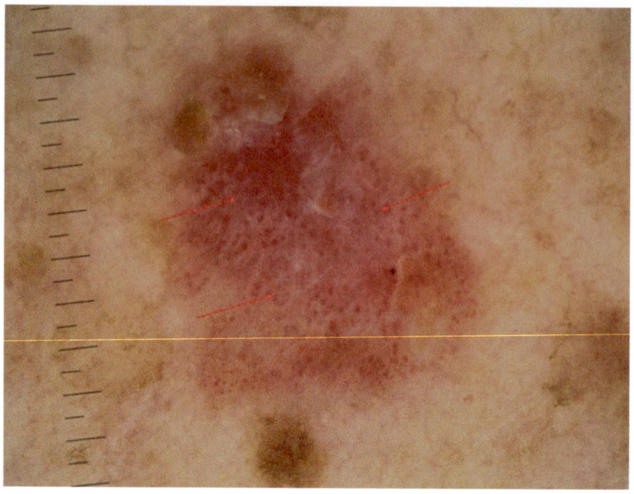

Fig. 29.3 Dermoscopy view: glomerular or spiral vessels, monomorphic pattern, focal distribution (red arrows)

Key Message

Diagnosis: Squamous cell carcinoma in situ—no pigmented Bowen's disease

Dermoscopy clues:

- Vessels
  - Glomerular or spiral vessels
  - Monomorphic pattern
  - Focal distribution
- Rough surface

Case 2: A.L.

Sex: female
Age: 61
Surface (flat/palpable/nodular): palpable
Maximum diameter: 1.7 cm
Duration of the lesion: 6 months
History of morphologic changes: yes, gradually enlarging
Personal history of skin cancer (if yes, please specify): no
Family history of skin cancer (if yes, please specify): no
Skin phototype: III
Total nevus count (<10, 10–50, 50–100, >100): 10–50
Other clinical findings (optional):

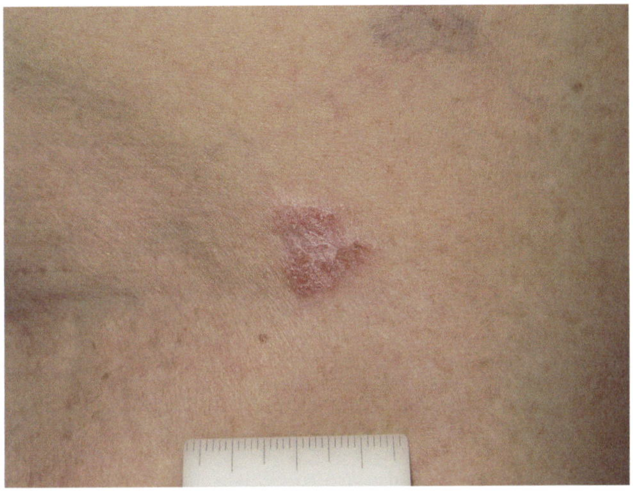

Fig. 29.4 Clinically, there is a solitary erythematous, scaly plaque with irregular borders and a small erosion on the right side located on the lower limbs

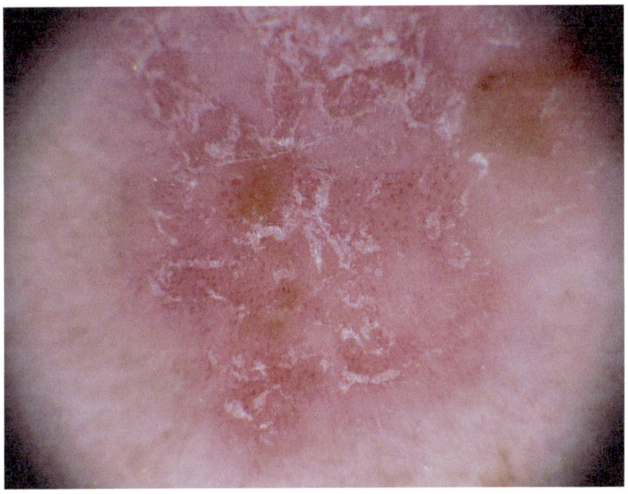

Fig. 29.5 From the dermoscopic point of view, the lesion appears glomerular and few dotted vessels together with white opaque scales and a red-yellowish background. On the right side, small erosion is also visible

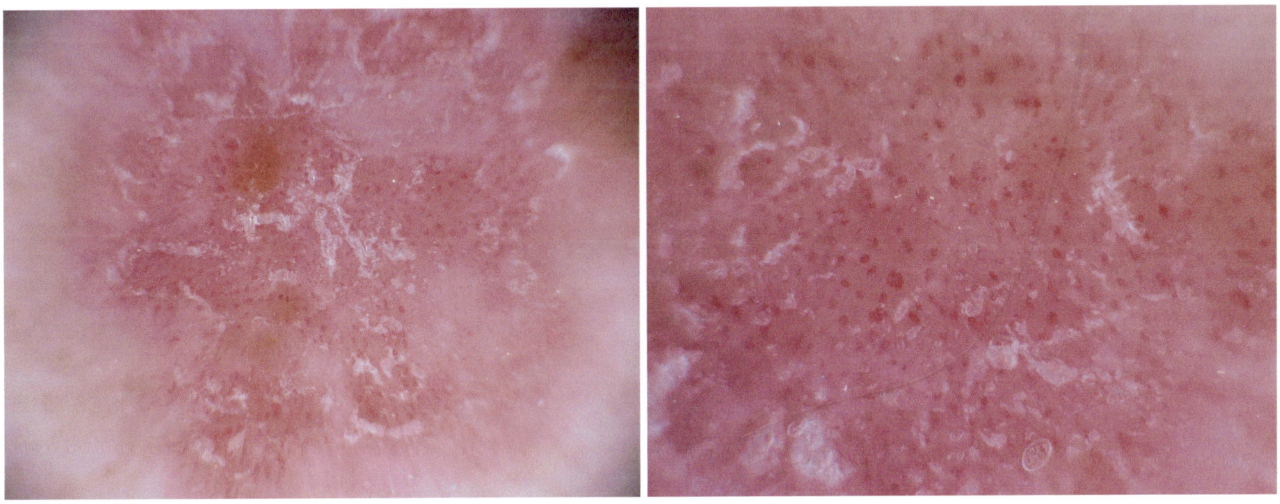

Figs. 29.6 and 29.7 In a higher magnification, glomerular vessels are even more apparent

Key Message

In this lesion, the presence of glomerular vessels combined with white scales is suggestive of Bowen's disease.

Nodular Nonpigmented Lesions on the Lower Limbs

30

Horacio Cabo, John Paoli, and Pedro Diego Zaballos

Case 1 H.C.

Sex: female
Age: 39
Surface: nodular
Maximum diameter: 9 mm
Duration of the lesion: < 8 months
History of morphologic changes: yes
Personal history of skin cancer: no
Family history of skin cancer: no
Skin photo type: III
Total nevus count: 10–50
Other clinical findings: the lesion is on the left heel and it is growing since 6 month ago

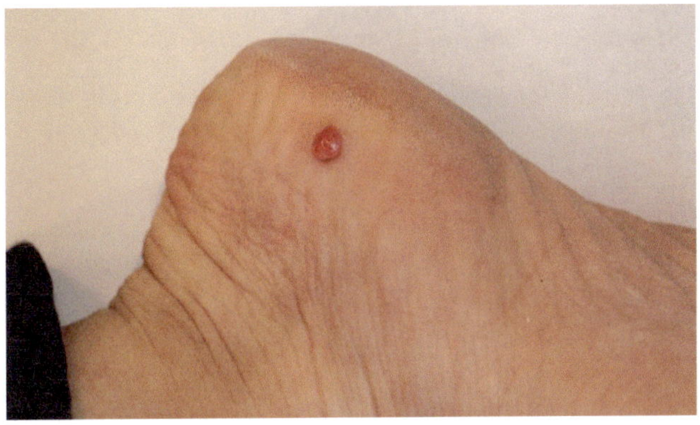

Fig. 30.1 Clinical view: pink acral nodular lesion on the left heel

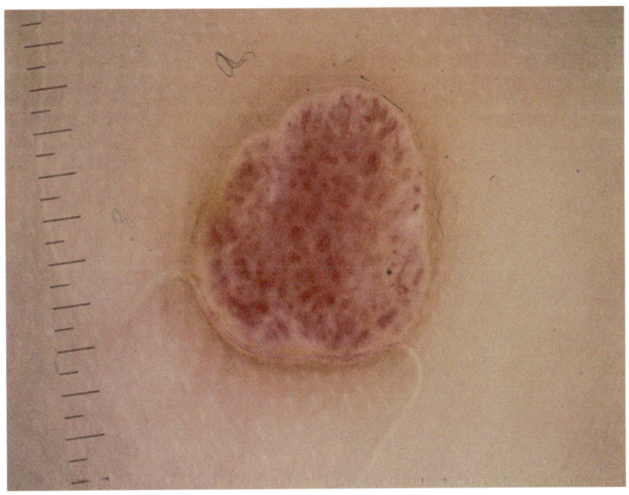

Fig. 30.2 Dermoscopy view

H. Cabo (✉)
Instituto de Investigaciones Medicas "A. Lanari". Dermatology Section, University of Buenos Aires, Buenos Aires, Argentina

J. Paoli
University of Gothenburg, Gothenburg, Sweden

P. D. Zaballos
Dermatology Department, Hospital Santa Tecla de Tarragona, University of Rovira i Virgili, Tarragona, Spain

H. Cabo, A. Lallas (eds.), *Comprehensive Atlas of Dermatoscopy Cases*, https://doi.org/10.1007/978-3-319-76932-5_30

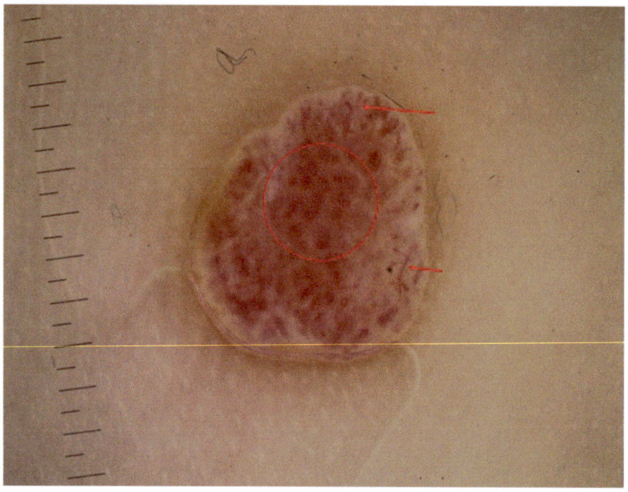

Fig. 30.3 Eccrine Poroma: Dermoscopy view: flower-like images (red arrows); frog eggs images (white circle)

Key Message

Diagnosis: Eccrine poroma

The main differential diagnosis is with pyogenic granuloma basal cell carcinoma and melanoma

Dermoscopy clues:

Vessels pattern

- Arborizing vessels, typically with a flower-like or grail-like appearance
- Pink lacunae surrounded by a whitish halo looking like "frog eggs"

Case 2 H.C.

Sex: male
Age: 12
Surface: nodular
Maximum diameter: 7 mm

Duration of the lesion: < 1 year
History of morphologic changes: yes
Personal history of skin cancer: no
Family history of skin cancer: no
Skin phototype: III
Total nevus count: < 10

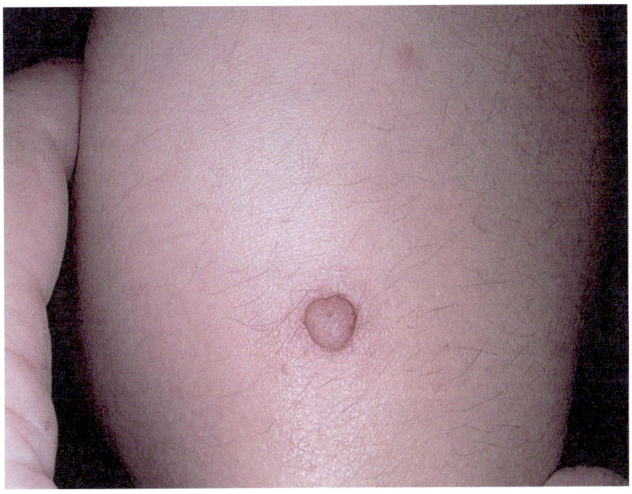

Fig. 30.4 Clinical view. Elevated pink lesion on the right leg

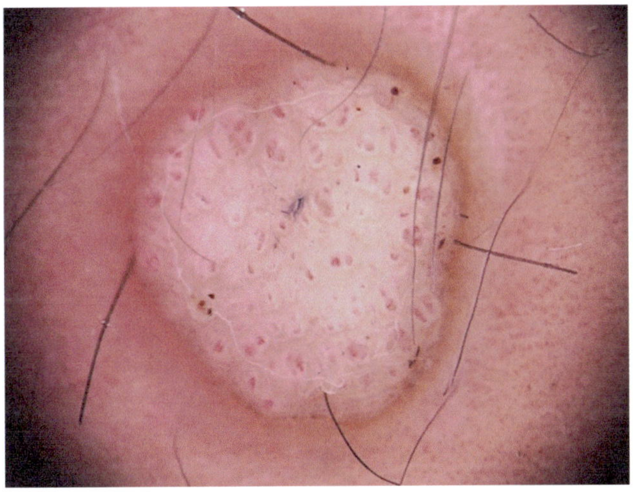

Fig. 30.5 Dermoscopy image

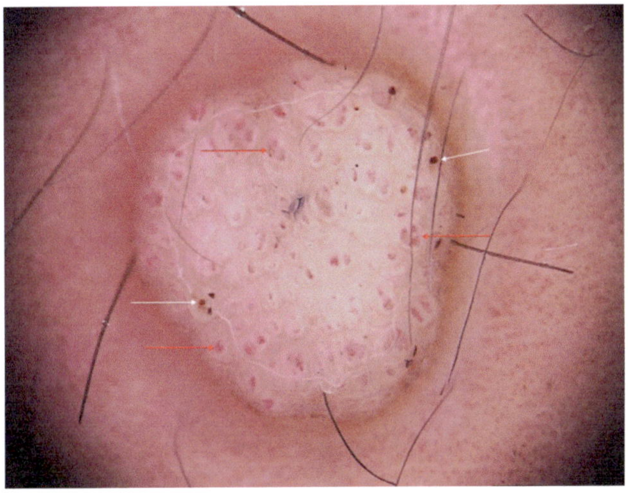

Fig. 30.6 Dermoscopy Image. Central vessels surrounded by a white halo (red arrows); thrombotic dilated vessels in multiple round or oval areas (white arrows)

Key Message
Diagnosis: Common wart

The main clue are central vessels surrounded by a white halo (vessels of the dermal papilla), and these are lineal irregular, comma, or hairpin vessels

Case 3 J.P.

Sex: female
Age: 70
Surface (flat/palpable/nodular): nodular
Maximum diameter: 15 mm
Duration of the lesion: 3–4 months
History of morphologic changes: growth during the past few months
Personal history of skin cancer (if yes, please specify): multiple actinic keratoses previously
Family history of skin cancer (if yes, please specify): none
Skin phototype: III
Total nevus count: (<10, 10–50, 50–100, >100): <10
Other clinical findings (optional):

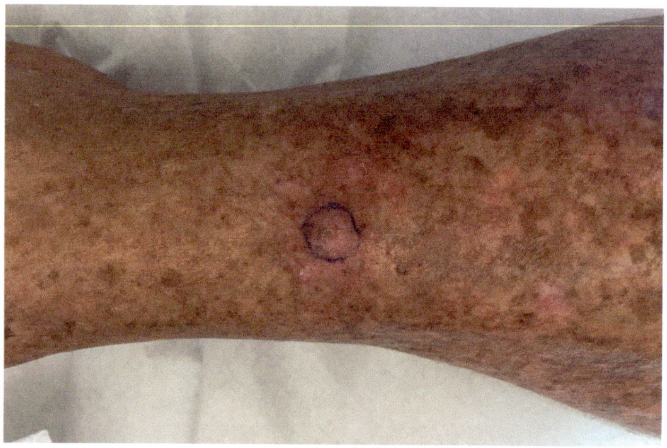

Fig. 30.7 In the clinical image, a pinkish white, slightly raised nodule with a hyperkeratotic surface is observed arising in UV-damaged skin on the anterior part of the lower leg. The patient had previously received over 200 PUVA treatments for psoriasis

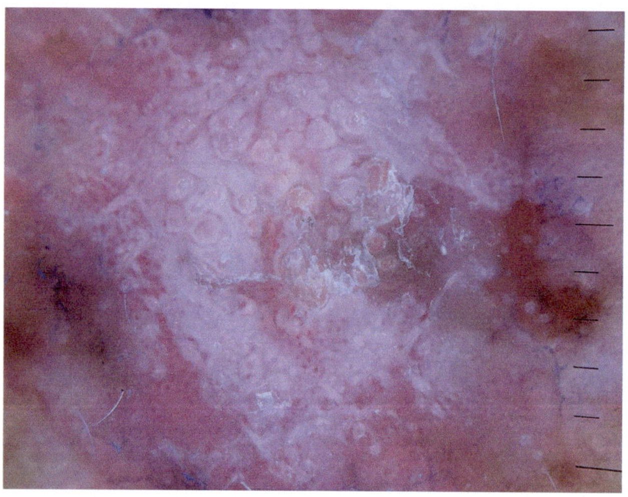

Fig. 30.8 In the dermoscopic image, white scales in the center of the lesion surrounded by multiple white circles and multiple areas with dotted or glomerular vessels. Some ulceration is observed at 6 o'clock

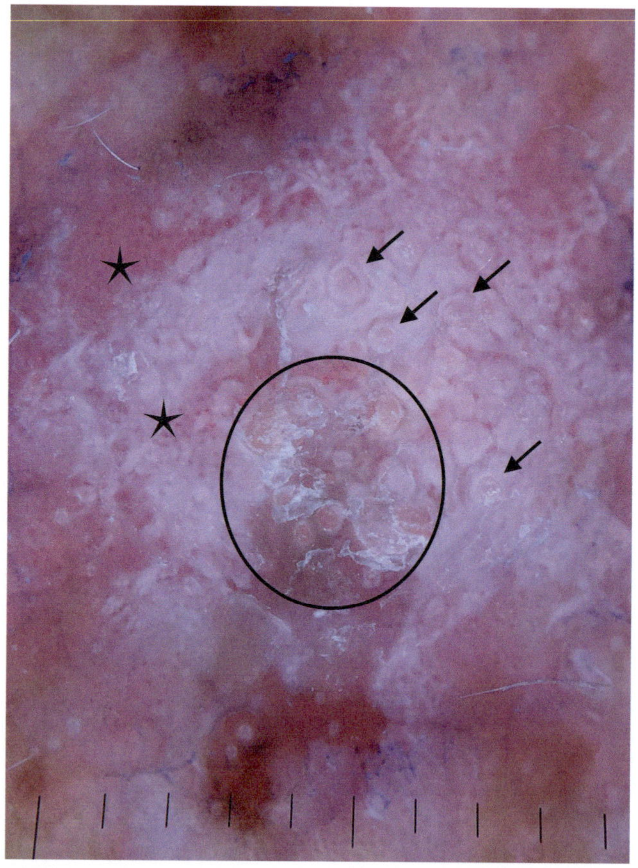

Fig. 30.9 Some of the white circles are highlighted with black arrows, the white scales are seen within the black circle in the center, and two of the areas with dotted/glomerular vessels are marked with a black star

Key Message

Histopathology confirmed the diagnosis of an early invasive squamous cell carcinoma. Although white scales and dotted or glomerular vessels are more indicative of Bowen's disease, white circles are highly specific for invasive squamous cell carcinoma.

Case 4 P.Z.

Sex: female
Age: 52
Surface (flat/palpable/nodular): nodular
Maximum diameter: 1 cm
Duration of the lesion: 3 years
History of morphologic changes: growing and bleeding
Personal history of skin cancer (if yes, please specify): none
Family history of skin cancer (if yes, please specify): none
Skin phototype: III
Total nevus count: (<10, 10–50, 50–100, >100): 10–50
Other clinical findings (optional):
Diagnosis: Clear cell acanthoma

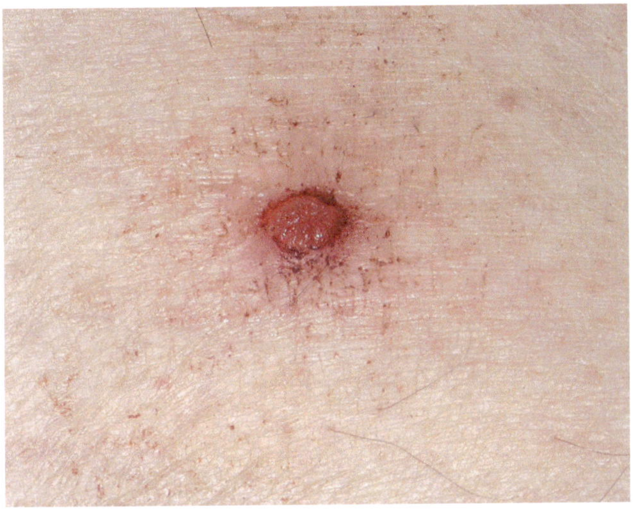

Fig. 30.10 Asymptomatic bleeding pinkish papule located on the leg of a 52-year-old-woman

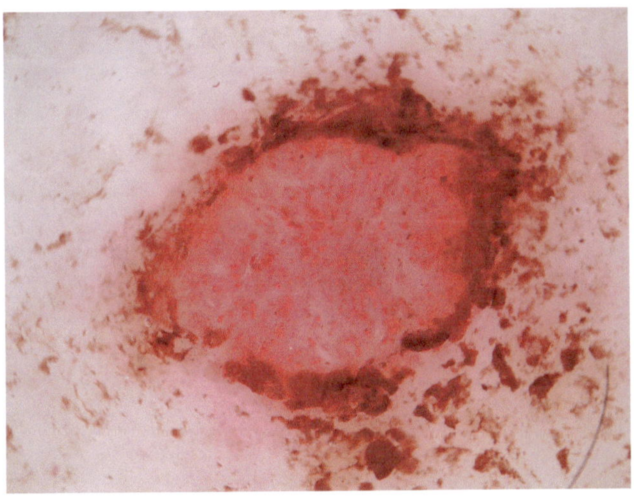

Fig. 30.11 Dermoscopically, we can observe a pinkish lesion with dotted and globular vessels in the center and hemorrhagic crusts at the periphery

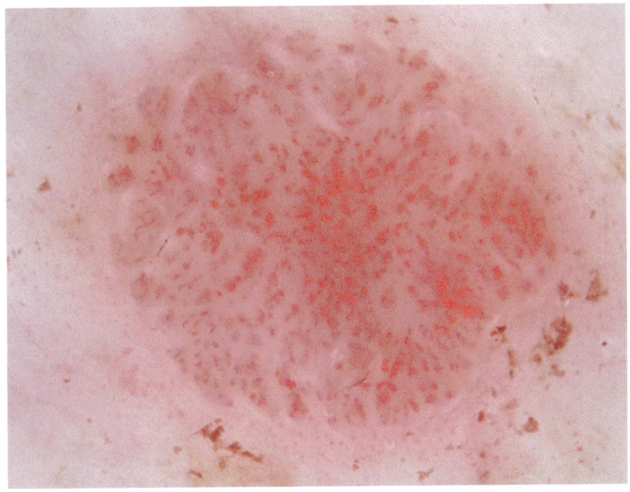

Fig. 30.12 After cleaning the lesion, we can observe mainly glomerular vessels in a linear or serpiginous distribution like a "string of pearls"

Key Message

- It is very important to clean the lesions before diagnosing.
- The pattern composed of dotted, globular, or glomerular vessels in a serpiginous distribution like a "string of pearls" is very characteristic of clear cell acanthomas.

Acral Lesions

31

Horacio Cabo, Aimilios Lallas, and Rainer Hofmann-Wellemhof

Case 1 H.C.

Sex: male
Age: 35
Surface: flat
Maximum diameter: 21 mm
Duration of the lesion: 3 weeks
History of morphologic changes: yes
Personal history of skin cancer: no
Family history of skin cancer: no
Skin phototype: III
Total nevus count: 10–50
Other clinical findings: practice running

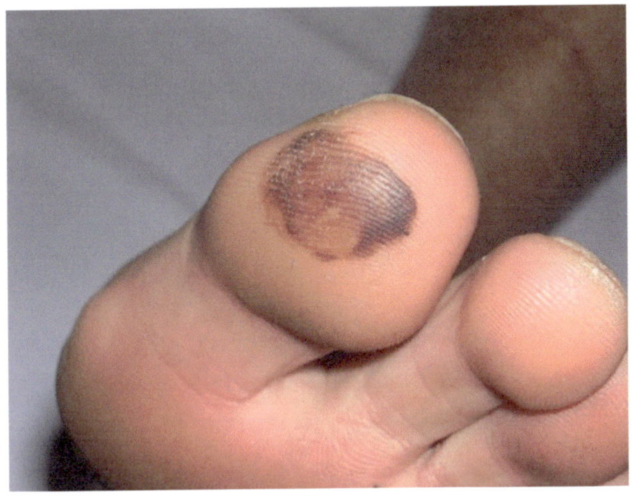

Fig. 31.1 Clinical view: flat lesion with different colors (light brown, dark brown, red, blue, and black)

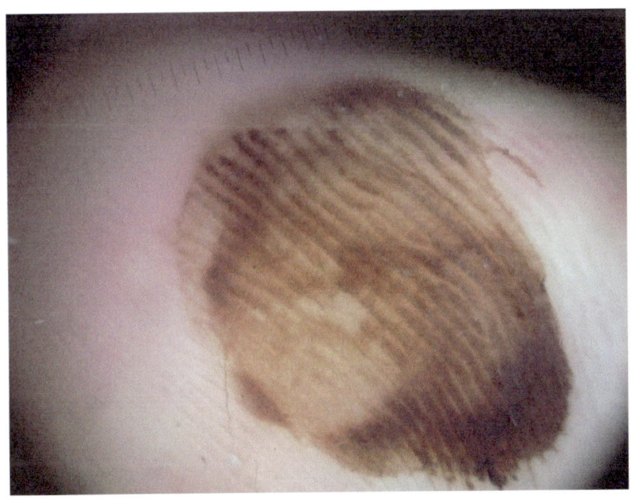

Fig. 31.2 Dermoscopy view

H. Cabo (✉)
Instituto de Investigaciones Medicas "A. Lanari". Dermatology Section, University of Buenos Aires, Buenos Aires, Argentina

A. Lallas
First Department of Dermatology, Aristotle University of Thessaloniki, Thessaloniki, Greece

R. Hofmann-Wellemhof
Department of Dermatology, Medical University of Graz, Graz, Austria

H. Cabo, A. Lallas (eds.), *Comprehensive Atlas of Dermatoscopy Cases*, https://doi.org/10.1007/978-3-319-76932-5_31

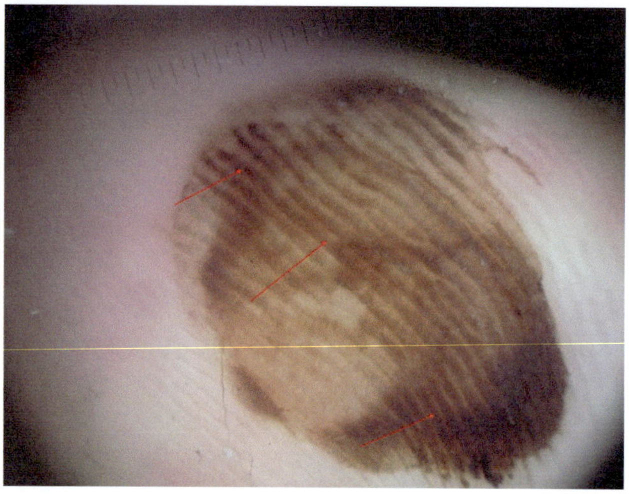

Fig. 31.3 Dermoscopy view: parallel ridge pattern (red arrows) with different shades of brown color and red, blue, and black color

Key Message

Diagnosis: Traumatic hematoma

Pseudo parallel ridge pattern. After trauma in palms and soles, the hemorrhage flows through the duct of the eccrine sweat gland and reaches the epidermis causing a pigmentation of the ridge due to hematic pigment.

As time goes on, the hematoma, due to degradation of hemoglobin, slowly changes color and they show different colors such as red, blue, black, and brown or yellow.

Case 2 H.C.

Sex: male

Age: 48

Surface: palpable

Maximum diameter: 18 mm

Duration of the lesion: >1 year

History of morphologic changes: yes

Personal history of skin cancer: no

Family history of skin cancer: no

Skin photo type: III

Total nevus count: 10–50

Other clinical findings: the lesion is in the sole of the right foot

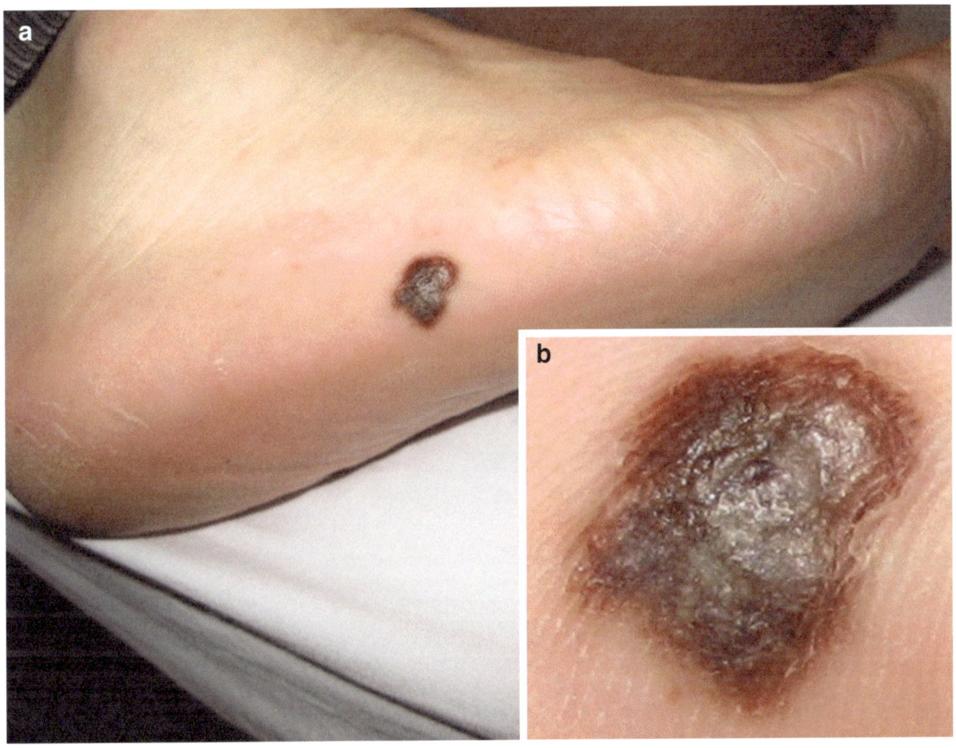

Fig. 31.4 Clinical view: (**a**) asymmetric pigmentary lesion with different colors; (**b**) close-up of the clinical view

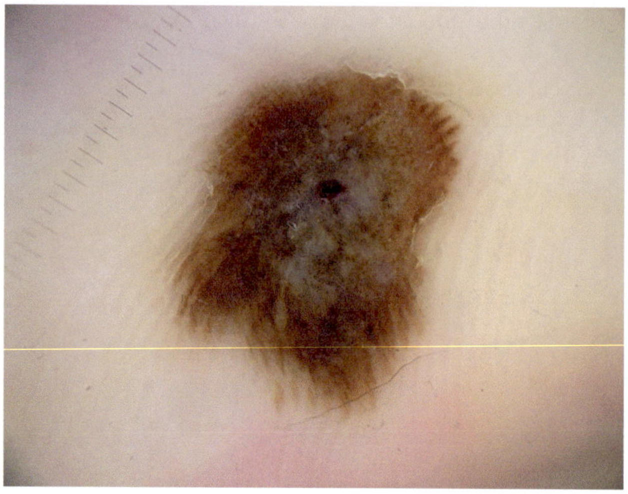

Fig. 31.5 Dermoscopy view

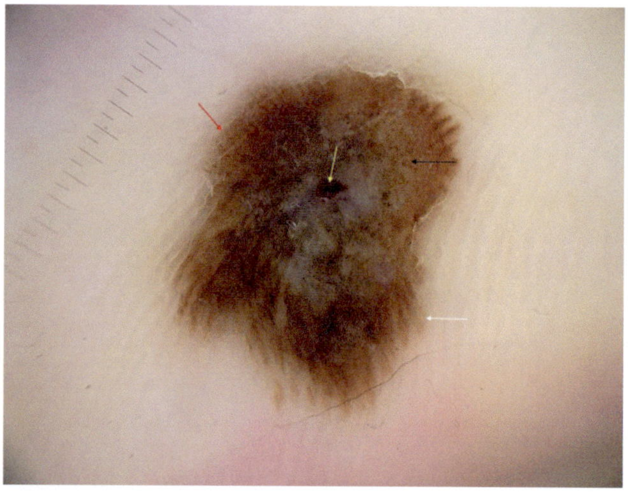

Fig. 31.6 Dermoscopy view: parallel ridge pattern (red arrow); irregular fibrillar pattern (white arrow); irregular globules (black arrow); ulceration (yellow arrow)

Key Message

Diagnosis: acral melanoma

Dermoscopy clues: parallel ridge pattern is highly specificity of acral melanoma (99%)

Case 3 A.L.

Sex: Male
Age: 31
Surface (flat/palpable/nodular): flat
Maximum diameter: 4 mm
Duration of the lesion: 3 years
History of morphologic changes: no
Personal history of skin cancer (if yes please specify): no
Family history of skin cancer (if yes please specify): no
Skin phototype: III
Total nevus count: (<10, 10–50, 50–100, >100): 50–100
Other clinical findings (optional):

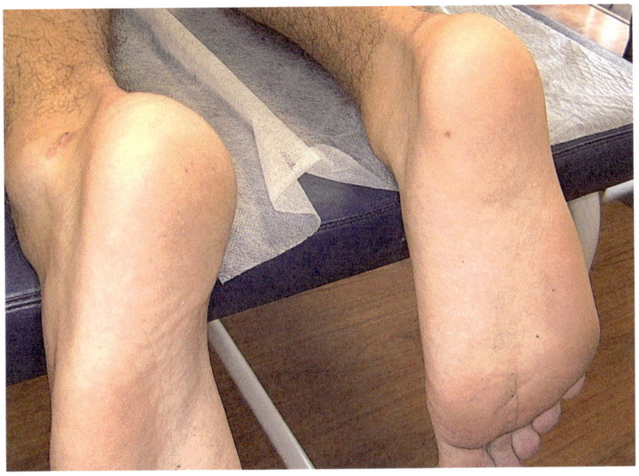

Fig. 31.7 Clinically, there is a symmetric flat pigmented lesion located on the right sole

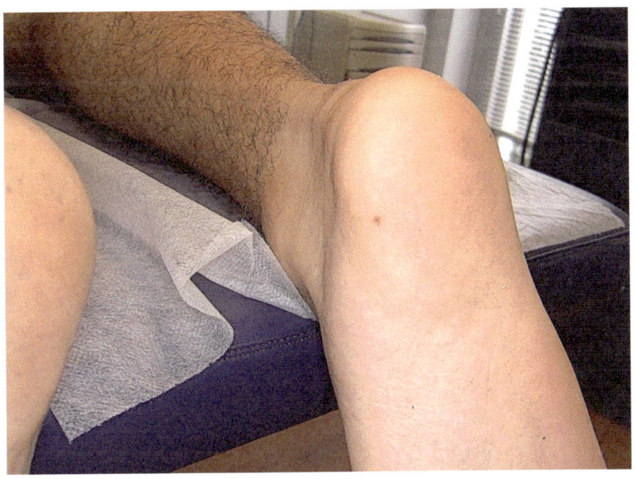

Fig. 31.8 Clinically, there is a symmetric flat pigmented lesion located on the right sole

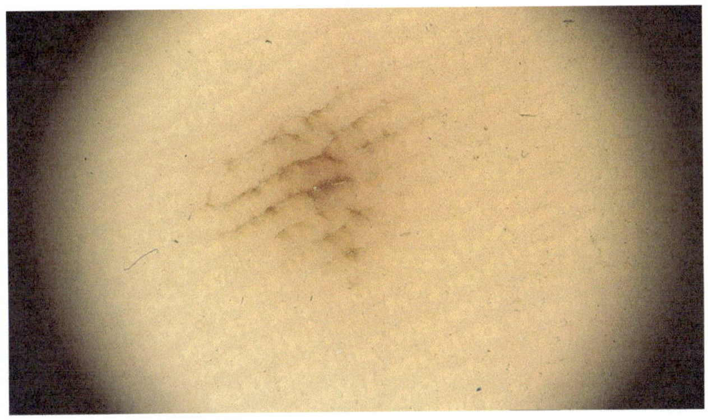

Fig. 31.9 Dermoscopically we can observe a linear pigmentation, predominantly localized to the furrows (known as parallel furrow pattern)

Key Message

Parallel furrow pattern is a pathognomonic feature of acral nevus.

Case 4 A.L.

Sex: female

Age: 7

Surface (flat/palpable/nodular): flat

Maximum diameter: 6 mm

Duration of the lesion: 1 year

History of morphologic changes: yes, growth

Personal history of skin cancer (if yes please specify): no

Family history of skin cancer (if yes please specify): no

Skin phototype: III

Total nevus count: (<10, 10–50, 50–100, >100): <10

Other clinical findings (optional):

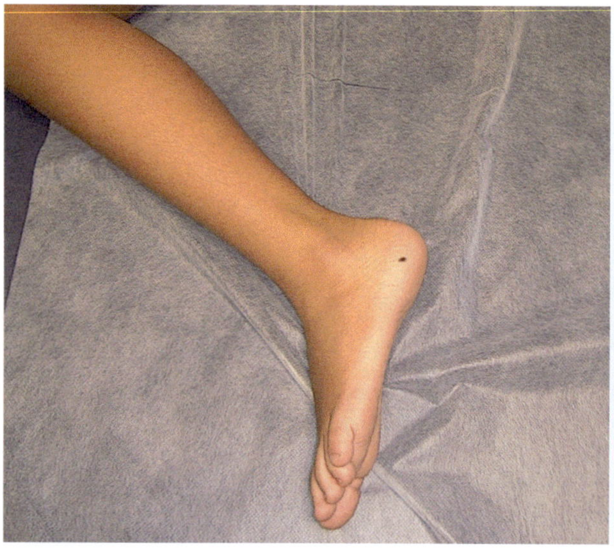

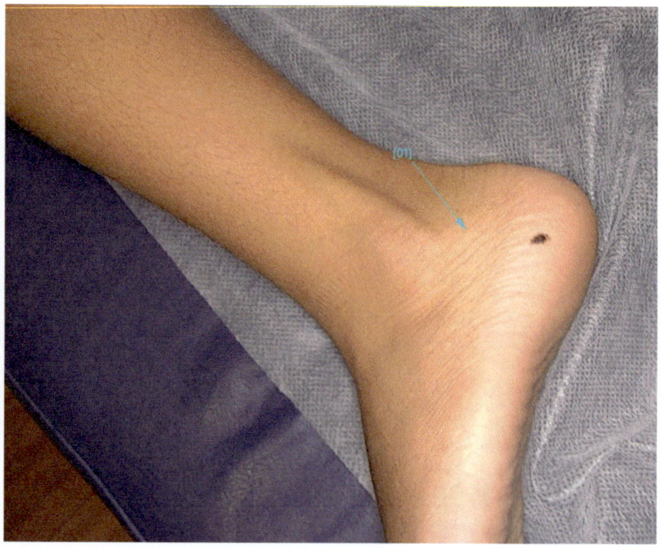

Fig. 31.10 and 31.11 On clinical examination, there is a pigmented flat lesion located on the left sole

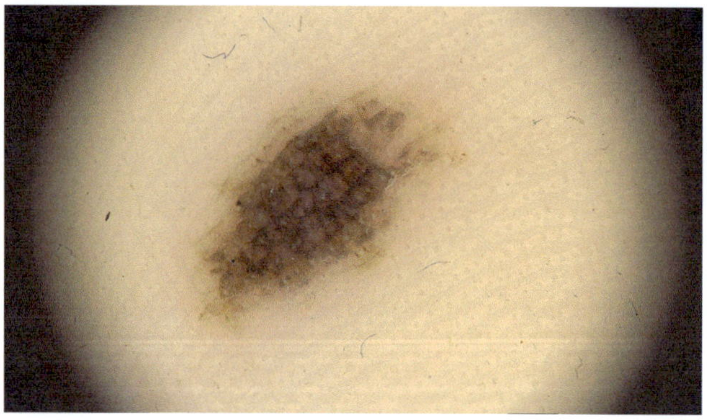

Fig. 31.12 On dermoscopic examination, the lesion is characterized not only by the parallel furrow pattern but also by parallel pigment bands that cross over the ridges from one furrow to the next (known as latticelike pattern)

Key Message

Latticelike pattern is a pathognomonic feature of acral nevus.

Case 5 R.H-W.

Sex: female
Age: 58
Surface (flat/palpable/nodular): flat
Maximum diameter: 8 mm
Duration of the lesion: 1 year
History of morphologic changes: change of color
Personal history of skin cancer (if yes please specify): no
Family history of skin cancer (if yes please specify): no
Skin phototype: I–II
Total nevus count: (<10, 10–50, 50–100, >100): 10–50
Other clinical findings (optional): Vitiligo axillar

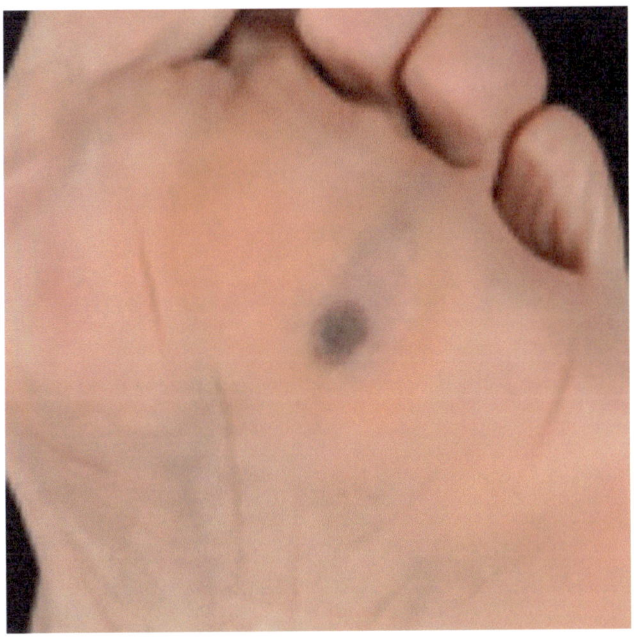

Fig. 31.13 Clinical view

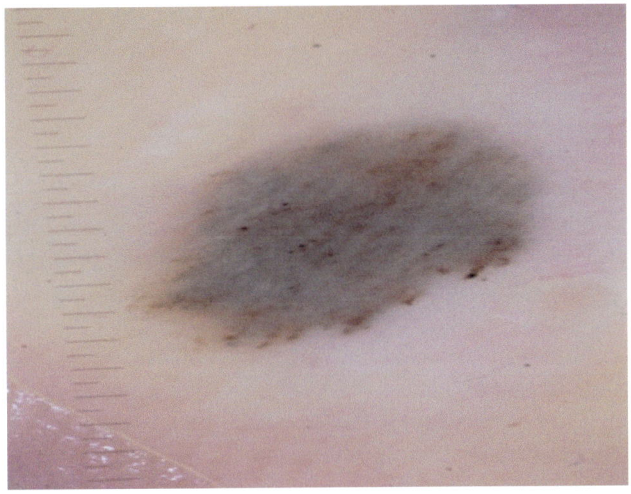

Fig. 31.14 Dermoscopy view

Key Message

Case 1
Diagnosis: acral melanoma in situ

Table 31.1 The checklist for the diagnosis of acral melanoma (1)

		Points
B	Irregular blotch	+1
R	Parallel ridge pattern	+3
A	Asymmetry of structures	+1
A	Asymmetry of colors	+1
F	Parallel furrow pattern	−1
F	Fibrillar pattern	−1

A total score of ≥1 is suspect for a diagnosis of melanoma

Table 31.2 Checklist, Case 1

		Points
B	No irregular blotch	0
R	Parallel ridge pattern	3
A	Asymmetry of structures	1
A	Asymmetry of colors	1
F	No parallel furrow pattern	0
F	No fibrillar pattern	0
	Total Score	5

Case 6 R.H-W.

Sex: male

Age: 27

Surface (flat/palpable/nodular): flat

Maximum diameter: 1 cm

Duration of the lesion: <1 month

History of morphologic changes: no changes

Personal history of skin cancer (if yes please specify): no

Family history of skin cancer (if yes please specify): no

Skin phototype: II

Total nevus count: (<10, 10–50, 50–100, >100): 10–50

Other clinical findings (optional):

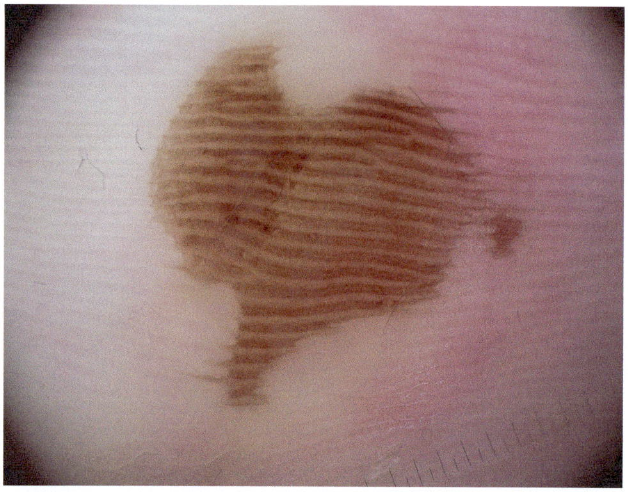

Fig. 31.15 Clinical view

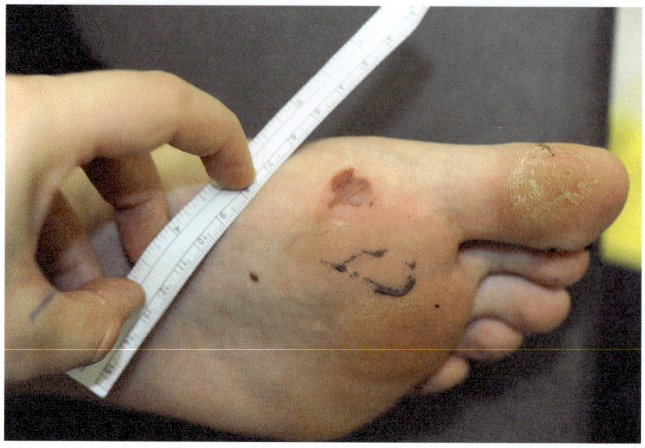

Fig. 31.16 Dermoscopy view

Key Message

Case 2

Diagnosis: subcorneal hemorrhage

Table 31.1 The checklist for the diagnosis of acral melanoma (1)

		Points
B	Irregular blotch	+1
R	Parallel ridge pattern	+3
A	Asymmetry of structures	+1
A	Asymmetry of colors	+1
F	Parallel furrow pattern	−1
F	Fibrillar pattern	−1

A total score of ≥1 is suspect for a diagnosis of melanoma

Table 31.2 Checklist, Case 2

		Points
B	Irregular blotch	1
R	Parallel ridge pattern	3
A	No asymmetry of structures	0
A	No asymmetry of colors	0
F	No parallel furrow pattern	0
F	No fibrillar pattern	0
	Total Score	4

32 Lesion on the Nails

Alon Scope, Antonella Tosti, Aimilios Lallas, Chryssoula Papageorgiou, and Luc Thomas

Case 1 A.S.

Sex: female
Age: 10
Surface (flat/palpable/nodular): flat
Maximum diameter: 10 mm
Duration of the lesion: 3 years
History of morphologic changes: When the patient was 7 years old, her parents noted a new pigmentation in the nail of the second fingernail of the right hand. At age 10, we performed a 4-month clinical and dermoscopic monitoring and noted significant darkening and dermoscopic change.
Personal history of skin cancer (if yes, please specify): negative
Family history of skin cancer (if yes, please specify): negative
Skin phototype: II
Total nevus count: (<10, 10–50, 50–100, >100): <10.

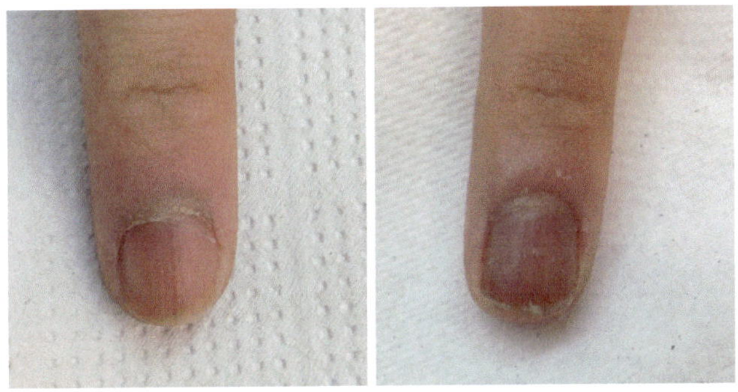

Fig. 32.1 Clinical image, at baseline (left) and at 4-months follow-up visit (right) showing nail-wide melanonychia that is getting diffusely darker. There is also slight erythema of the proximal nail fold and scaling of the nail plate at follow-up

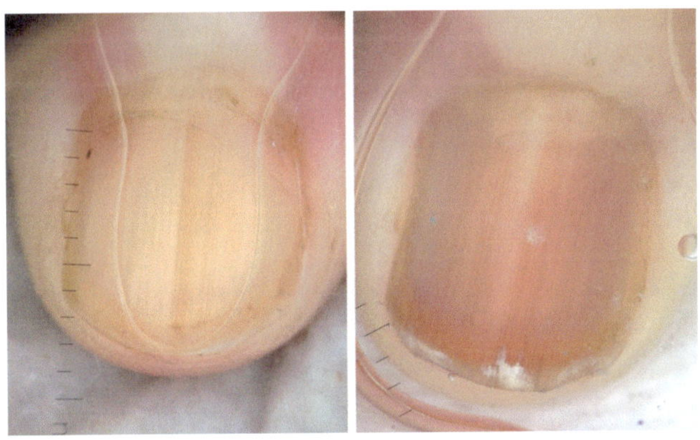

Fig. 32.2 Short-term dermoscopic monitoring. At baseline (left), there is nail-wide melanonychia with parallel pigmented lines that are slightly darker at the center. At follow-up (right), the nail band is darker, with variability in the spacing and thickness of the lines. Scaling of the nail plate can also be observed

A. Scope (✉)
Melanoma and Pigmented Lesion Clinic, Chaim Sheba Medical Center, Ramat-Gan, Israel

Faculty of Medicine, Tel Aviv University, Tel Aviv, Israel
e-mail: scopea1@gmail.com

A. Tosti
Department of Dermatology, Miller School of Medicine, University of Miami, Miami, FL, USA

A. Lallas · C. Papageorgiou
First Department of Dermatology, Aristotle University of Thessaloniki, Thessaloniki, Greece

L. Thomas
Department of Dermatology, Lyons Cancer Research Center (Pr Puisieux) INSERM U1052, CNRS UMR5286 Lyon 1 University Centre Hospitalier Lyon Sud, Lyon, France

H. Cabo, A. Lallas (eds.), *Comprehensive Atlas of Dermatoscopy Cases*, https://doi.org/10.1007/978-3-319-76932-5_32

Key Message
Due to the breadth of the melanonychia and the rapid evolution, a lateral longitudinal nail biopsy including the matrix was performed. Histopathology reported a melanoma in situ. Subsequently, the entire nail apparatus and surrounding distal phalangeal skin were surgically removed, with clear margins histopathologically confirmed.

This is a rare case of pediatric nail matrix in situ melanoma. A clue to the diagnosis is probably the late age of onset. Broad melanonychia may be seen in congenital nevi of the matrix that usually appear before the age of 5 years. The appearance of nail-wide melanonychia and the rapid clinical and dermoscopic evolution after the age of 7 years are unusual and warrant a nail matrix biopsy.

Acknowledgment I would like to thank Prof. Luc Thomas for his excellent insights in this rare case.

Case 2 A.T.

Sex: male
Age: 42
Duration of the lesion: 3 years
History of morphologic changes: Progressive nail thickening and discoloration of the medial side of his 1st left toenail, recently he developed in growing and granulomatous growth on the opposite site
Personal history of skin cancer (if yes, please specify): no
Family history of skin cancer (if yes, please specify): no
Skin phototype: III
Total nevus count: NA
Other clinical findings (optional):

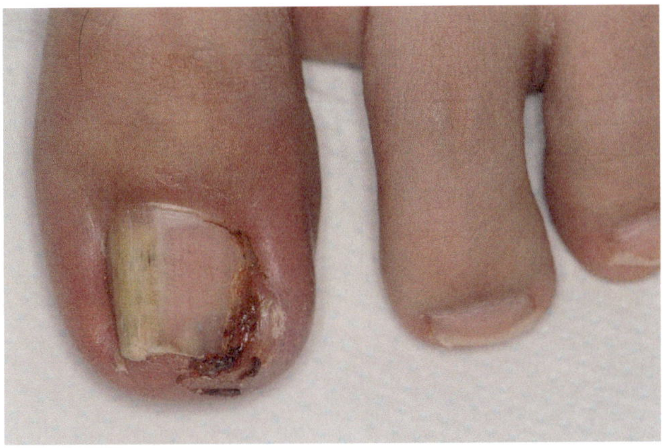

Fig. 32.3 The 1st left toenail shows longitudinal thickening and yellow discoloration of its medial part and stage 2 lateral in growing on the opposite site

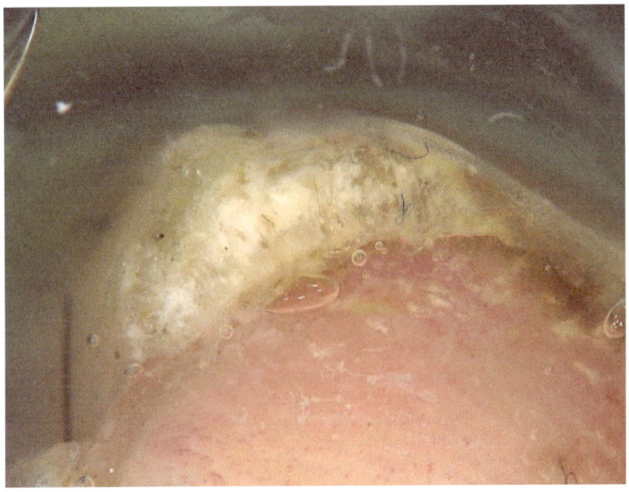

Fig. 32.5 Frontal view showing multiple holes in the nail free margin

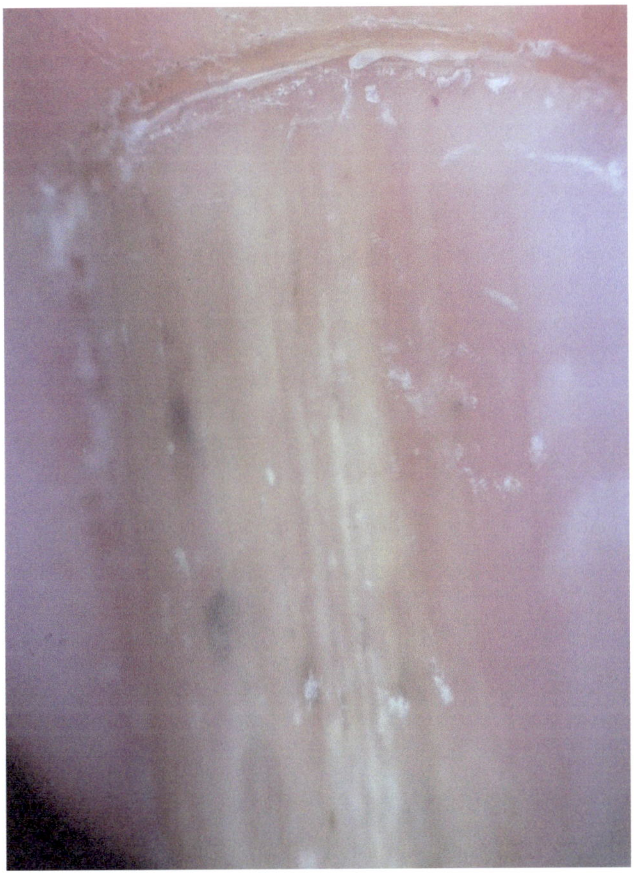

Fig. 32.4 Nail plate dermoscopy showing longitudinal white lines and splinter hemorrhages

Key Message

Onychomatricoma is a benign tumor of the nail matrix that extends with projections within the nail plate. The tunnels containing the tumor projections appear as white longitudinal lines at dermoscopy of the nail plate. These tunnels reach the free margin of the nail. Dermoscopy of the free edge of the nail plate shows holes looking as woodworm-like cavities.

Case 3 A.T.

Sex: female
Age:67
Duration of the lesion: 1 year
History of morphologic changes: Longitudinal band of black discoloration of her right thumb that is slightly enlarging

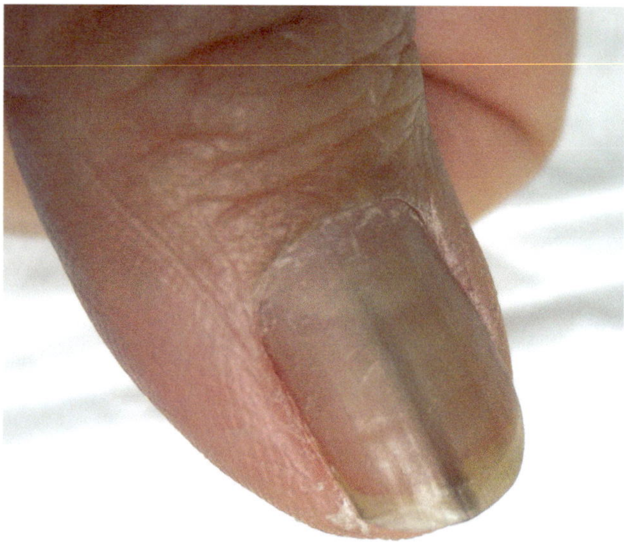

Fig. 32.6 Band of longitudinal melanonychia extending from the lunula region to the free margin

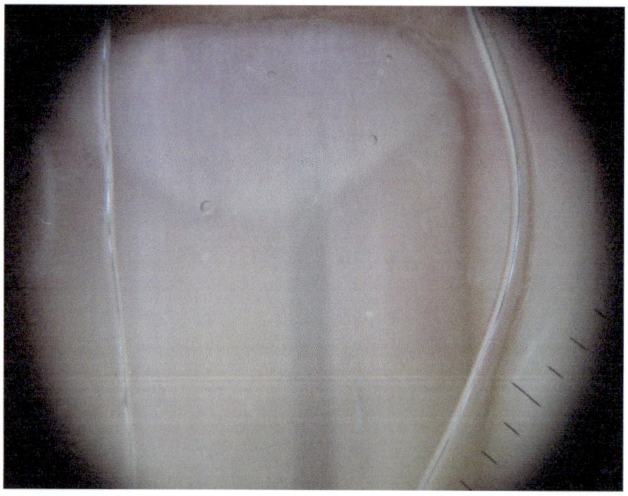

Fig. 32.7 At dermoscopy, the band is homogeneous color with a gray hue. There are not longitudinal lines

Personal history of skin cancer (if yes, please specify): no
Family history of skin cancer (if yes, please specify): no
Skin phototype: IV
Total nevus count: NA
Other clinical findings (optional):

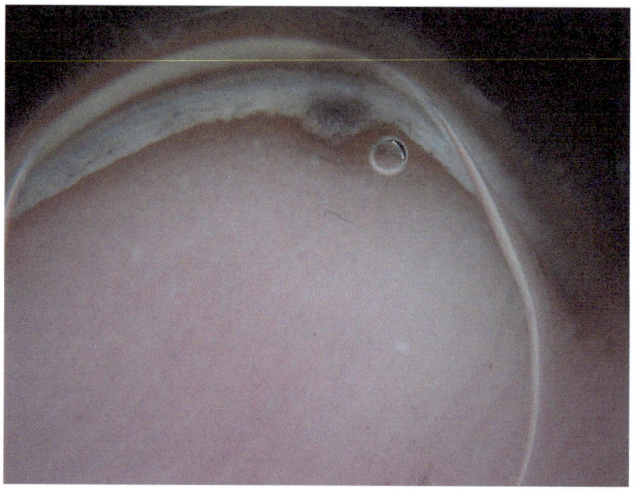

Fig. 32.8 Frontal view showing a focal keratotic mass under the free edge of nail plate

Key Message

Onychopapilloma is a frequent benign tumor of the nail matrix and bed. It most commonly causes longitudinal erythronychia, but it can cause melanonychia due to melanocyte activation in patients with dark phototypes. In this case, nail plate dermoscopy showed characteristic features of activation (gray band without longitudinal lines). Diagnosis of onychopapilloma was suggested by the presence of a focal keratotic mass at free edge dermoscopy and confirmed by pathology.

Case 4 A.L.

Sex: female
Age: 56
Surface (flat/palpable/nodular): flat
Maximum diameter: 6 mm
Duration of the lesion: 7 months
History of morphologic changes: yes
Personal history of skin cancer (if yes, please specify): no
Family history of skin cancer (if yes, please specify): no
Skin phototype: III
Total nevus count: (<10, 10–50, 50–100, >100): 10–50
Other clinical findings (optional):

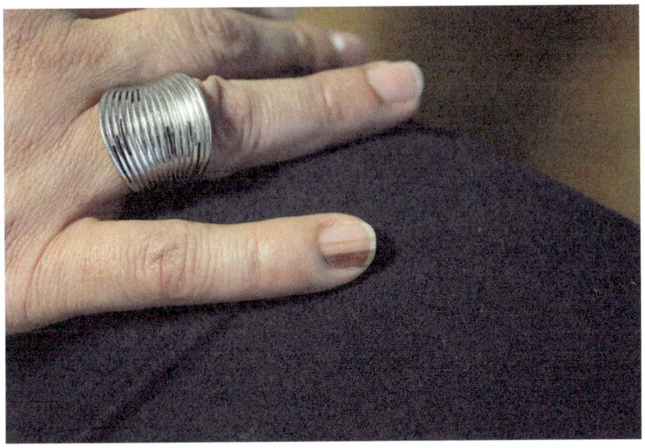

Fig. 32.9 Macroscopically, we can see a longitudinal melanonychia on one fingernail of the right hand. The black/brown pigmentation runs across the nail plate from the matrix to the free edge

Key Message

The presence of brown to black longitudinal lines totally asymmetrical and irregular in color, spacing, and width along with the history and the age of the patient is indicative of a subungual melanoma.

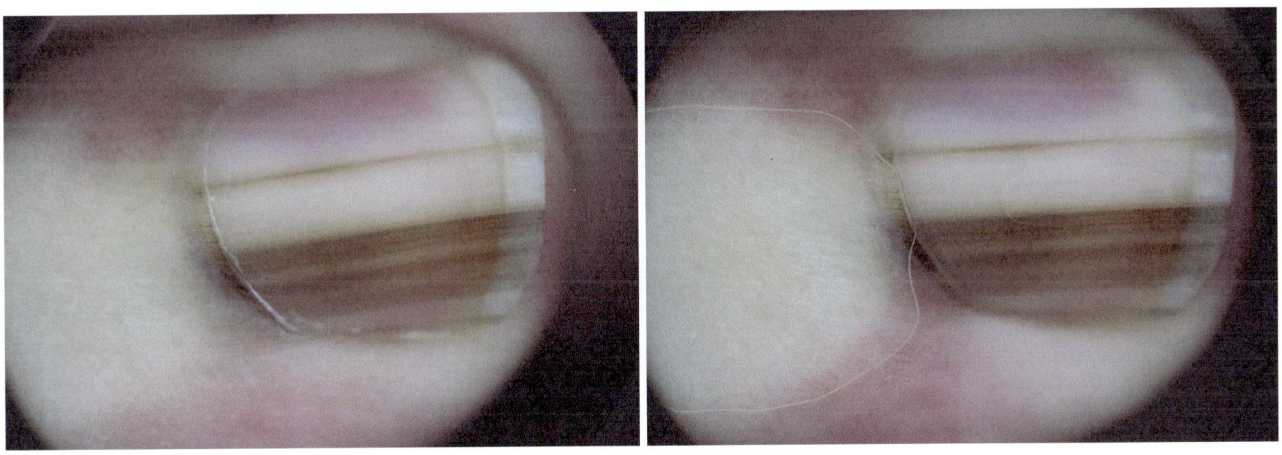

Figs. 32.10 and 32.11 Dermoscopy reveals brown to black longitudinal lines, characterized by irregularity in terms of color, spacing, and width. Hutchinson's sign is also evident

Case 6 L.T.

Sex: male
Age: 64 years old
Surface (flat/palpable/nodular): changes of the right thumbnail aspect in a right-handed person. Other nails are uninvolved.
Maximum diameter: length, the whole nail plate; width, 4 mm
Duration of the lesion: about 3 years yet history not very clear
History of morphologic changes: lesion was initially pink/red. Recently occurrence of a black discoloration at the distal part of the plate
Personal history of skin cancer (if yes, please specify): none
Family history of skin cancer (if yes, please specify): none
Skin phototype: IIIa
Total nevus count: (<10, 10–50, 50–100, >100): less than 10
Other clinical findings (optional): Lesion is not painful. Final histopathological diagnosis was invasive 0.7 mm thick squamous cell carcinoma of the nail matrix and nail bed. Patient was treated by complete excision of the nail unit and is in complete remission after 2,5 years.

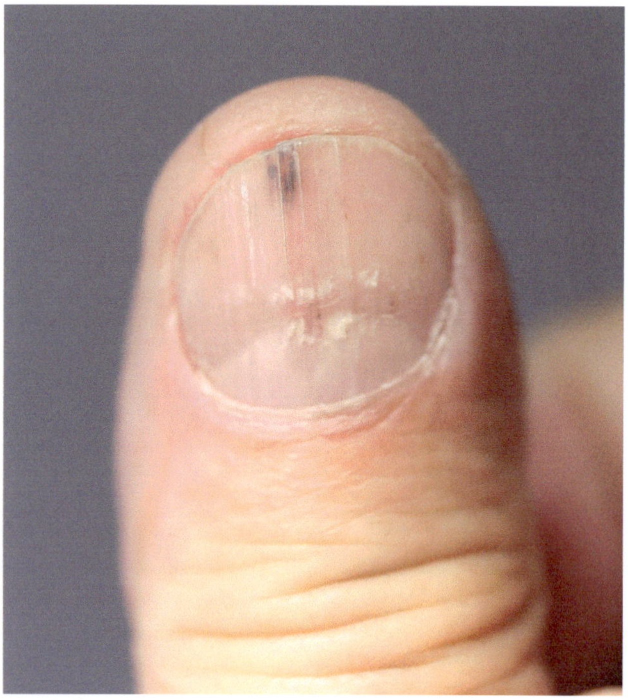

Fig. 32.12 Clinical view shows erythronychia with purpuric changes at the distal part of the plate

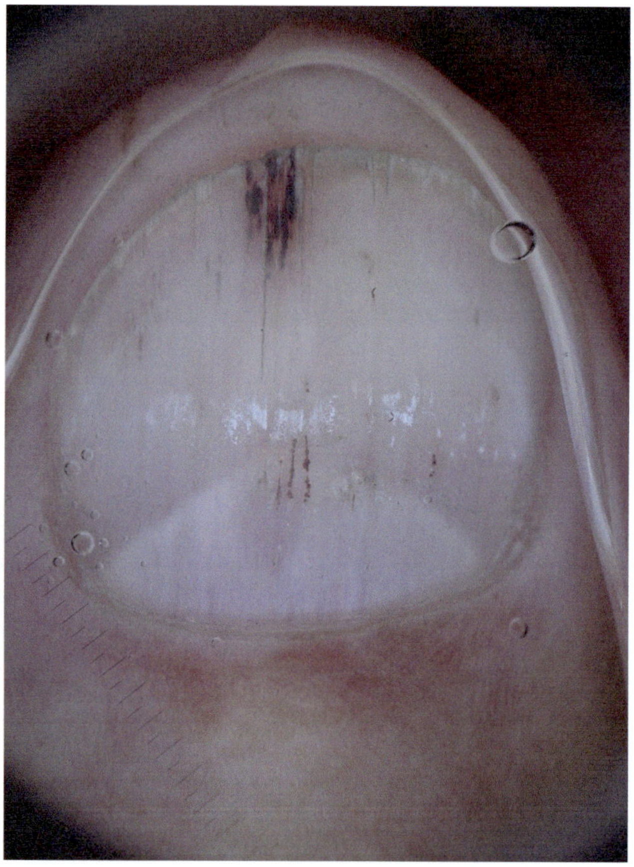

Fig. 32.13 Dermoscopy shows longitudinal erythronychia with splinter hemorrhages, lateral limits are barely visible, and lesion does not seem to be sharply demarcated longitudinally. In the lunula (distal matrix), a pink triangular-shaped spot is visible

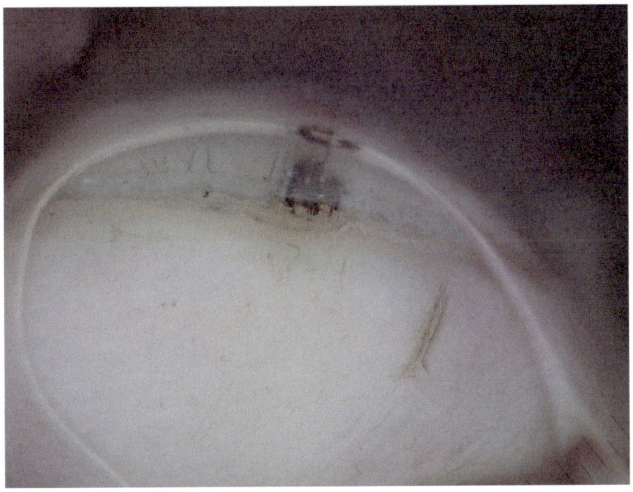

Fig. 32.14 Free edge dermoscopic examination shows that hyperkeratotic material is present underneath the nail plate in the area corresponding to the linear abnormalities of the plate. Purpura is also observed there. The nail plate is thinner above and convexically distorted

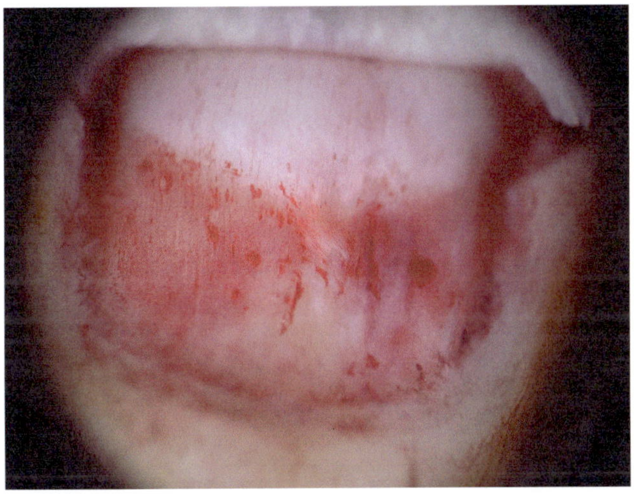

Fig. 32.15 Per-operative dermoscopy of the nail bed and matrix objectives a whitish irregular and asymmetrical tumor mainly located on the nail bed with very subtle vascular changes in the distal matrix

Key Message

Longitudinal erythronychia with or without purpuric changes deserves dermoscopical examination of the nail plate but also of the free edge. If hyperkeratotic material is present underneath the nail plate and if the lesion shows irregular and ill-defined lateral borders, the diagnosis of squamous cell carcinoma should be considered.

Case 7 L.T.

Sex: female
Age: 16 years old
Surface (flat/palpable/nodular): *melanonychia striata* discovered at age 14 progressively enlarging
Maximum diameter: length, all table/width, 4.5 mm
Duration of the lesion: 2 years
History of morphologic changes: progressively enlarging but with recent change of the pigmentation (became darker in the center)
Personal history of skin cancer (if yes, please specify): none
Family history of skin cancer (if yes, please specify): none
Skin phototype: IV
Total nevus count: (<10, 10–50, 50–100, >100): 10–50
Other clinical findings (optional): other nails not involved, no pigmentation-inducing drug intake, no family history of nail pigmentation, and no other signs of lentiginosis of any type

Diagnosis of in situ acral lentiginous melanoma of the nail matrix was suggested extemporaneously by per-operative confocal microscopy of the nail matrix and confirmed by definitive histiopathological examination of the lesion. Patient has been treated by complete excision of the nail unit and is in complete remission after 2.5 years.

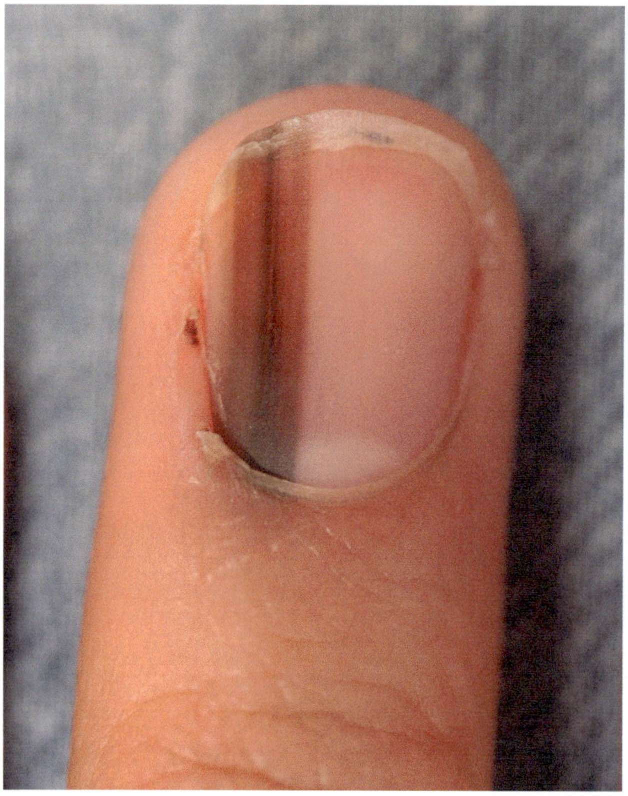

Fig. 32.16 Clinical examination shows an irregularly pigmented melanonychia striata with pseudo-Hutchinson sign (visibility of the pigmentation through the cuticle)

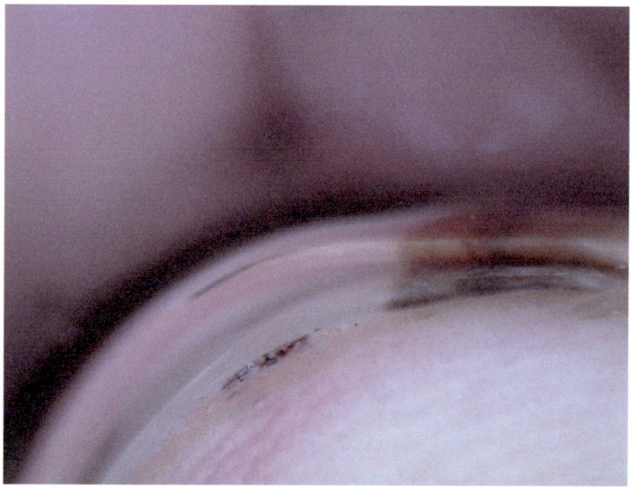

Fig. 32.17 Dermoscopy of the nail plate shows a brown background and irregular longitudinal lines in their thickness spacing and color with a triangular shape of some of them in the center (parallelism disruption). Note some unrelated (trauma-induced) purpuric changes on the distal plate

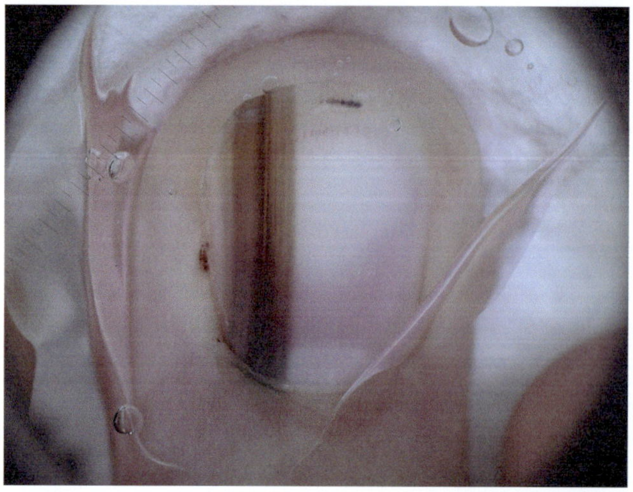

Fig. 32.18 Free edge dermoscopy shows a pigmentation mainly in the lower part of the nail plate indicating a distal matrix origin of the lesion. Unrelated purpuric changes are also visible

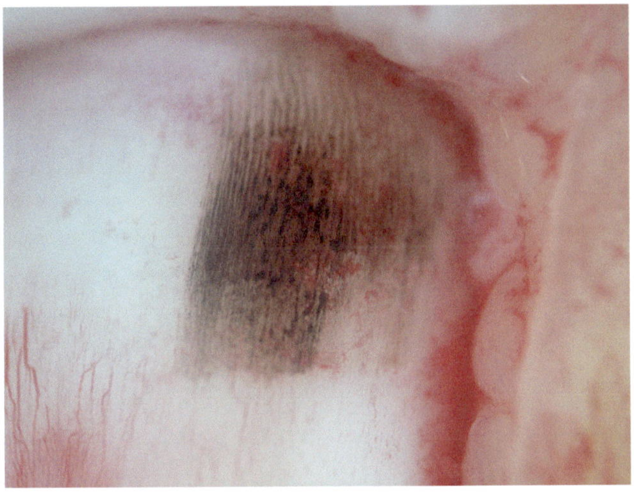

Fig. 32.19 Per-operative nail matrix and bed dermoscopy shows irregular pigmentation (irregular thickness and various color of the lines and irregular size and asymmetrical disposition of the blotches) mainly localized in the distal matrix

Key Message

Melanonychia striata, even in young post-puberty patients, can correspond to melanoma; early diagnosis indeed warrants better prognosis but also allows conservative treatment options. Dermoscopy gives precious indications for the management and should include plate, free edge, and (per-operative) nail matrix examination.

Lesions on Specific Sites (Areola, Genital, Mucosa, etc.)

33

Horacio Cabo, Aimilios Lallas, Chryssoula Papageorgiou, and Wilhelm Stolz

Case 1: H.C.

Sex: female
Age: 30
Surface: flat
Maximum diameter: 7 mm
Duration of the lesion: <1 year
History of morphologic changes: no
Personal history of skin cancer: no
Family history of skin cancer: no
Skin photo type: III
Total nevus count: 10–50

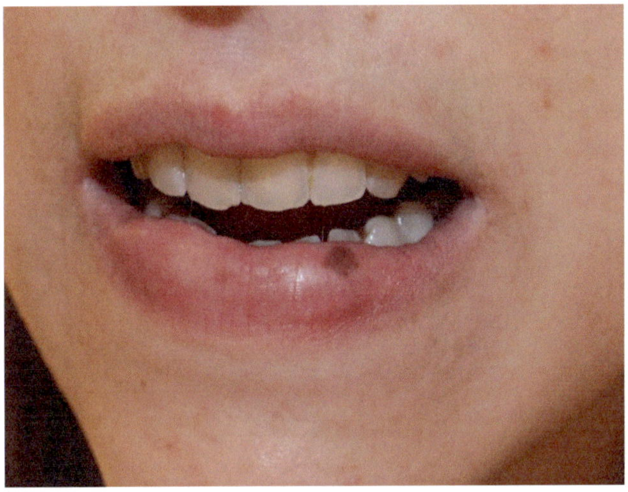

Fig. 33.1 Clinical view

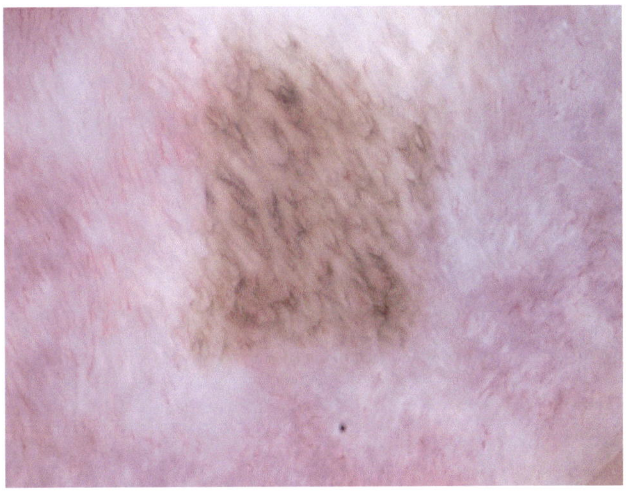

Fig. 33.2 Dermoscopy view

H. Cabo (✉)
Instituto de Investigaciones Medicas "A. Lanari". Dermatology Section, University of Buenos Aires, Buenos Aires, Argentina

A. Lallas · C. Papageorgiou
First Department of Dermatology, Aristotle University of Thessaloniki, Thessaloniki, Greece

W. Stolz
Dermatology Department, Klinikum Schwabing, Munich, Germany

H. Cabo, A. Lallas (eds.), *Comprehensive Atlas of Dermatoscopy Cases*, https://doi.org/10.1007/978-3-319-76932-5_33

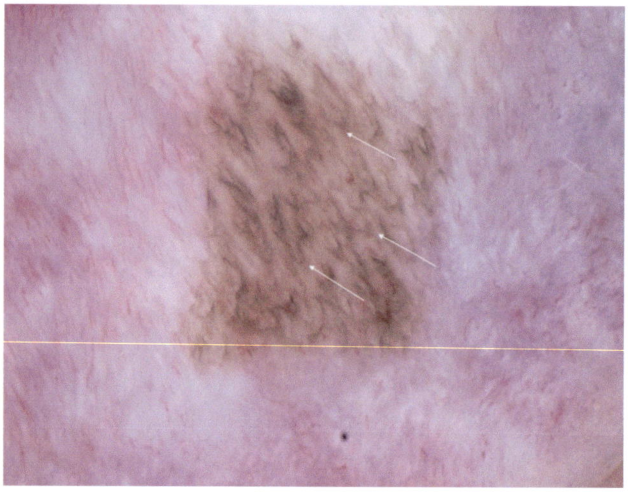

Fig. 33.3 Dermoscopy view: fish scale-like pattern (arrows)

Key Message

Diagnosis: Labial melanotic macule

Dermoscopy clues:

Fish scale-like pattern is one of the dermoscopy features of benign lesion of the mucosa.

The other criteria are the following:

- Dotted-globular pattern
- Homogeneous pattern
- Fingerprint-like pattern
- Hyphal pattern
- Ring-like pattern

Case 2: A.L.

Sex: female
Age: 42
Surface (flat/palpable/nodular): flat
Maximum diameter: 10 mm
Duration of the lesion: unknown
History of morphologic changes: no
Personal history of skin cancer (if yes, please specify): no
Family history of skin cancer (if yes, please specify): no
Skin phototype: III
Total nevus count (<10, 10–50, 50–100, >100): 10–50
Other clinical findings (optional):

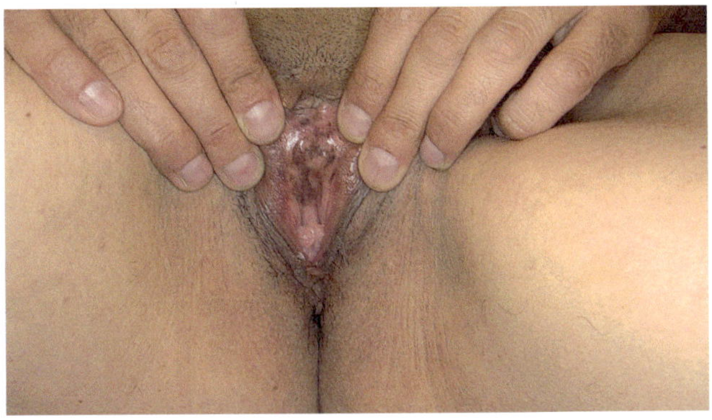

Fig. 33.4 On clinical examination, we can observe diffuse, irregularly outlined, brownish-grayish confluent macules that form a speckled pattern

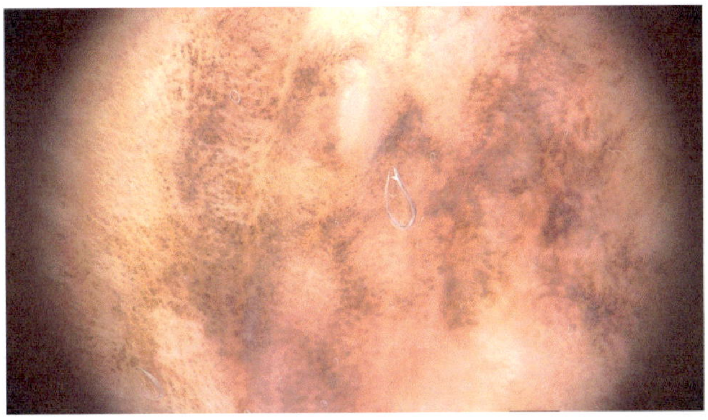

Fig. 33.5 On dermoscopic examination, brown-gray is the predominant color. The main dermoscopic characteristics are the parallel curved lines as well as a structureless pattern

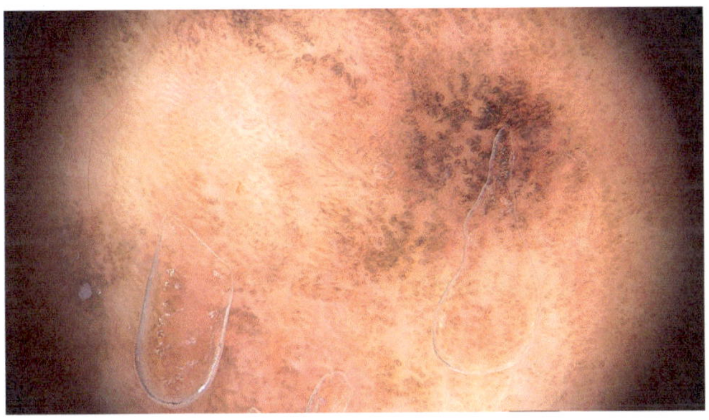

Fig. 33.6 In the upper-right side of the lesion, brown-gray roundish to oval circles are also apparent

Key Message

Parallel curved lines that might form incomplete or complete circles are highly suggestive of mucosal melanosis. In contrast, detection of blue, gray, or white color in combination with structureless areas, atypical pigment network or irregular black dots and globules should always be considered suspicious and warrant histopathological examination in order to rule out melanoma.

Case 3: W.S.

Sex: male
Age: 80
Surface: flat
Maximum diameter: 6 cm
Duration of the lesion: unknown
History of morphologic changes: unknown
Personal history of skin cancer: no
Family history of skin cancer: no
Skin photo type: III
Total nevus count: <10
Other clinical findings: the patient refers itching in this area

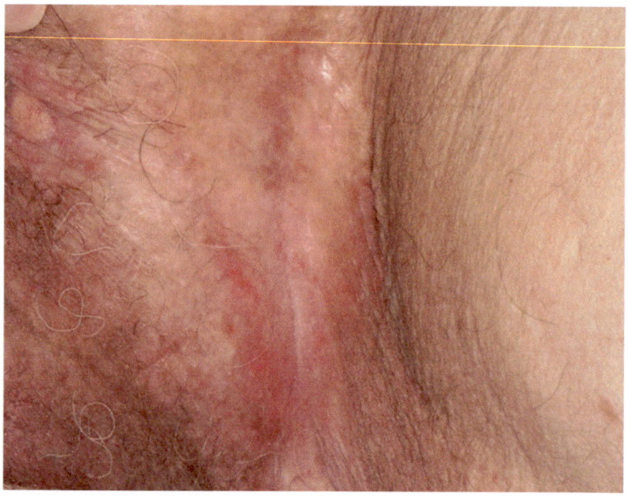

Fig. 33.7 Clinical view: left groin

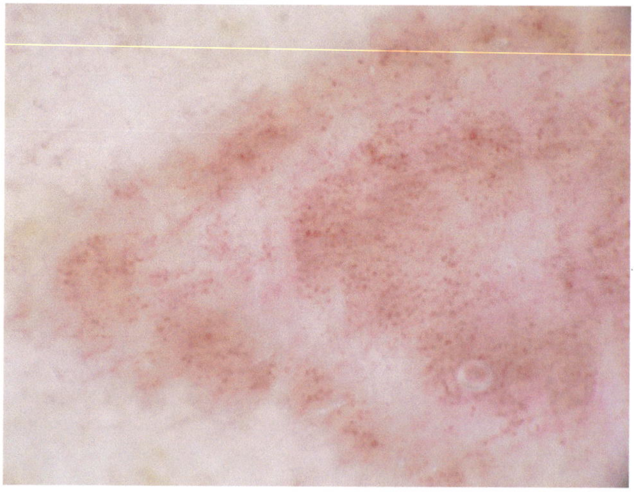

Fig. 33.8 Dermoscopy view

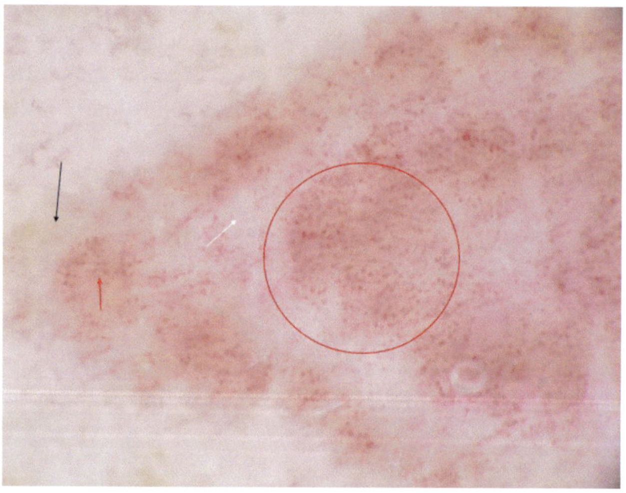

Fig. 33.9 Dermoscopy view: dotted vessels in line (red circle and red arrow); hypopigmented (white or whitish areas) (white arrows); trace of pigmentation (black arrow)

Key Message
Diagnosis: Morbus Paget
Dermoscopy clues:

- Dotted vessels in line
- Hypopigmented (white or whitish areas)
- Trace of pigmentation

Other Lesions

34

Aimilios Lallas, Chryssoula Papageorgiou,
Roberta Giuffrida, Romana Kupsa, Fabrizio Favero,
and Iris Zalaudek

Case 1: A.L.

Sex: female
Age: 62
Surface (flat/palpable/nodular): palpable
Maximum diameter:
Duration of the lesion: 8 months
History of morphologic changes: yes, gradually expanding
Personal history of skin cancer (if yes, please specify): no
Family history of skin cancer (if yes, please specify): no
Skin phototype: III
Total nevus count (<10, 10–50, 50–100, >100): 10–50
Other clinical findings (optional):

A. Lallas (✉) · C. Papageorgiou
First Department of Dermatology,
Aristotle University of Thessaloniki, Thessaloniki, Greece

R. Giuffrida
Department of Clinical and Experimental Medicine, Section of Dermatology, University of Messina, Messina, Italy

R. Kupsa · I. Zalaudek
Department of Dermatology, Medical University of Graz,
Graz, Austria

F. Favero
Department of Dermatology and Venereology,
Medical University of Graz, Graz, Austria

H. Cabo, A. Lallas (eds.), *Comprehensive Atlas of Dermatoscopy Cases*, https://doi.org/10.1007/978-3-319-76932-5_34

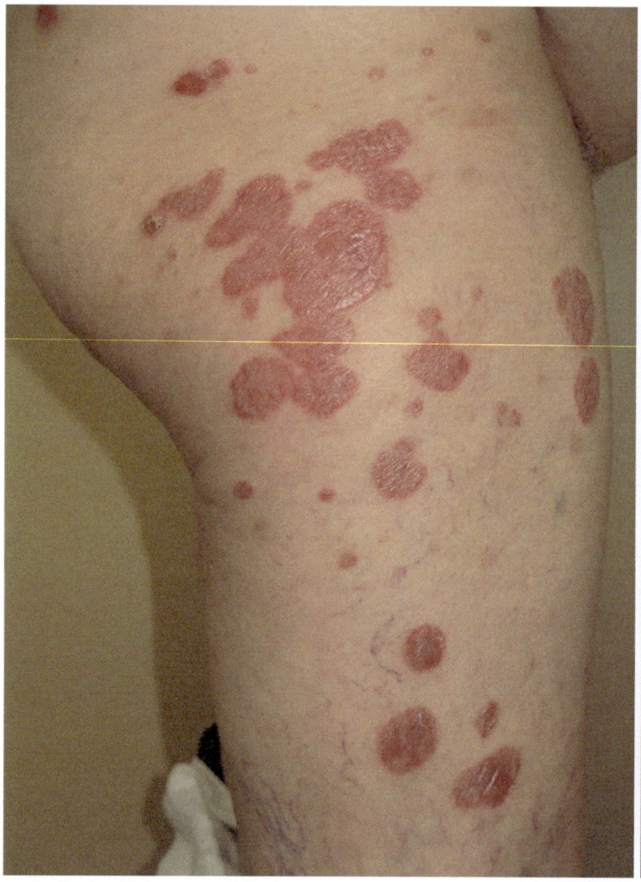

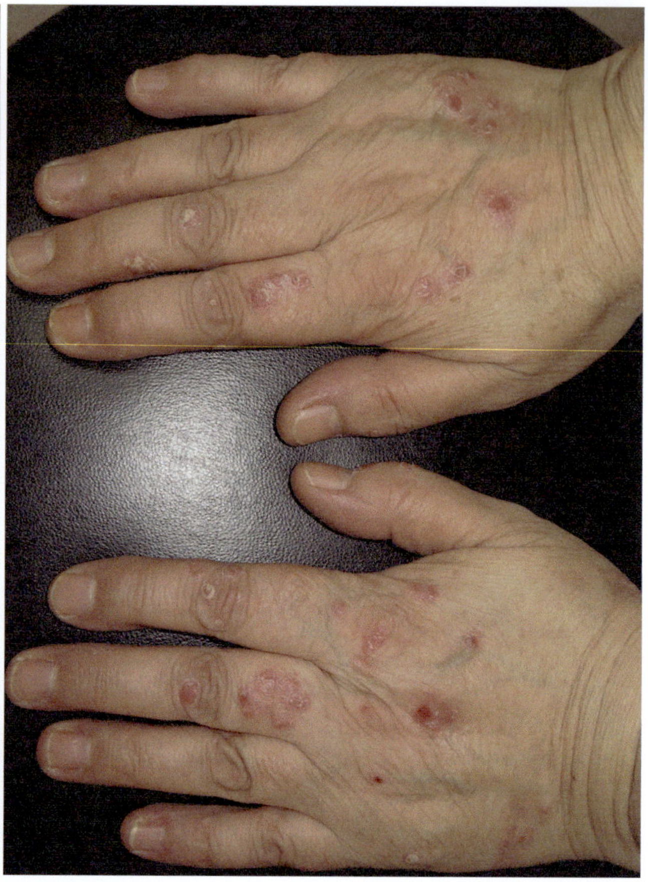

Figs. 34.1 and 34.2 Clinically, there are numerous erythematous papulosquamous lesions on the trunk, lower extremities, and the dorsal surface of the hands, some of them coalescing to form plaques. The lesions appear as well circumscribed, circular, red papules and plaques with a silvery-white scale

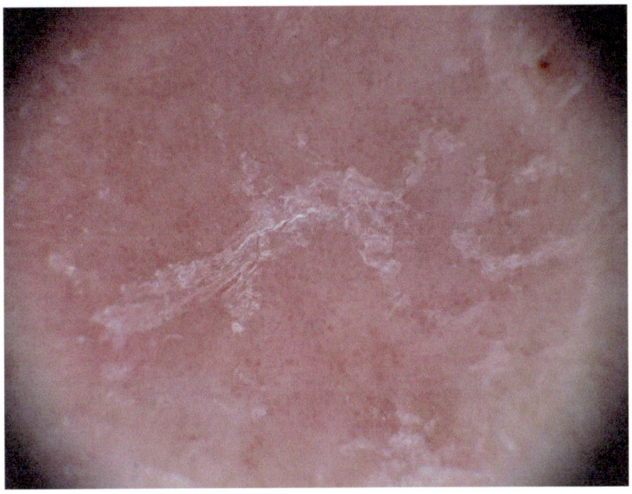

Fig. 34.3 Dermoscopy highlights the dotted and glomerular vessels in a regular distribution. Additionally, a light red background and white superficial scales are also seen

Key Message

The combination of dotted and glomerular vessels in a symmetric and homogenous arrangement with white scales represents the dermoscopic hallmark of psoriasis.

Case 2: A.L.

Sex: male
Age: 30
Surface (flat/palpable/nodular): palpable
Maximum diameter:
Duration of the lesion: 1 month

History of morphologic changes: yes
Personal history of skin cancer (if yes, please specify): no
Family history of skin cancer (if yes, please specify): no
Skin phototype: III
Total nevus count (<10, 10–50, 50–100, >100): 10–50
Other clinical findings (optional):

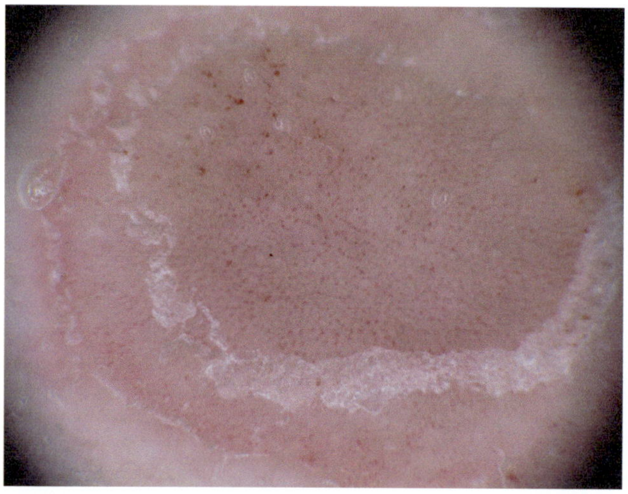

Fig. 34.4 In the upper-left side of the lesion, scale removal reveals tiny red blood drops (Auspitz sign). The characteristic vascular pattern is still clearly visible

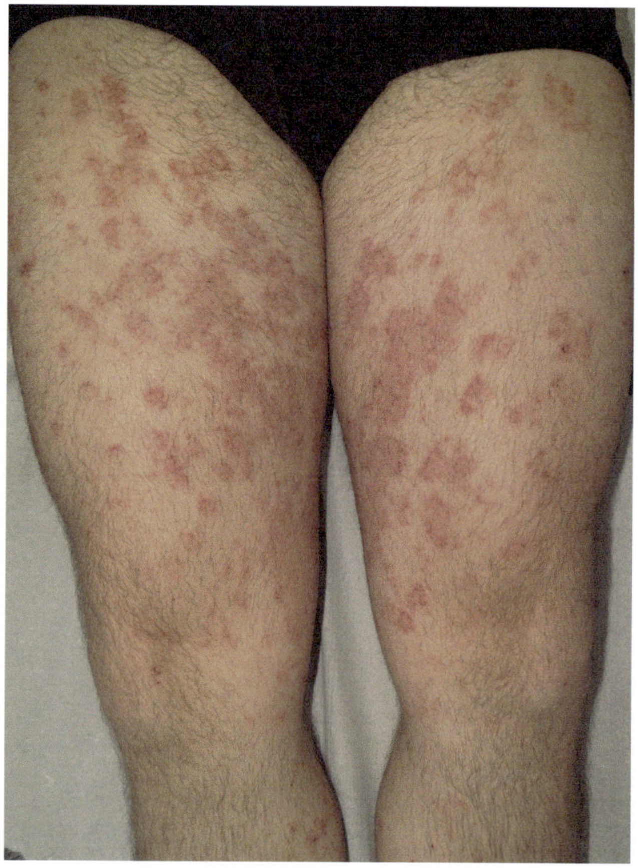

Fig. 34.5 Macroscopically, there are numerous erythematous papulo-squamous lesions on the lower extremities, some of them coalescing to form plaques

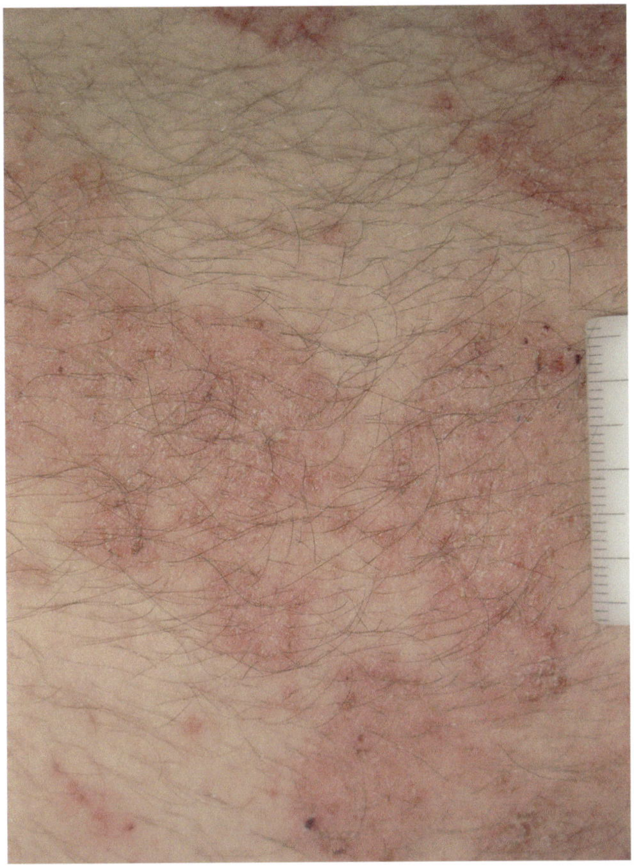

Fig. 34.6 In a closer view, we can see red papules and plaques with a scaly surface and signs of itching

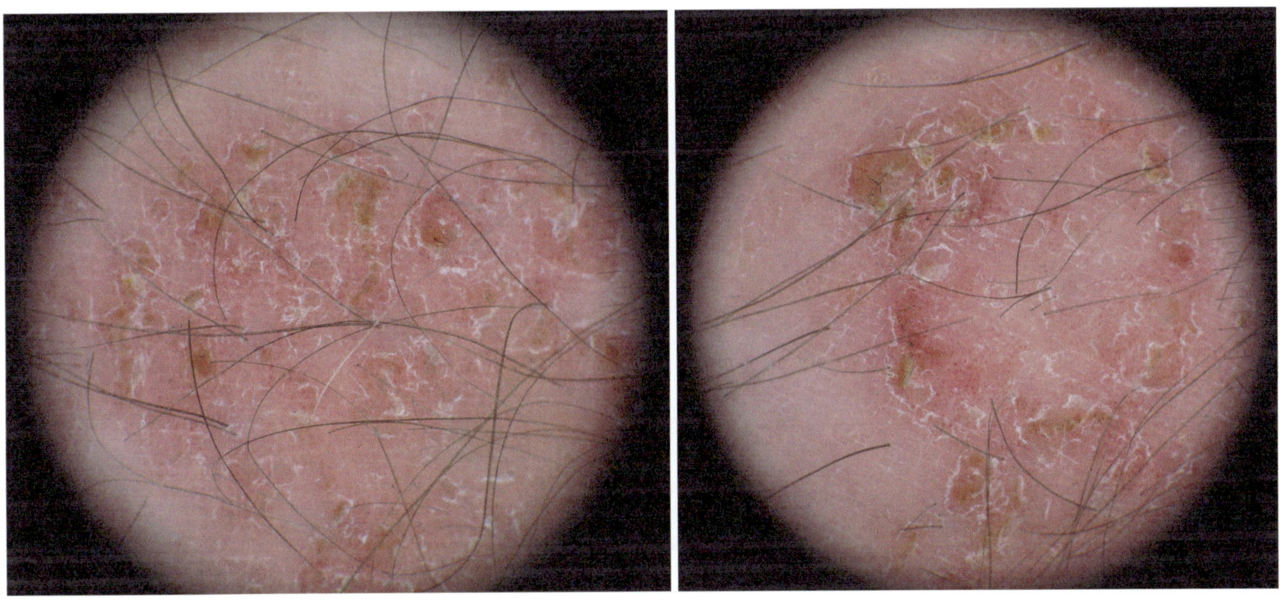

Fig. 34.7 and 34.8 Dermoscopically, the lesions exhibit red dots in a patchy distribution, diffuse yellowish and white scales, and yellowish-orange crusts

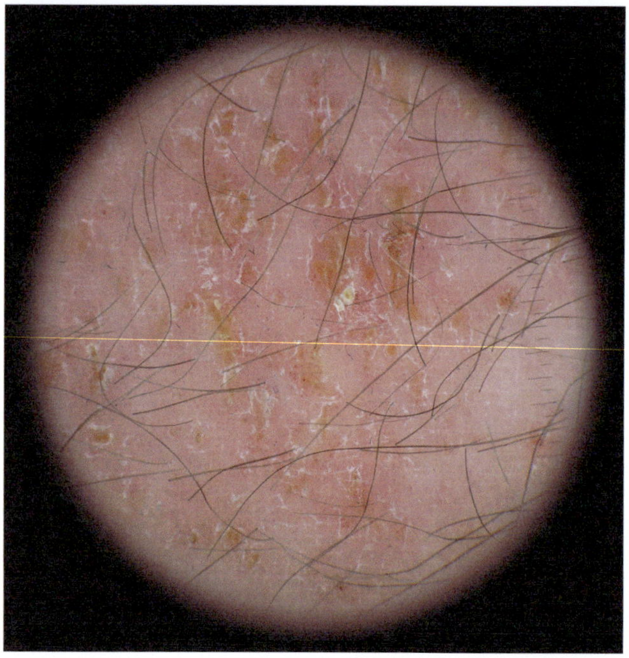

Fig. 34.9 Note that there are sites of the lesion in which vessels are not detectable at all as a result of the asymmetric arrangement

Key Message

Although dotted vessels are also seen in psoriasis, in this case of dermatitis, they are distributed in an asymmetric and patchy pattern in contrast with the regular distribution of the first. Moreover, the presence of yellow scale color favors dermatitis and differentiates it from psoriasis in which the scales are white by definition.

Case 3: A.L.

Sex: female
Age: 67
Surface (flat/palpable/nodular): palpable
Maximum diameter:
Duration of the lesion: 2 months
History of morphologic changes: yes
Personal history of skin cancer (if yes, please specify): no
Family history of skin cancer (if yes, please specify): no
Skin phototype: III
Total nevus count (<10, 10–50, 50–100, >100): 10–50
Other clinical findings (optional):

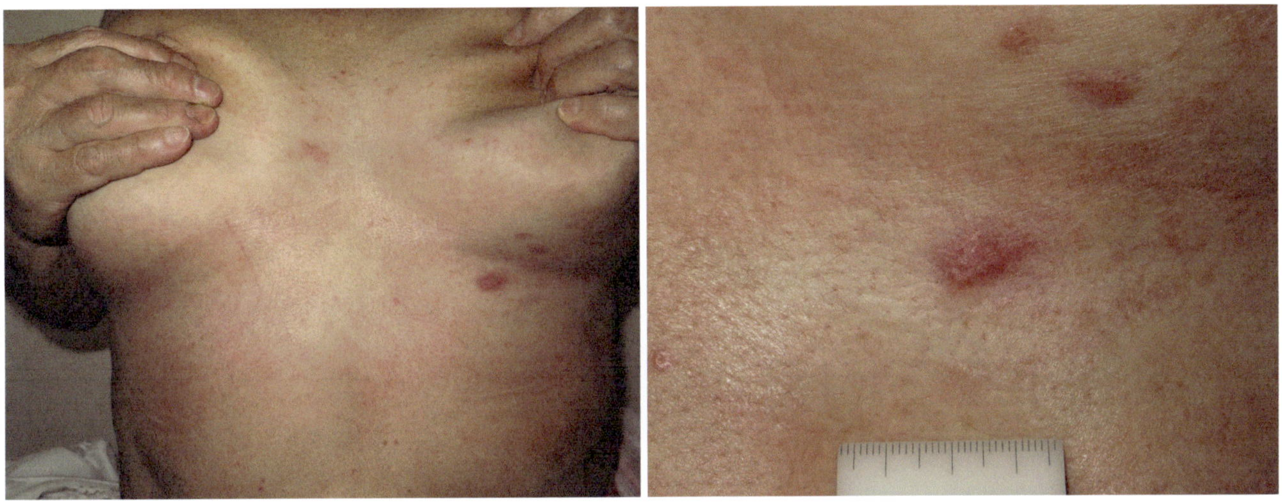

Fig. 34.10 and 34.11 On clinical examination, there are numerous pruritic erythematous papules located on the trunk

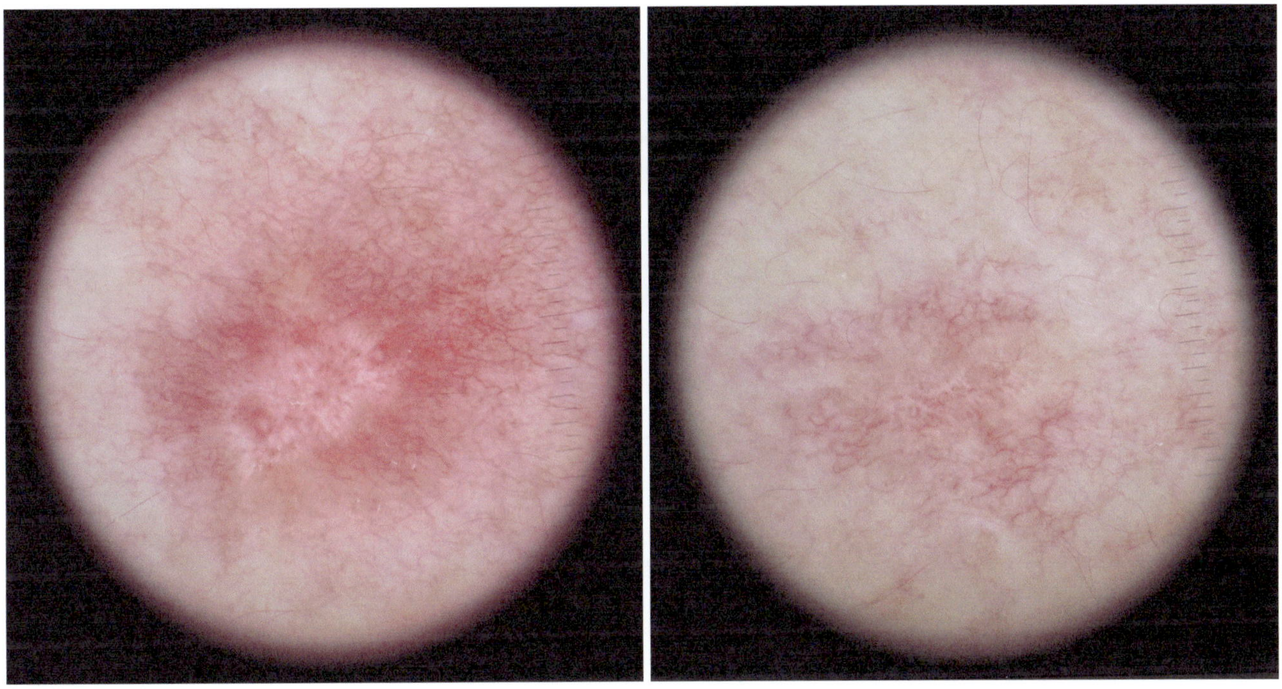

Fig. 34.12 and 34.13 Application of dermoscopy reveals white crossing lines (the so-called Wickham striae), along with dotted and short linear vessels

Key Message

The presence of the so-called Wickham striae allows a straightforward diagnosis of lichen planus.

Case 4: A.L.

Sex: male
Age: 48
Surface (flat/palpable/nodular): palpable
Maximum diameter:
Duration of the lesion: 3 weeks
History of morphologic changes: yes, a solitary macule that gradually expanded
Personal history of skin cancer (if yes, please specify): no
Family history of skin cancer (if yes, please specify): no
Skin phototype: III
Total nevus count (<10, 10–50, 50–100, >100): 10–50
Other clinical findings (optional):

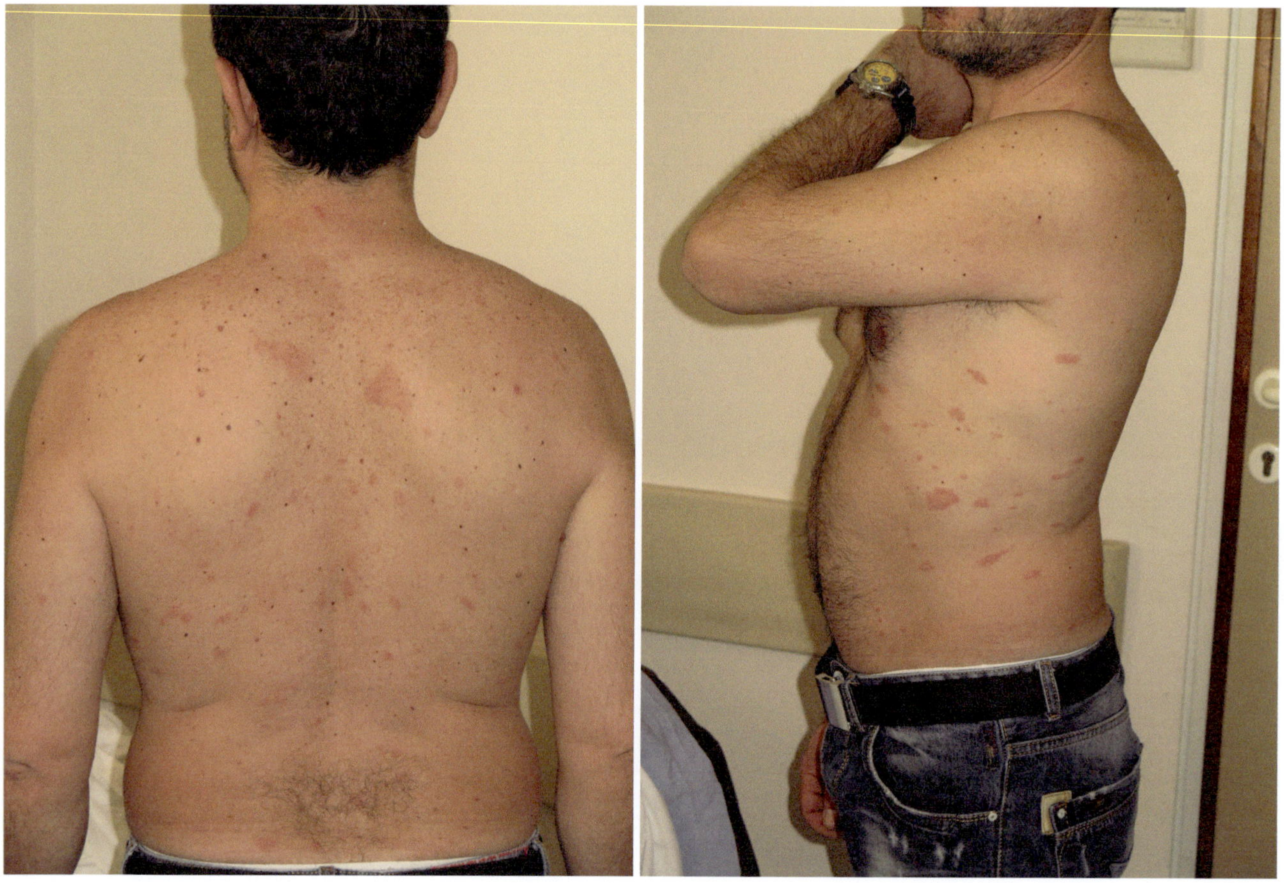

Figs. 34.14 and 34.15 Clinically, we can see a generalized papulosquamous eruption located mainly on the trunk

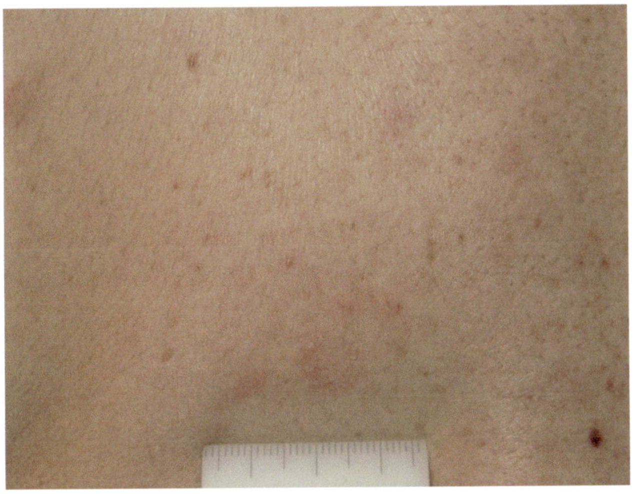

Fig. 34.16 In a closer view, we can see scaly round to oval macules and papules characterized by a collarette appearance of the scales

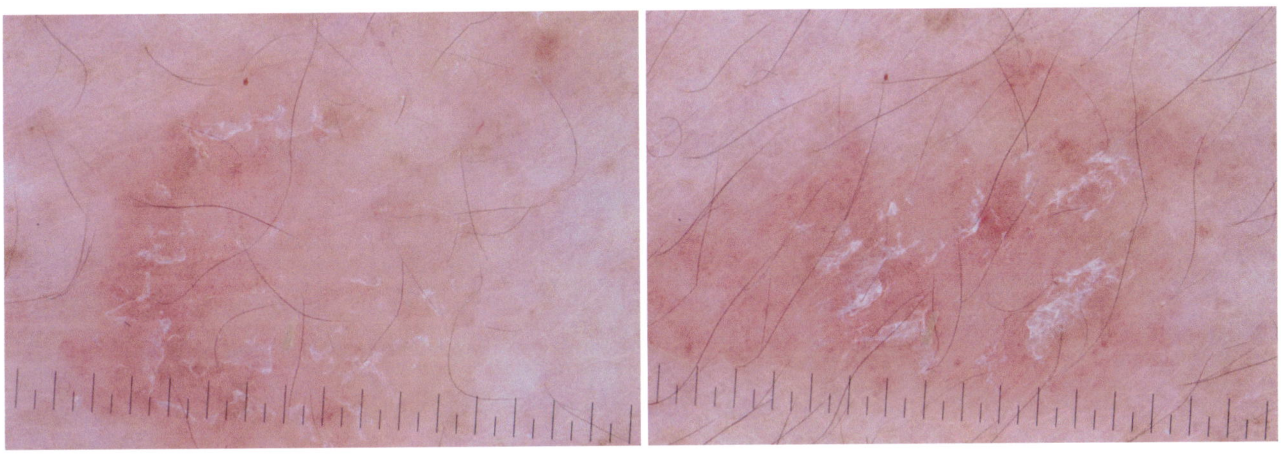

Figs. 34.17 and 34.18 Dermoscopically, the peripheral whitish (collarette) scales and a yellowish background are highlighted. Few dotted vessels are also observed in a focal distribution

Key Message
The combination of history with the clinical and dermoscopic images (peripheral collarette whitish scales and yellowish background) is the key for a safe diagnosis of pityriasis rosea.

Case 5: A.L.

Sex: female
Age: 27
Surface (flat/palpable/nodular): palpable
Maximum diameter:
Duration of the lesion: 3 months
History of morphologic changes: yes, gradually enlarging
Personal history of skin cancer (if yes, please specify): no
Family history of skin cancer (if yes, please specify): no
Skin phototype: III
Total nevus count (<10, 10–50, 50–100, >100): 10–50
Other clinical findings (optional):

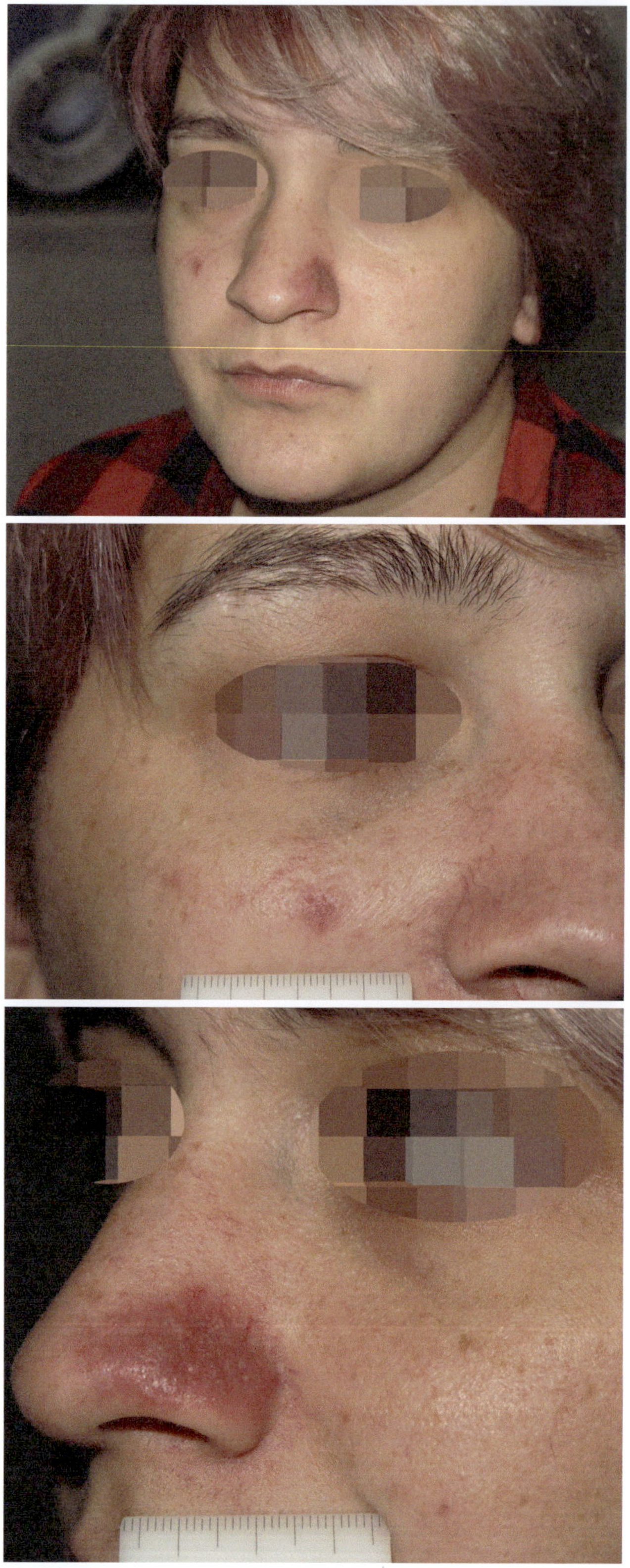

Figs. 34.19 , 34.20, and 34.21 On clinical examination, there are two erythematous, slightly infiltrated plaques located on the cheek and nose

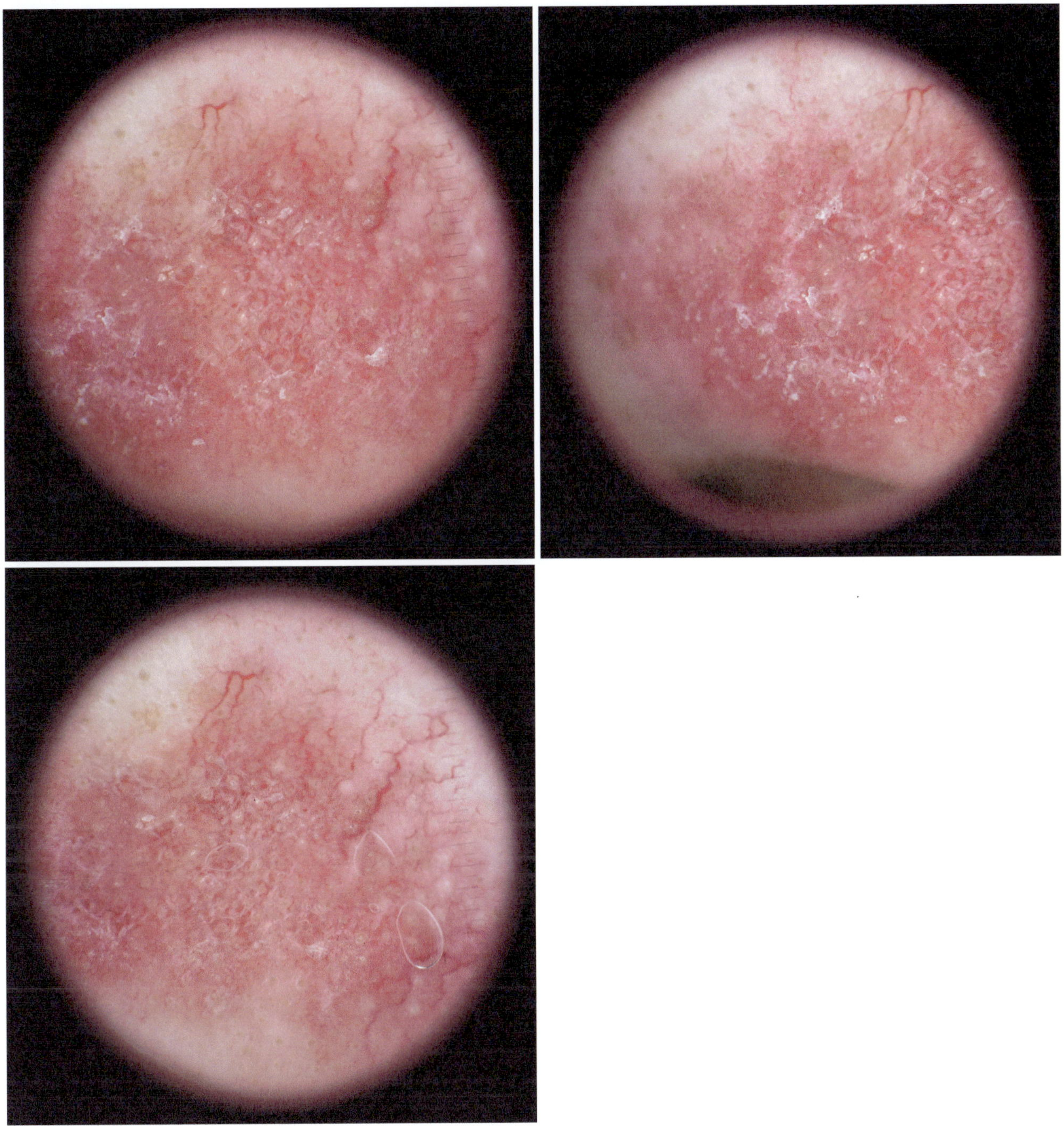

Figs. 34.22, 34.23, and 34.24 Dermoscopy of both lesions revealed numerous follicular openings surrounded by a white halo, white scales, and follicular plugs

Key Message

The clinical and dermoscopic images allow the recognition of discoid lupus erythematosus. Note that these dermoscopic characteristics (i.e., perifollicular whitish halo, follicular plugs, and white scales) are seen in early lesions, while long-standing lesions exhibit pigmented structures, linear telangiectasias, and whitish structureless areas.

Case 6: A.L.

Sex: female
Age: 44
Surface (flat/palpable/nodular): flat
Maximum diameter: 35 mm
Duration of the lesion: 6 months
History of morphologic changes: yes, slowly enlarging
Personal history of skin cancer (if yes, please specify): no
Family history of skin cancer (if yes, please specify): no
Skin phototype: III
Total nevus count (<10, 10–50, 50–100, >100): 10–50
Other clinical findings (optional):

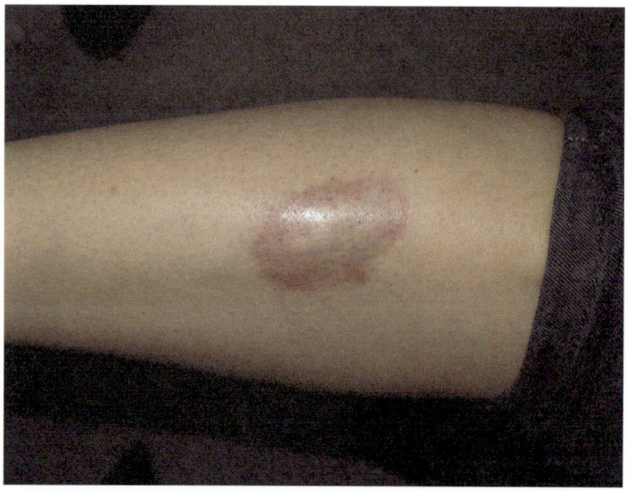

Fig. 34.25 Macroscopically, there is a solitary oval reddish patch with a yellowish brown center located on the right limb

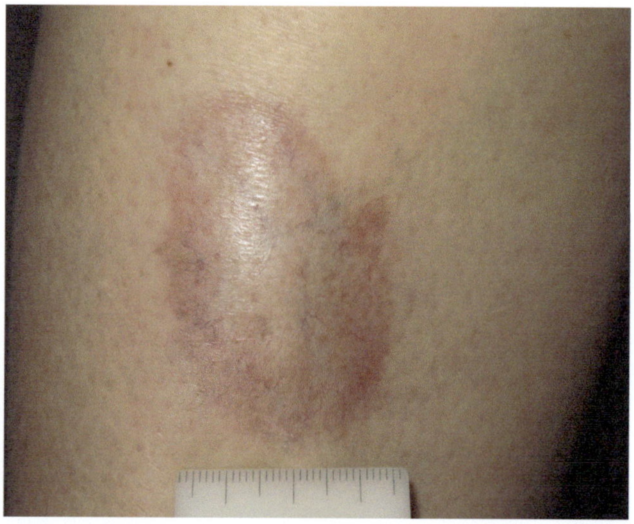

Fig. 34.26 In a closer view, we can observe the shiny and thinned center of the patch as well as the prominent blood vessels (telangiectasia)

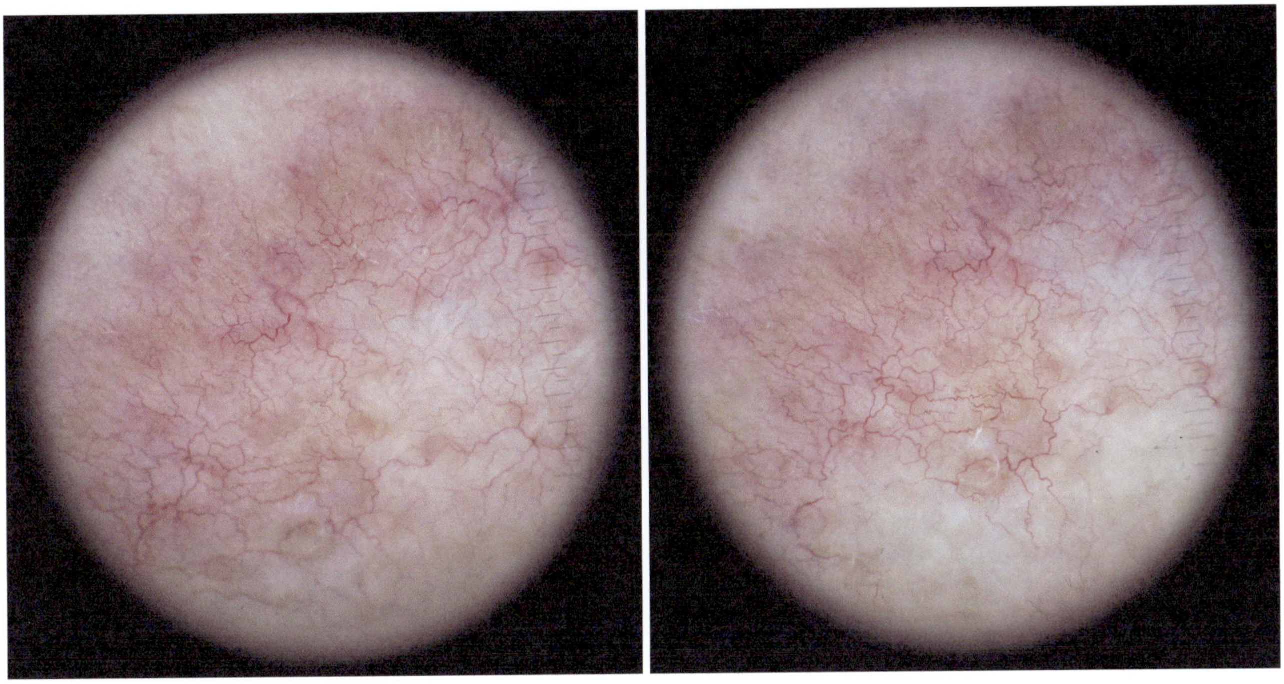

Fig. 34.27 and 34.28 Application of dermoscopy revealed a prominent network of linear branching vessels on a yellowish background

Key Message

The presence of yellow-orange color in dermatoscopy is suggestive of a granulomatous skin disease. Necrobiosis lipoidica typically displays, in addition to the orange-yellow color, a dense plexus of linear serpentine vessels.

Case 6: R.G., R. K., F. F., I. Z.

Sex: female
Age: 19
Surface (flat/palpable/nodular): palpable
Maximum diameter: 1.2 cm
Duration of the lesions: 2 months
History of morphologic changes: the lesions developed on the legs, bilaterally, as pruritic erythematous small papules and vesicles that in few weeks joined to form eczematous circular patches, different in size.
Personal history of skin cancer (if yes, please specify): none
Family history of skin cancer (if yes, please specify): none
Skin phototype: 3
Total nevus count (<10, 10–50, 50–100, >100): <10
Other clinical findings (optional): fungal infection was excluded by negative microscopic and cultural exams.

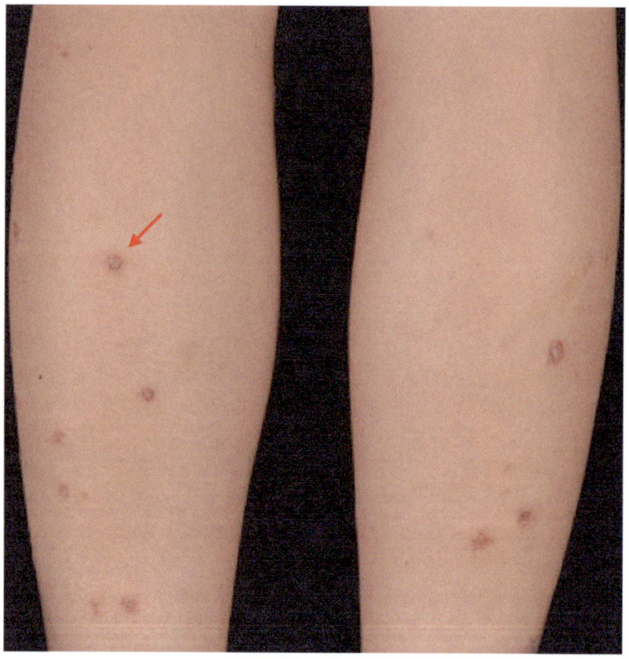

Fig. 34.29 Clinical presentation: multiple erythematous roundish, slightly scaly, well-circumscribed patches, located on the lower legs

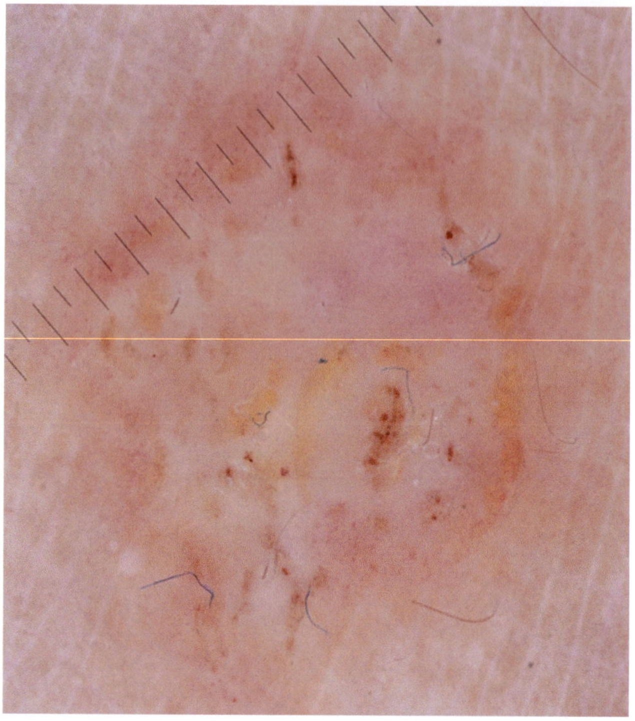

Fig. 34.30 Dermoscopy of the lesion indicated by the red arrow in Fig. 34.1

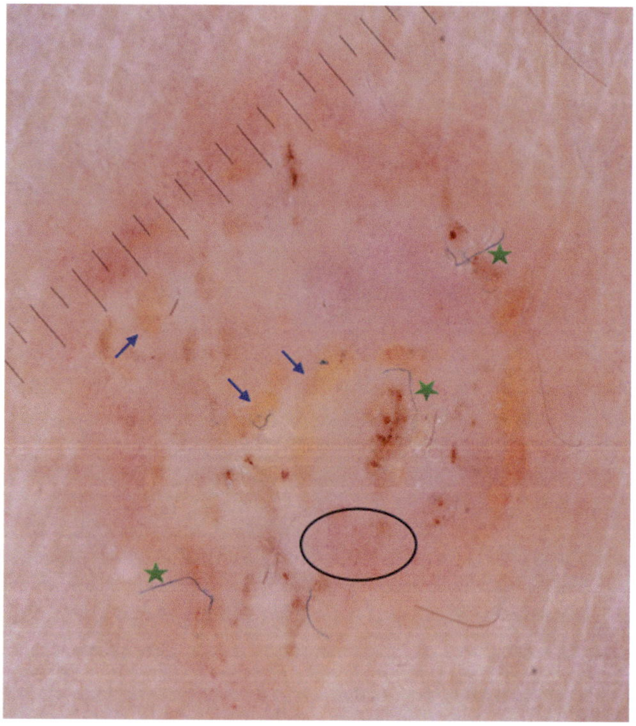

Fig. 34.31 Dermoscopy of the lesion indicated by the red arrow in Fig. 34.1 shows dotted vessels in a patchy distribution (black circle) together with yellowish serocrusts (blue arrows) and discrete whitish scales. In addition, multiple fibers visible under dermoscopy are an indirect sign of erosion (green stars)

Key Message

Dermoscopy helps in the differential diagnosis of clinical erythrosquamous inflammatory patches by disclosing specific patterns to allow an accurate diagnosis in many cases. In the case of eczema, dermoscopy typically shows yellow serocrusts and dotted vessels in a patchy distribution.

MIX
Papier aus verantwortungsvollen Quellen
Paper from responsible sources
FSC® C105338

If you have any concerns about our products,
you can contact us on
ProductSafety@springernature.com

In case Publisher is established outside the EU,
the EU authorized representative is:
Springer Nature Customer Service Center GmbH
Europaplatz 3, 69115 Heidelberg, Germany

Printed by Libri Plureos GmbH
in Hamburg, Germany